Lecture Notes in Computer Science 11040

Commenced Publication in 1973
Founding and Former Series Editors:
Gerhard Goos, Juris Hartmanis, and Jan van Leeuwen

More information about this series at http://www.springer.com/series/7412

Danail Stoyanov · Zeike Taylor
Bernhard Kainz · Gabriel Maicas
Reinhard R. Beichel et al. (Eds.)

Image Analysis for Moving Organ, Breast, and Thoracic Images

Third International Workshop, RAMBO 2018
Fourth International Workshop, BIA 2018
and First International Workshop, TIA 2018
Held in Conjunction with MICCAI 2018
Granada, Spain, September 16 and 20, 2018
Proceedings

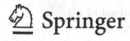

Springer

Editors
Danail Stoyanov
University College London
London, UK

Gabriel Maicas
University of Adelaide
Adelaide, SA, Australia

Zeike Taylor
University of Leeds
Leeds, UK

Reinhard R. Beichel
University of Iowa
Iowa City, IA, USA

Bernhard Kainz ⓘ
Imperial College London
London, UK

Additional Workshop Editors *see next page*

ISSN 0302-9743   ISSN 1611-3349   (electronic)
Lecture Notes in Computer Science
ISBN 978-3-030-00945-8   ISBN 978-3-030-00946-5   (eBook)
https://doi.org/10.1007/978-3-030-00946-5

Library of Congress Control Number: 2018955275

LNCS Sublibrary: SL6 – Image Processing, Computer Vision, Pattern Recognition, and Graphics

This Springer imprint is published by the registered company Springer Nature Switzerland AG
The registered company address is: Gewerbestrasse 11, 6330 Cham, Switzerland

Additional Workshop Editors

Tutorial and Educational Chair

Anne Martel
University of Toronto
Toronto, ON
Canada

Workshop and Challenge Co-chair

Lena Maier-Hein
German Cancer Research Center (DKFZ)
Heidelberg
Germany

Third International Workshop on Reconstruction and Analysis of Moving Body Organs, RAMBO 2018

Kanwal K. Bhatia
Visulytix Limited
London
UK

Ozan Oktay
Imperial College London
London
UK

Tom Vercauteren
King's College London
London
UK

Fourth International Workshop on Breast Image Analysis, BIA 2018

Gustavo Carneiro
University of Adelaide
Adelaide, SA
Australia

Jacinto C. Nascimento
Instituto Superior Técnico
Lisboa
Portugal

Andrew P. Bradley
Queensland University of Technology
Brisbane, QLD
Australia

Hang Min
University of Queensland
Brisbane, QLD
Australia

First International Workshop on Thoracic Image Analysis, TIA 2018

Matthew S. Brown
David Geffen School of Medicine
at UCLA
Los Angeles, CA
USA

Colin Jacobs ⓘ
Radboud University Medical Center
Nijmegen
The Netherlands

Bianca Lassen-Schmidt
Fraunhofer Institute for Medical Image
Computing (MEVIS)
Bremen
Germany

Kensaku Mori
Nagoya University
Nagoya
Japan

Jens Petersen ⓘ
University of Copenhagen
Copenhagen
Denmark

Raúl San José Estépar ⓘ
Harvard Medical School
Boston, MA
USA

Alexander Schmidt-Richberg ⓘ
Philips Research Laboratories
Hamburg
Germany

Catarina Veiga ⓘ
University College London
London
UK

RAMBO 2018 Preface

Physiological motion is an important factor in several medical imaging applications. The speed of motion may inhibit the acquisition of high-resolution images needed for effective visualization and analysis, for example, in cardiac or respiratory imaging or in functional magnetic resonance imaging (fMRI) and perfusion applications. Additionally, in cardiac and fetal imaging, the variation in the frame of reference may confound automated analysis pipelines. The underlying motion may also need to be characterized either to enhance images or for clinical assessment. Techniques are therefore needed for faster or more accurate reconstruction or for analysis of time-dependent images. Despite the related concerns, few meetings have focused on the issues caused by motion in medical imaging, without restriction on the clinical application area or methodology used.

After a very successful international workshop on Reconstruction and Analysis of Moving Body Organs (RAMBO) at MICCAI 2016 in Athens, Greece, and MICCAI 2017 in Quebec, Canada, we are proud to have organized this meeting for the third time in conjunction with MICCAI 2018 in Granada, Spain.

RAMBO was set up to provide a discussion forum for researchers for whom motion and its effects on image analysis or visualization is a key aspect of their work. By inviting contributions across all application areas, the workshop aimed to bring together ideas from different areas of specialization, without being confined to a particular methodology. In particular, the recent trend to move from model-based to learning-based methods of analysis has resulted in increased transferability between application domains. A further goal of this workshop series is to enhance the links between image analysis (including computer vision and machine learning techniques) and image acquisition and reconstruction, which generally tends to be addressed in separate meetings.

The presented contributions cover registration and tracking to image reconstruction and information retrieval techniques, while application areas include cardiac, pulmonary, abdominal, fetal, and renal imaging, showing the breadth of interest in the topic. Research from both academia and industry was presented and keynote lectures from Dr. Leo Grady (Senior Vice President of Engineering at HeartFlow Inc.) and Dr. Elisenda Eixarch (Consultant and Associate Professor, Fetal and Perinatal Medicine Research Group, Hospital Clínic de Barcelona) gave an overview of recent developments.

We believe that this workshop fosters the cross-fertilization of ideas across application domains while tackling and taking advantage of the problems and opportunities arising from motion in medical imaging.

August 2018

Bernhard Kainz
Kanwal Bhatia
Tom Vercauteren
Ozan Oktay

BIA 2018 Preface

Welcome to the fourth edition of the Breast Image Analysis (BIA) workshop held in conjunction with MICCAI. The aim of BIA is to bring together the growing number of researchers in the field given the significant amount of effort in the development of tools that can automate the analysis and synthesis of breast imaging. The main purpose of the workshop is to provide a stimulating environment for an in-depth discussion of important recent developments among experts in the field that enables future research impact in the field. For the keynote talks, we invited Prof. Anne Martel from Sunnybrook Health Sciences Centre, Assist. Prof. Orcun Goksel from ETH Zurich and Dr. Markus Wenzel from Fraunhofer Institute for Medical Image Computing MEVIS - they represent three prominent researchers in the field of breast image analysis.

The first call for papers for the 4th BIA was released on April 4, 2018 and the last call was done on June 5, 2018, with the paper deadline set to June 18, 2018. The submission site of BIA received 22 papers registrations, from which 18 papers turned into full paper submissions. Each submission was reviewed by three or four reviewers. The chairs decided to select nine out of the 18 submissions (50% acceptance rate) based on the majority voting of three meta-reviewers. Meta-reviewers decided on acceptance or rejection based on the scores and comments made by the reviewers. Finally, we would like to acknowledge the support from the Australian Research Council for the realisation of this workshop (discovery project DP180103232). We would also like to thank the program committee members of BIA.

July 2018   BIA Workshop Chairs

TIA 2018 Preface

The First International Workshop on Thoracic Image Analysis was held at the Medical Image Computing and Computer-Assisted Intervention Conference (MICCAI) in Granada, Spain, 2018. Building on the history of the Pulmonary Image Analysis workshop, a roughly biannual event at MICCAI going back 10 years, the aim of the workshop was to bring together medical image analysis researchers in the area of thoracic imaging to discuss recent advances in this rapidly developing field. Cardiovascular disease, lung cancer, and chronic obstructive pulmonary disease (COPD), three diseases all visible on thoracic imaging, are among the top causes of death worldwide. Many imaging modalities are currently available to study the pulmonary and cardiac system, including radiography, computed tomography (CT), positron emission tomography (PET) and magnetic resonance imaging (MRI). Papers dealing with all aspects of image analysis of thoracic data, including but not limited to segmentation, registration, quantification, modelling of the image acquisition process, visualization, validation, statistical modelling biophysical modelling (computational anatomy), deep learning, image analysis in small animals, and novel applications were invited. Good-sized independent validation studies on the use of deep learning models in the area of thoracic imaging, despite having possibly little technical novelty, were particularly invited.

The 21 papers submitted to the workshop were reviewed in a double-blind manner with at least two reviewers per paper, whose affiliations and recent publications were checked to avoid conflicts of interests. Finally, 20 papers were accepted for presentation as either oral or poster. Of the accepted papers, 18 were long format (8–12 pages) and two were short format (4–7 pages). The papers were grouped into four topics, which are reflected in the structure of this volume: Image Acquisition and Enhancement (3), Image Segmentation (7), Image Registration (4), and Computer-Aided Diagnosis (6). Deep learning is undoubtedly a hot topic in the community, with techniques like transfer learning and generative adversarial networks being in the focus of recent research activities. We were pleased to note that the majority (70%) of the submissions were on the use of such state-of-the-art methods for a variety of important clinical applications – some examples include enhancement of chest radiographs, image registration of the lungs, lung cancer screening, and segmentation of airways. The imaging modalities used were a good mixture of 2D X-ray, 3D CT, 4D CT, and functional MRI, demonstrating the complementary information brought together by different modalities used to study the thoracic system.

We would like to express our gratitude to all the authors for submitting papers to the First International Workshop on Thoracic Image Analysis, as well as to everyone involved in the organization and peer review process.

July 2018   TIA Workshop Chairs

Organization

RAMBO 2018 Organizing Committee

Bernard Kainz	Imperial College London, UK
Kanwal Bhatia	Visulytix, UK
Tom Vercauteren	King's College London, UK
Ozan Oktay	Imperial College London, UK

BIA 2018 Organizing Committee

Gabriel Maicas	University of Adelaide, Australia
Gustavo Carneiro	University of Adelaide, Australia
Andrew P. Bradley	University of Queensland, Australia
Jacinto C. Nacimento	Instituto Superior Tecnico, Portugal
Hang Min	University of Queensland, Australia

TIA 2018 Organizing Committee

Reinhard R. Beichel	The University of Iowa, USA
Matthew S. Brown	David Geffen School of Medicine at UCLA, USA
Colin Jacobs	Radboud University Medical Center, The Netherlands
Bianca Lassen-Schmidt	Fraunhofer Institute for Medical Image Computing MEVIS, Germany
Kensaku Mori	Nagoya University, Japan
Jens Petersen	University of Copenhagen, Denmark
Raúl San José Estépar	Brigham and Women's Hospital, Harvard Medical School, USA
Alexander Schmidt-Richberg	Philips Research Laboratories Hamburg, Germany
Catarina Veiga	University College London, UK

Contents

First International Workshop on Thoracic Image Analysis, TIA 2018

Third International Workshop on Reconstruction and Analysis of Moving Body Organs, RAMBO 2018

Resection-Based Demons Regularization for Breast Tumor Bed Propagation

Marek Wodzinski[✉][iD] and Andrzej Skalski[iD]

Department of Measurement and Electronics,
AGH University of Science and Technology, Krakow, Poland
wodzinski@agh.edu.pl

Abstract. A tumor resection introduces a problem of missing data into the image registration process. The state-of-the-art methods fail while attempting to recover the real deformations when the structure of interest is missing. In this work, we propose an empirical, greedy regularization term which promotes the tumor contraction. The proposed method is simple but very effective. It is based on a priori medical knowledge about the scar localization to promote the direction of the tumor propagation. The proposed method is compared to the Demons algorithm using both the artificially generated data with a known ground-truth and a real, medical data. A relative tumor volume reduction, a Hausdorff distance between the tumor beds, a RMSE between the deformation fields, and a visual inspection are used as the evaluation methods. The proposed method models the tumor resection accurately in the target data and improves the potential dose distribution for the radiotherapy planning.

Keywords: Image registration · Missing data · Demons
Cancer surgery · Breast cancer

1 Introduction

The breast tumor surgery and the following radiotherapy are usually planned using the computed tomography (CT). This fact can be exploited to use the image registration techniques to improve the estimation of the radiation dose margins. However, an alignment of the pre-operative to the post-operative scans is a challenging task. The tumor resection introduces the problem of missing data which leads to several difficulties which are not present in the typical image registration procedures.

Related Work: The majority of recent research about the image registration was dedicated to ensuring that the calculated deformation field is a diffeomorphism. Since the diffeomorphic deformation field is inherently invertible and smooth, it is desirable for majority of the image registration tasks. However, for the tumor resection problem, the deformation field nearby the structure of interest is obviously not invertible and not smooth. There were much less research

© Springer Nature Switzerland AG 2018
D. Stoyanov et al. (Eds.): RAMBO 2018/BIA 2018/TIA 2018, LNCS 11040, pp. 3–12, 2018.
https://doi.org/10.1007/978-3-030-00946-5_1

about the image registration with missing data compared to ensuring the diffeo-morphic properties. One of the first works used the thin-plate splines to estimate the brain tumor propagation [1]. However, the author assumed that there is still a partial correspondence between the structures which could be used as control points. For the full tumor resection, it is not true. An interesting work about algorithm based on local affine transformations was presented in [2]. Nonethe-less, the main assumption was that the structure of interest is not missing, only its surroundings. The TV-L^1 was a promising algorithm [3], however it turned out that its global optimization procedure makes it fail during the tumor bed propagation in the CT. The reason for this was a low influence of the similarity cost gradient nearby the resected tumor. Moreover, the deformation can be very large so an attempt to use local realization of this technique failed. There were even attempts to localize the tumor bed using the rigid registration based on surgical clips which is inherently wrong because the rigid transformation is an isometry preserving the tumor volume [4,5]. Interesting works were introduced in the context of missing data as a result of the brain tumor resection. A fully automatic method based on the level-set segmentation of intensity disagreements and anisotropic diffusion filter modeling the resection area as a diffusion sink was proposed in [6]. An improved Demons algorithm based on a fourth dimension in order to separate removed tissues from others was proposed in [7]. There was also a work related to an atlas-based segmentation of brain images which used mod-ified bijective Demons to model the tumor growth process with an assumption about a radial growth of the tumor [8]. The model is similar to our method with the difference about ability to reconstruct larger deformations. Our method still uses the Demons force inside the tumor which makes is possible to reconstruct, usually large, breast deformations.

Contribution: In this work, we propose a simple but very effective regulariza-tion term for the greedy version of the Demons algorithm. The proposed method is based on the *a priori* knowledge about the cancer resection. Since we know that the tumor is resected, its volume in the target image significantly decreases. The proposed regularization uses this knowledge to promote the tumor volume reduction. We evaluate the proposed method using artificially generated data, artificial deformations resembling the tumor resection and real, medical data representing women with the breast cancer before and after the tumor surgery. We show that the proposed method greatly decreases the breast tumor volume and improves the tumor bed localization.

2   Methods

The proposed method is based on the greedy, implicit version of the Demons algorithm. For the further reference and the comparison purposes, we present a shortened algorithmic summary of the compositive, symmetric Demons in Algorithm 1.

The proposed method consists of an empirical, greedy regularization term which enforces the tumor contraction and a scheme to automatically

---

Algorithm 1. Demons Algorithm

Input : M (moving image), F (fixed image), σ_f (fluid sigma), σ_d (diffusion sigma), u_i (initial deformation field - optionally) number of resolutions, convergence indicator

Output: u (calculated deformation field)

1 **Ms, Fs** = create moving and fixed images for each resolution
2 **u** = initialize the deformation field
3 **foreach** *resolution* **do**
4      $G(\sigma_d)$, $G(\sigma_f)$ = initialize convolution kernels (typically Gaussian)
5   **while** *not converged* **do**
6          $v = -\dfrac{F-M\circ u}{||\nabla F||^2+(F-M\circ u)^2}\nabla F - \dfrac{F-M\circ u}{||\nabla M\circ u||^2+(F-M\circ u)^2}\nabla M \circ u$
7          $v = G(\sigma_f) \star v$
8          $u = u \circ v$
9          $u = G(\sigma_d) \star u$
10      $u = $ upsample_deformation_field(u)
11 **return u**

---

determine an optimal regularization step. Its algorithmic summary is presented in Algorithm 2. The presented algorithm requires a binary mask of the segmented tumor as an additional parameter. The binary mask is usually obtained during the surgery planning and therefore is easily available. The tumor can be segmented manually or automatically. The method does not require any additional parameter tunning (only the smoothing sigmas σ_d, σ_f must be chosen). The regularization is added as an additional greedy step during the Demons algorithm, between the deformation field update and the diffusion regularization.

The direction structure d_s can be defined as a binary mask with a single point or a structure representing the expected tumor bed shape. Its localization is defined relative to the initial tumor position and transformed during each iteration. In the experiments performed, the direction structure is defined as a center of mass of the tumor because both the source and the target are acquired for the same patient position. Conceptually, it can be compared to the mean shift algorithm. During each iteration, both the tumor and the structure are being transformed, until convergence. In practice, the direction structure is defined using the *a priori* knowledge, usually with help of the surgical protocol.

The regularization term **c** (a vector field) is based on the direction of a difference between coordinates of the direction structure and the image domain (a grid) with the minimum distance to a given coordinate. It is simply a coordinates subtraction, which can be defined as:

$$c = \arg\min(D(d_s, T_m \circ u)) - Id_u, \tag{1}$$

where Id_u denotes the image domain, the $T_m \circ u$ is the transformed tumor and D denotes an Euclidean distance calculation. What is important, the calculation needs to be performed only for the segmented tumor. Then, the vector field **c** is normalized to unit length, which is later compensated by the tumor volume and the average velocity field vector length. The distance calculation must include the knowledge about physical voxel size which is, for clarity, omitted in the algorithm description.

Algorithm 2. Resection-based Demons Algorithm

Input : $\mathbf{M}$ (moving image), $\mathbf{F}$ (fixed image), $\mathbf{T_m}$ (tumor mask), $\mathbf{d_s}$ (direction structure) σ_f (fluid sigma), σ_d (diffusion sigma), $\mathbf{u_i}$ (initial deformation field - optionally), expected tumor volume after the resection, number of resolutions, convergence indicator

Output: $\mathbf{u}$ (calculated deformation field)

1 $\mathbf{Ms, Fs, Ts_m}$ = create moving, fixed and mask images for each resolution
2 $\mathbf{u}$ = initialize the deformation field
3 **foreach** *resolution* **do**
4 $\quad$ $\mathbf{G}(\sigma_d), \mathbf{G}(\sigma_f)$ = initialize convolution kernels (typically Gaussian)
5 $\quad$ **while** *not converged* **do**
6 $\quad\quad$ $\mathbf{v} = -\frac{\mathbf{F}-\mathbf{M}\circ\mathbf{u}}{||\nabla\mathbf{F}||^2+(\mathbf{F}-\mathbf{M}\circ\mathbf{u})^2}\nabla\mathbf{F} - \frac{\mathbf{F}-\mathbf{M}\circ\mathbf{u}}{||\nabla\mathbf{M}\circ\mathbf{u}||^2+(\mathbf{F}-\mathbf{M}\circ\mathbf{u})^2}\nabla\mathbf{M}\circ\mathbf{u}$
7 $\quad\quad$ $\mathbf{v} = \mathbf{G}(\sigma_f) \star \mathbf{v}$
8 $\quad\quad$ $\mathbf{u} = \mathbf{u} \circ \mathbf{v}$
9 $\quad\quad$ $\mathbf{c} = \arg\min(D(\mathbf{d_s}, \mathbf{T_m} \circ \mathbf{u})) - \mathrm{Id}_u$
$\quad\quad$ /* a vector field with a minimum distance between the
$\quad\quad\quad\quad$ transformed tumor and the direction structure   */
10 $\quad\quad$ $\kappa = \frac{1}{s}$ (volume($\mathbf{T_m} \circ \mathbf{u}$) − expected_volume)
$\quad\quad$ /* s - an average velocity vector length   */
11 $\quad\quad$ $\mathbf{u} = \mathbf{u} \circ \kappa\mathbf{c}$
12 $\quad\quad$ $\mathbf{u} = \mathbf{G}(\sigma_d) \star \mathbf{u}$
13 $\quad$ $\mathbf{u}$ = upsample_deformation_field($\mathbf{u}$)
14 **return u**

The optimal regularization step κ controls the tumor contraction size during each iteration. It consists of two steps. Firstly, an average length of velocity vectors s is being calculated. If the velocity field magnitude is significant, the contraction term should have lower influence. It is necessary because enforcing strong contraction during the initial alignment phase leads to medically not reliable deformations. Secondly, the remaining tumor volume is being calculated to make the algorithm more stable. The influence of the regularization term linearly depends on the current tumor volume. The final regularization step is defined as:

$$\kappa = \frac{1}{s}(\text{volume}(\mathbf{T_m} \circ \mathbf{u}) - \text{expected\_volume}), \tag{2}$$

where s is the average length of the velocity vectors. Usually, the expected volume after the resection is zero. Adding this term makes to possible to model less idealized scenario, e.g. when the cavity area it not completely filled with the surrounding tissues. However, it is not a common event because the time between the breast tumor surgery and the radiotherapy planning usually is long enough.

The proposed method can be compared to an explicit volume regularization where the gradient of tumor volume with respect to the deformation field is being calculated. However, this method is extremely computationally inefficient. We have compared the results obtained by both approaches and they were very similar, both for the tumor and the tumor bed. However, the proposed method is computationally efficient. It increases the overall Demons algorithm computation time by about 4% using the CPU implementation which is absolutely acceptable. For the explicit volume regularization the computation time depends strongly on the tumor volume and for an average tumor size increases the computation time by about an order of magnitude.

3   Experiments and Results

Three experiments were performed to show the influence of the proposed algorithm on the tumor bed localization. The proposed method was compared to the compositive, symmetric Demons because our previous study has shown that, among the state-of-the-art methods (B-Splines FFD, Demons, TV-L^1, and others), the Demons method provided the best results [9]. The data spatial resolution was equal to 0.97 mm x 0.97 mm x 3 mm. The σ_d, σ_f were set to 0.5 mm and 3.0 mm respectively. The proposed method is abbreviated as RB Demons (Resection-based Demons).

3.1   Artificial Data

The first experiment used an artificially generated data. This experiment was necessary because the ground-truth about tumor bed localization is unknown for the real, medical data. The artificial data made it possible to state an exact tumor bed localization and shape in both the source and the target. We created 10 artificial cases with breast tumors in different localizations and with different shapes. The artificial cases were synthesized based on the real CT data. Small, big, symmetric, asymmetric convex and concave tumors were introduced. Then, the target image was created with the explicitly stated tumor bed localization and deformed using a known deformation based on the B-Splines transformation. We assumed that the volume of surrounding soft tissues in the source data and the volume of tumor bed in the target data is equal. The artificial data were synthesized using the ASTRA Toolbox [10]. The registration results were evaluated using the relative tumor volume and the Hausdorff distance between the ground-truth and transformed tumor beds. The relative tumor volume (defined as the ratio of the transformed tumor volume to the initial tumor volume) was used because we know that in the ideal case the tumor volume in the target volume is equal to zero. The Hausdorff distance was applied because it directly shows the potential improvement for the radiotherapy planning where the maximum margins are a crucial factor. The results are presented in Fig. 1. The proposed method models the tumor resection and significantly decreases the maximum margin. This confirms that ensuring the tumor resection improves the tumor

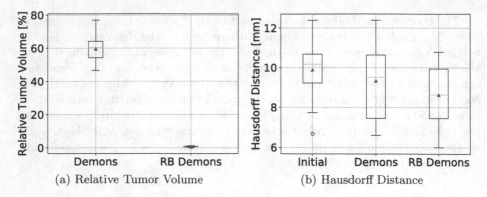

(a) Relative Tumor Volume   (b) Hausdorff Distance

Fig. 1. The relative tumor volume and the Hausdorff distance for the artificially generated breast tumor CT data. Initial - the original source and target. Demons - the compositive, symmetric Demons. RB Demons - the proposed method.

bed localization. The margin is still above 8 mm because the artificial data uses the same intensity value for the tumor bed and other surrounding soft tissues. This assumption seems valid because in the real CT data the tumor bed in the target is indistinguishable from other soft tissues. As a consequence, the alignment of the tumor bed is not driven by the intensity difference but the proposed regularization term.

3.2   Artificial Deformations

The second experiment was based on an artificial but real-like deformation fields resembling the tumor resection process. The applied deformation fields were proposed in [9]. The applied deformations significantly decreased the tumor volume and smoothly deformed the surrounding soft tissues. However, please notice that a real tumor resection cannot be modeled by the artificial deformation field because then it should point outside the image. The applied vector lengths and the calculated RMSE for both the original Demons and the proposed RB Demons are shown in Fig. 2a. The RMSE for the proposed method is lower and the relative improvement on average is equal to 15.25%.

3.3   Real Data

The final experiment used a real, medical data. We acquired 20 CT scans acquired before the breast cancer surgery, and after, during the radiotherapy planning. The tumors were manually segmented by a medical expert with more than 20 years experience in the breast cancer radiotherapy. The images were firstly rigidly registered based on bones segmentation, SIFT and RANSAC algorithms. For the real data, the ground-truth about the tumor bed is unknown. Therefore, a quantitative assessment of the tumor bed propagation is impossible. However, we can still use the relative tumor volume reduction to evaluate

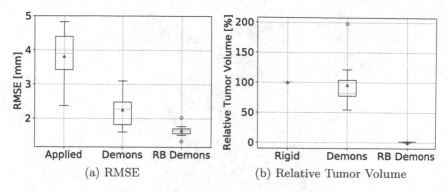

(a) RMSE

(b) Relative Tumor Volume

Fig. 2. The RMSE [mm] for artificially applied deformation fields and the relative tumor volume [%] for real data using different registration methods. The applied deformation fields resemble the tumor resection process. The rigid registration is shown to present the influence of warping error which is negligible. Please note that (a) and (b) are from different experiments.

the calculated deformation fields. If the method is unable to model the complete tumor resection, it is certainly incorrect. The calculated relative tumor volumes are shown in Fig. 2b. The original Demons algorithm is incorrect (for one case it even doubled the tumor volume) while the proposed method resembled all the resections well. Moreover, a visual assessment is crucial for the correctness evaluation. An example of the tumor propagation using different methods is shown in Fig. 3. An exemplary 3D visualization of the tumor propagation is shown in Fig. 4.

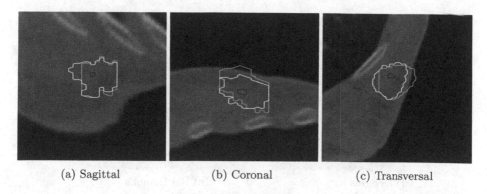

(a) Sagittal   (b) Coronal   (c) Transversal

Fig. 3. An exemplary visualization of the propagated tumor in the CT target using three image registration algorithms. The data is shown on the sagittal, coronal and transversal planes respectively. The colors indicate following methods: ■ - Rigid Registration ■ - Original Demons ■ - Proposed RB Demons. Please note that for the rigid registration the tumor is not even inside the body. (Color figure online)

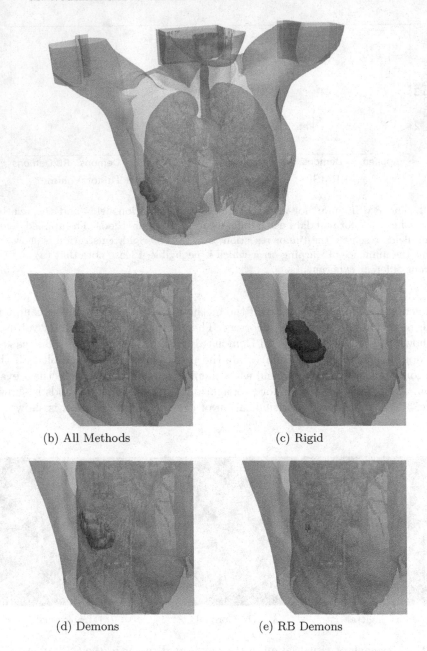

(b) All Methods   (c) Rigid

(d) Demons   (e) RB Demons

Fig. 4. An exemplary 3D visualization of the propagated tumor in the CT target for real, medical data. The colors indicate following methods: ■ - Rigid Registration ■ - Original Demons ■ - Proposed RB Demons. Please note the significant volume decrease of the tumor using the proposed method. (Color figure online)

4 Discussion and Conclusion

The experiments presented a significant volume reduction for the propagated tumors with different sizes and shapes. The evaluation based on the tumor volume reduction is able to show just the evaluated algorithm wrongness. A volume greater than zero clearly indicates the incorrectness of the registration method. The proposed method modeled a complete resection of tumors for both the artificial and real data while the original Demons failed. The proposed algorithm not only improved the tumor propagation but also the tumor bed localization which is the structure of interest for the radiotherapy planning.

The Hausdorff distance shows the potential improvement on the radiotherapy. The 1.5 mm decrease of Hausdorff distance (compared to the original Demons algorithm), for an average tumor size, can lead to the reduction of the irradiated volume by 32.5%. This value is significant and can decrease the risk of both the secondary carcinogenesis and tumor recurrence.

Moreover, the proposed method is independent of the registration forces calculation which makes it useful in the multi-modal registration. Therefore, this technique can be easily extended to multi-modal problems, like e.g. a real-time imaging system for the tumor surgery. This method, without any modifications, can be used in the MIND-based [11] or the NMI-based Demons [12].

The proposed method can be extended to incorporate the mechanical properties of the tissues being deformed. A biomechanical model of the breast will be used in the further study to better model the propagation destination for large deformations. Moreover, the calculated vector directions can be changed to more complex shape to make it useful for complex, concave and anisotropic shapes.

To conclude, we proposed a greedy, empirical regularization term for the Demons algorithm which ensures an appropriate tumor resection. The proposed method not only improved the tumor propagation but also the tumor bed localization. In the further research, we will incorporate this technique into multi-modal registration e.g. for the real-time surgery based on MRI-USG scans. Moreover, we will extend this technique to a structure-based contraction which should improve the tumor bed localization even more. We will perform a research about reliable, quantitative evaluation methods for image registration algorithms dedicated to the missing data problem.

Acknowledgments. This work was funded by the Ministry of Science and Higher Education in Poland (Dean's Grant no. 15.11.120.699 and Statutory Activity no. 11.11.120.774). We would like to thank P. Kedzierawski, I. Ciepiela and T. Kuszewski for providing the real, medical CT data and the tumor outlines.

References

1. Fornefett, M., Rohr, K., Stiehl, H.: Radial basis functions with compact support for elastic registration of medical images. Image Vis. Comput. **19**(1–2), 87–96 (2001)
2. Periaswamy, S., Farid, H.: Medical image registration with partial data. Med. Image Anal. **10**(3 Spec. Iss.), 452–464 (2006)

3. Pock, T., Urschler, M., Zach, C., Beichel, R., Bischof, H.: A duality based algorithm for TV-L^1-optical-flow image registration. In: Ayache, N., Ourselin, S., Maeder, A. (eds.) MICCAI 2007. LNCS, vol. 4792, pp. 511–518. Springer, Heidelberg (2007). https://doi.org/10.1007/978-3-540-75759-7_62
4. Kirova, Y., et al.: How to boost the breast tumor bed? A multidisciplinary approach in eight steps. Int. J. Radiat. Oncol. Biol. Phys. **72**(2), 494–500 (2008)
5. Kirova, Y., et al.: Improving the definition of tumor bed boost with the use of surgical clips and image registration in breast cancer patients. Int. J. Radiat. Oncol. Biol. Phys. **78**(5), 1352–1355 (2010)
6. Risholm, P., et al.: Validation of a non-rigid registration framework that accommodates tissue resection. In: Medical Imaging 2010: Image Processing - SPIE, pp. 1–11 (2010)
7. Nithiananthan, S., et al.: Extra-dimensional Demons: a method for incorporating missing tissue in deformable image registration. Med. Phys. **39**(9), 5718–5731 (2012)
8. Bach, M., et al.: Atlas-based segmentation of pathological MR brain images using a model of lesion growth. IEEE Trans. Med. Imaging **23**(10), 1301–1314 (2004)
9. Wodzinski, M., et al.: Improving oncoplastic breast tumor bed localization for radiotherapy planning using image registration algorithms. Phys. Med. Biol. **63**(3), 035024 (2018)
10. Van Aarle, W., et al.: Fast and flexible X-ray tomography using the ASTRA toolbox. Opt. Express **24**(22), 25129–25147 (2016)
11. Reaungamornrat, S., et al.: MIND Demons: symmetric diffeomorphic deformable registration of MR and CT for image-guided spine surgery. IEEE Trans. Med. Imaging **35**(11), 2413–2424 (2016)
12. Lu, H., et al.: Multi-modal diffeomorphic demons registration based on point-wise mutual information, pp. 372–375 (2010)

Linear and Deformable Image Registration with 3D Convolutional Neural Networks

Christodoulidis Stergios[1]($\boxtimes$), Sahasrabudhe Mihir[2], Vakalopoulou Maria[2], Chassagnon Guillaume[2,3], Revel Marie-Pierre[3], Mougiakakou Stavroula[1], and Paragios Nikos[4]

[1] ARTORG Center, University of Bern, Murtenstrasse 50, 3008 Bern, Switzerland
{stergios.christodoulidis,stavroula.mougiakakou}@artorg.unibe.ch
[2] CVN, CentraleSupélec, Université Paris-Saclay, 91190 Gif-sur-Yvette, France
{mihir.sahasrabudhe,maria.vakalopoulou,
guillaume.chassagnon}@centralesupelec.fr
[3] Groupe Hospitalier Cochin-Hôtel Dieu, Université Paris Descartes, Paris, France
marie-pierre.revel@aphp.fr
[4] TheraPanacea, Paris, France
n.paragios@therapanacea.eu

Abstract. Image registration and in particular deformable registration methods are pillars of medical imaging. Inspired by the recent advances in deep learning, we propose in this paper, a novel convolutional neural network architecture that couples linear and deformable registration within a unified architecture endowed with near real-time performance. Our framework is modular with respect to the global transformation component, as well as with respect to the similarity function while it guarantees smooth displacement fields. We evaluate the performance of our network on the challenging problem of MRI lung registration, and demonstrate superior performance with respect to state of the art elastic registration methods. The proposed deformation (between inspiration & expiration) was considered within a clinically relevant task of interstitial lung disease (ILD) classification and showed promising results.

Keywords: Convolutional neural networks · Deformable registration
Unsupervised learning · Lungs · Breathing · MRI
Interstitial lung disease

1 Introduction

Image registration is the process of aligning two or more sources of data to the same coordinate system. Through all the different registration methods used in medical applications, deformable registration is the one most commonly used due to its richness of description [15]. The goal of deformable registration is to calculate the optimal non-linear dense transformation G to align in the best

© Springer Nature Switzerland AG 2018
D. Stoyanov et al. (Eds.): RAMBO 2018/BIA 2018/TIA 2018, LNCS 11040, pp. 13–22, 2018.
https://doi.org/10.1007/978-3-030-00946-5_2

possible way, a source (moving) image S to a reference (target) image R [2,6]. Existing literature considers the mapping once the local alignment has been performed and therefore is often biased towards the linear component. Furthermore, state of the art methods are sensitive to the application setting, involve multiple hyper-parameters (optimization strategy, smoothness term, deformation model, similarity metric) and are computationally expensive.

Recently, deep learning methods have gained a lot of attention due to their state of the art performance on a variety of problems and applications [4,12]. In computer vision, optical flow estimation—a problem highly similar to deformable registration—has been successfully addressed with numerous deep neural network architectures [9]. In medical imaging, some methods in literature propose the use of convolutional neural networks (CNNs) as robust methods for image registration [5,14]. More recently, adversarial losses have been introduced with impressive performance [16]. The majority of these methods share two limitations: *(i)* dependency on the linear component of the transformation and *(ii)* dependency on ground truth displacement which is used for supervised training.

In this paper, we address the previous limitations of traditional deformable registration methods and at the same time propose an unsupervised method for efficient and accurate registration of 3D medical volumes that determines the linear and deformable parts in a single forward pass. The proposed solution outperforms conventional multi-metric deformable registration methods and demonstrates evidence of clinical relevance that can be used for the classification of patients with ILD using the transformation between the extreme moments of the respiration circle.

The main contributions of the study are fourfold: *(i)* coupling linear and deformable registration within a single optimization step/architecture, *(ii)* creating a modular, parameter-free implementation which is independent of the different similarity metrics, *(iii)* reducing considerably the computational time needed for registration allowing real-time applications, *(iv)* associating deformations with clinical information.

2   Methodology

In this study, we propose the use of an unsupervised CNN for the registration of pairs of medical images. A source image S and a reference image R are presented as inputs to the CNN while the output is the deformation G along with the registered source image D. This section presents details of the proposed architecture as well as the dataset that we utilized for our experiments. Please note that henceforth, we will use the terms *deformation*, *grid*, and *transformation* interchangeably.

2.1   Linear and Deformable 3D Transformer

One of the main components of the proposed CNN is the 3D transformer layer. This layer is part of the CNN and is used to warp its input under a deformation G. The forward pass for this layer is given by

$$D = \mathcal{W}(S, G), \tag{1}$$

where $\mathcal{W}(\cdot, G)$ indicates a sampling operation $\mathcal{W}$ under the deformation G. G is a dense deformation which can be thought of as an image of the same size as D, and which is constructed by assigning for every output voxel in D, a sampling coordinate in the input S.

In order to allow gradients to flow backwards though this warping operation and facilitate back-propagation training, the gradients with respect to the input image as well as the deformation should be defined. Similar to [10], such gradients can be calculated for a backward trilinear interpolation sampling. The deformation is hence fed to the transformer layer as sampling coordinates for backward warping. The sampling process is illustrated by

$$D(\mathbf{p}) = \mathcal{W}(S, G)(\mathbf{p}) = \sum_{\mathbf{q}} S(\mathbf{q}) \prod_d \max\left(0, 1 - |[G(\mathbf{p})]_d - \mathbf{q}_d|\right), \tag{2}$$

where $\mathbf{p}$ and $\mathbf{q}$ denote pixel locations, $d \in \{x, y, z\}$ denotes an axis, and $[G(\mathbf{p})]_d$ denotes the d-component of $G(\mathbf{p})$.

Our modeling of the deformation G offers a choice of the type of deformation we wish to use—linear, deformable, or both. The linear (or affine) part of the deformation requires the prediction of a 3×4 affine transformation matrix A according to the relation $[\hat{x}, \hat{y}, \hat{z}]^T = A[x, y, z, 1]^T$, where $[x, y, z, 1]^T$ represents the augmented points to be deformed, whereas $[\hat{x}, \hat{y}, \hat{z}]^T$ represents their locations in the deformed image. The matrix A can then be used to build a grid, G_A, which is the affine component of the deformation G.

To model the deformable part G_N, a simple and straightforward approach is to generate sampling coordinates for each output voxel ($G_N(\mathbf{p})$). We can let the network calculate these sampling points directly. Such a choice would however require the network to produce feature maps with large value ranges which complicates training. Moreover without appropriate regularization, non-smooth and even unconnected deformations could be produced. In order to circumvent this problem, we adopt the approach proposed by [13] and predict spatial gradients Φ of the deformation along each dimension instead of the deformation itself. This quantity measures the displacements of consecutive pixels. By enforcing these displacements to have positive values and subsequently applying an integration operation along each dimension, the spatial sampling coordinates can be retrieved. This integration operation could be approximated by simply applying a cumulative sum along each dimension of the input (i.e. integral image). In such a case, for example, when $\Phi_{\mathbf{p}_d} = 1$ there is no change in the distance between the pixels $\mathbf{p}$ and $\mathbf{p} + 1$ in the deformed image along the axis d. On the other hand, when $\Phi_{\mathbf{p}_d} < 1$, the distance between these consecutive pixels along d will decrease, while it will increase when $\Phi_{\mathbf{p}_d} > 1$. Such an approach ensures the generation of smooth deformations that avoid self-crossings, while allows the control of maximum displacements among consecutive pixels.

Finally, to compose the two parts we apply the deformable component to a moving image, followed by the linear component. When operating on a fixed image S, this step can be written as

$$\mathcal{W}(S,G) = \mathcal{W}\left(\mathcal{W}(S,G_N),G_A\right). \tag{3}$$

During training, the optimization of the decoders of A and G_N is done jointly, as the network is trained end-to-end. We also impose regularization constraints on both these components. We elaborate on the importance of this regularization for the joint training in Sect. 2.3.

2.2 Architecture

The architecture of the CNN is based on an encoder-decoder framework presented in [1] (Fig. 1). The encoder adopts dilated convolutional kernels along with multi-resolution feature merging, while the decoder employs non-dilated convolutional layers and up-sampling operations. Specifically, a kernel size of $3 \times 3 \times 3$ was set for the convolutional layers while LeakyReLU activation was employed for all convolutional layers except the last two. Instance normalization was included before most of the activation functions. In total five layers are used in the encoder and their outputs are merged along with the input pair of image to form a feature map of 290 features with a total receptive field of $25 \times 25 \times 25$. In the decoder, two branches were implemented—one for the spatial deformation gradients and the other for the affine matrix. As far as the former is concerned, a squeeze-excitation block [8] was added in order to weigh the most important features for the spatial gradients calculation while for the latter a simple global average operation was used to reduce the spatial dimensions

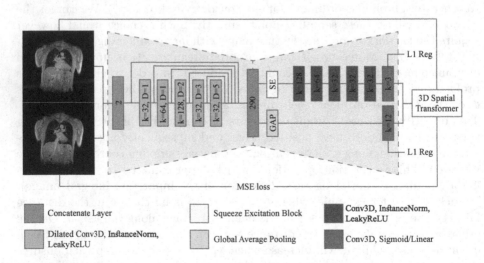

Fig. 1. The overall CNN architecture. The network uses a pair of 3D images and calculates the optimal deformations from the one image to the other.

to one. For the affine parameters and the spatial deformation gradients, a linear layer and sigmoid activation were respectively used. Finally to retrieve Φ, the output of the sigmoid function should be scaled by a factor of 2 in order to fall in the range $[0, 2]$ and hence allow for consecutive pixels to have larger distance than the initial.

2.3 Training

The network was trained by minimizing the mean squared error (MSE) between the R and D image intensities as well as the regularization terms of the affine transformation parameters and the spatial deformation gradients using the Adam optimizer [11]. Our loss is defined as

$$\text{Loss} = \|R - \mathcal{W}(S, G)\|^2 + \alpha \|A - A_I\|_1 + \beta \|\Phi - \Phi_I\|_1, \tag{4}$$

where A_I represents the identity affine transformation matrix, Φ_I is the spatial gradient of the identity deformation, and α and β are regularization weights. As mentioned before, regularization is essential to the joint optimization. To elaborate, without the L1 regularization on A, the network might get stuck in a local minimum where it aligns only high-level features using the affine transformation. This will result in a high reconstruction error. On the other hand, without the smoothness regularizer on Φ, the spatial gradients decoder network can predict very non-smooth grids which again makes it prone to fall in a local minimum. Having both linear and deformable components is helpful to the network because these two components now share the work. This hypothesis aligns with [13] and is also evaluated in Sect. 3.

The initial learning rate is 10^{-3} and subdued by a factor of 10 if the performance on the validation set does not improve for 50 epochs while the training procedure stops when there is no improvement for 100 epochs. The regularization weights α and β were set to 10^{-6} so that neither of the two components has an unreasonably large contribution to the final loss. As training samples, random pairs among all cases were selected with a batch size of 2 due to the limited memory resources on the GPU. The performance of the network was evaluated every 100 batches, and both proposed models—with and without affine components—converged after nearly 300 epochs. The overall training time was calculated to $\sim$16 h.

2.4 Dataset

MRI exams were acquired as a part of a prospective study aiming to evaluate the feasibility of pulmonary fibrosis detection in systemic sclerosis patients by using magnetic resonance imaging (MRI) and an elastic registration-driven biomarker. This study received institutional review board approval and all patients gave their written consent. The study population consisted of 41 patients (29 patients with systemic sclerosis and 12 healthy volunteers). Experienced radiologists annotated the lung field for the total of the 82 images and provided information about the pathology of each patient (healthy or not). Additionally, eleven characteristic landmarks inside the lung area had been provided by two experienced radiologists.

All MRI examinations were acquired on a 3T-MRI unit (SKYRA magneton, Siemens Healthineers) using an 18-phased-array-body coil. All subjects were positioned in the supine position with their arms along the body. Inspiratory and expiratory MRI images were acquired using an ultrashort time of echo (UTE) sequence, the spiral VIBE sequence, with the same acquisition parameters (repetition time 2.73 ms, echo time 0.05 ms, flip angle 5°, field-of-view 620×620 mm, slice thickness 2.5 mm, matrix 188×188, with an in-plane resolution of 2.14×2.14 mm).

As a pre-processing step, the image intensity values were cropped within the window $[0, 1300]$ and mapped to $[0, 1]$. Moreover, all the images were scaled down along all dimensions by a factor of $2/3$ with cubic interpolation resulting to an image size of $64 \times 192 \times 192$ to compensate GPU memory constraints. A random split was performed and 28 patients (56 pairs of images) were selected for the training set, resulting to 3136 training pairs, while the rest 13 were used for validation.

3   Experimental Setup and Results

3.1   Evaluation

We evaluated the performance of our method against two different state-of-the-art methods, namely, Symmetric Normalization (SyN) [2], using its implementation on the ANTs package [3] and the deformable method presented in [6,7] for a variety of similarity metrics (normalized cross correlation (NCC), mutual information (MI) and discrete wavelet metric (DWM), and their combination). For the evaluation we calculated the Dice coefficient metric, measured on the lung masks, after we applied the calculated deformation on the lung mask of the moving image. Moreover, we evaluate our method using the provided landmark locations. For comparison reasons we report the approximate computational time each of these methods needed to register a pair of images. For all the implementations we used a GeForce GTX 1080 GPU except for SyN implementation where we used a CPU implementation running on 4 cores of an i7-4700HQ CPU.

3.2   Results and Discussion

Starting with the quantitative evaluation, in Table 1 the mean Dice coefficient values along with their standard deviations are presented for different methods. We performed two different types of tests. In the first set of experiments (Table 1: Inhale-Exhale), we tested the performance of the different methods for the registration of the MRI images, between the inhale and exhale images, for the 13 validation patients. The SyN implementation reports the lowest Dice scores while at the same time, it is computationally quite expensive due to its CPU implementation. Moreover, we tested three different similarity metrics along with their

Table 1. Dice coefficient scores (%) calculated over the deformed lung masks and the ground truth.

Method	Inhale-exhale	All combinations	Time/subject (s)
Unregistered	75.62 ± 10.89	57.22 ± 12.90	–
Deformable with NCC [6]	84.25 ± 6.89	76.10 ± 7.92	$\sim$1 (GPU)
Deformable with DWM [6]	88.63 ± 4.67	75.92 ± 8.81	$\sim$2 (GPU)
Deformable with MI [6]	88.86 ± 5.13	76.33 ± 8.74	$\sim$2 (GPU)
Deformable with all above [6]	88.81 ± 5.85	78.71 ± 8.56	$\sim$2 (GPU)
SyN [2]	83.86 ± 6.04	–	$\sim$2500 (CPU)
Proposed w/o Affine	91.28 ± 2.47	81.75 ± 7.88	$\sim$0.5 (GPU)
Proposed	$\mathbf{91.48 \pm 2.33}$	$\mathbf{82.34 \pm 7.68}$	$\sim$0.5 (GPU)

combinations using the method proposed in [6] as described earlier. In this specific setup, the MI metric seam to report the best Dice scores. However, the scores reported by the proposed architecture are superior by at least $\sim$2.5% to the ones reported by the other methods. For the proposed method, the addition of a linear component to the transformation layer does not change the performance of the network significantly in this experiment. Finally, we calculated the errors over all axes in predicted locations for eleven different manually annotated landmark points on inhale volumes after they were deformed using the decoded deformation for each patient. We compare the performance of our method against the inter-observer (two different medical experts) distance and the method presented in [6] in Table 2. We observe that both methods perform very well considering the inter-observer variability, with the proposed one reporting slightly better average euclidean distances.

For the second set of experiments (Table 1: All combinations), we report the Dice scores for all combinations of the 13 different patients, resulting on 169 validation pairs. Due to the large number of combinations, this problem is more challenging since the size of the lungs in the extreme moments of the respiratory circles can vary significantly. Again, the performance of the proposed architecture is superior to the tested baselines, highlighting its very promising results. In this experimental setup, the linear component plays a more important part by boosting the performance by $\sim$0.5%.

Concerning the computation time, both [6] and the proposed method report very low inference time, due to their GPU implementations, with the proposed method reaching $\sim$0.5 s per subject. On the other hand, [2] is computationally quite expensive, making it difficult to test it for all the possible combinations on the validation set.

Finally, in Fig. 2, we present the deformed image produced by the proposed method on coronal view for a single patient in the two different moments of the respiratory cyrcle. The grids were superimposed on the images, indicating the displacements calculated by the network. The last column shows the difference

Table 2. Errors measured as average euclidean distances between estimated landmark locations and ground truth marked by two medical experts. We also report as *inter-observer*, the average euclidean distance between same landmark locations marked by the two experts. dx, dy, and dz denote distances along x-, y-, and z- axes, respectively, while ds denotes the average error along all axes.

Method	dx	dy	dz	ds
Inter-observer	1.664	2.545	1.555	3.905
Deformable with NCC, DWM, and MI [6]	1.855	3.169	2.229	4.699
Proposed w/o Affine	2.014	2.947	1.858	4.569
Proposed	**1.793**	**2.904**	**1.822**	**4.358**

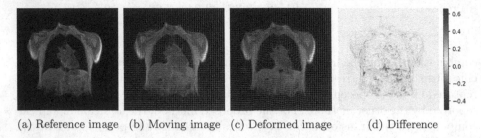

(a) Reference image   (b) Moving image   (c) Deformed image   (d) Difference

Fig. 2. A visualized registration of a pair of images, generated by the proposed architecture. The initial and deformed grids are superimposed on the images.

between the reference and deformed image. One can observe that the majority of the errors occur on the boundaries, as the network fails to capture large local displacements.

3.3   Evaluation of the Clinical Relevance of the Deformation

To asses the relevance of the decoded transformations in a clinical setting, we trained a small classifier on top of the obtained residual deformations to classify patients as healthy or unhealthy. The residual deformation associated with a pair of images indicates voxel displacements, written as $G_\delta = G - G_I$, where G is the deduced deformation between the two images, and G_I is the identity deformation.

We trained a downsampling convolutional kernel followed by a multi-layer perceptron (MLP) to be able to predict whether a case is healthy or not. The network architecture is shown in Fig. 3. The model includes batch normalization layers, to avoid overfitting, as we have few training examples at our disposal. Further, a Tanh activation function is used in the MLP. The downsampling kernel is of size $3 \times 3 \times 3$, with a stride of 2 and a padding of 1. The number of units in the hidden layer of the MLP was set to 100. We trained with binary cross entropy loss, with an initial learning rate of 10^{-4}, which is halved every

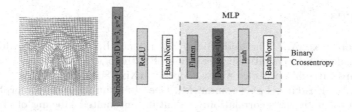

Fig. 3. The neural network trained as a classifier on top of the transformations.

fifty epochs. Training five models in parallel took about 2 h on two GeForce GTX 1080 GPUs.

We cross-validate five models on the training set of 28 patients, and report the average response of these models on the rest 13 patients. We conduct the same experiment for deformations obtained using [6] and all similarity measures (NCC, DWM, MI). The results on the test set using a threshold of 0.5 on the predicted probability are reported in Table 3, suggesting that indeed the deformations between inhale and exhale carry information about lung diseases.

Table 3. Results on disease prediction using deformations on the test set. The reported accuracy is in percentage points.

Method	Accuracy
Deformable with NCC, DWM, and MI [6]	69.23
Proposed	**84.62**

4   Conclusion

In this paper, we propose a novel method which exploits the 3D CNNs to calculate the optimal transformation (combining a linear and a deformable component within a coupled framework) between pair of images that is modular with respect to the similarity function, and the nature of transformation. The proposed method generates deformations with no self-crossings due to the way the deformation layer is defined, efficient due to the GPU implementation of the inference and reports high promising results compared to other unsupervised registration methods. Currently, the proposed network was tested on the challenging problem of lung registration, however, its evaluation on the registration of other modalities, and other organs is one of the potential directions of our method.

References

1. Anthimopoulos, M., Christodoulidis, S., Ebner, L., Geiser, T., Christe, A., Mougiakakou, S.: Semantic segmentation of pathological lung tissue with dilated fully convolutional networks. arXiv preprint arXiv:1803.06167 (2018)
2. Avants, B., Epstein, C., Grossman, M., Gee, J.: Symmetric diffeomorphic image registration with cross-correlation: evaluating automated labeling of elderly and neurodegenerative brain. Med. Image Anal. **12**, 26–41 (2008)
3. Avants, B.B., Tustison, N.J., Song, G., Cook, P.A., Klein, A., Gee, J.C.: A reproducible evaluation of ants similarity metric performance in brain image registration. NeuroImage **54**, 2033–2044 (2011)
4. Chandra, S., Usunier, N., Kokkinos, I.: Dense and low-rank Gaussian CRFs using deep embeddings. In: 2017 IEEE International Conference on Computer Vision (ICCV) (2017)
5. Cheng, X., Zhang, L., Zheng, Y.: Deep similarity learning for multimodal medical images (2016)
6. Ferrante, E., Dokania, P.K., Marini, R., Paragios, N.: Deformable registration through learning of context-specific metric aggregation. In: Wang, Q., Shi, Y., Suk, H.-I., Suzuki, K. (eds.) MLMI 2017. LNCS, vol. 10541, pp. 256–265. Springer, Cham (2017). https://doi.org/10.1007/978-3-319-67389-9_30
7. Glocker, B., Sotiras, A., Komodakis, N., Paragios, N.: Deformable medical image registration: setting the state of the art with discrete methods. Ann. Rev. Biomed. Eng. **13**, 219–244 (2011)
8. Hu, J., Shen, L., Sun, G.: Squeeze-and-excitation networks. In: IEEE Conference on Computer Vision and Pattern Recognition (CVPR) (2018)
9. Hui, T.W., Tang, X., Loy, C.C.: Liteflownet: A lightweight convolutional neural network for optical flow estimation. In: IEEE Conference on Computer Vision and Pattern Recognition (CVPR) (2018)
10. Jaderberg, M., Simonyan, K., Zisserman, A., et al.: Spatial transformer networks. In: Advances in Neural Information Processing Systems, pp. 2017–2025 (2015)
11. Kingma, D.P., Ba, J.: Adam: a method for stochastic optimization. arXiv preprint arXiv:1412.6980 (2014)
12. Riza, A., Neverova, N., Kokkinos, I.: DensePose: dense human pose estimation in the wild. arXiv (2018)
13. Shu, Z., Sahasrabudhe, M., Güler, R.A., Samaras, D., Paragios, N., Kokkinos, I.: Deforming autoencoders: unsupervised disentangling of shape and appearance. In: 2018 IEEE European Conference on Computer Vision (ECCV) (2018)
14. Simonovsky, M., Gutiérrez-Becker, B., Mateus, D., Navab, N., Komodakis, N.: A deep metric for multimodal registration. In: Ourselin, S., Joskowicz, L., Sabuncu, M.R., Unal, G., Wells, W. (eds.) MICCAI 2016. LNCS, vol. 9902, pp. 10–18. Springer, Cham (2016). https://doi.org/10.1007/978-3-319-46726-9_2
15. Sotiras, A., Davatzikos, C., Paragios, N.: Deformable medical image registration: a survey. IEEE Trans. Med. Imaging **32**, 1153–1190 (2013)
16. Yan, P., Xu, S., Rastinehad, A.R., Wood, B.J.: Adversarial image registration with application for MR and TRUS image fusion (2018). http://arxiv.org/abs/1804.11024

Super Resolution of Cardiac Cine MRI Sequences Using Deep Learning

Nicolas Basty$^{(\boxtimes)}$ and Vicente Grau

Institute of Biomedical Engineering, Department of Engineering Science,
University of Oxford, Oxford, UK
nicolas.basty@eng.ox.ac.uk

Abstract. Cardiac cine MRI facilitates structural and functional analysis of the heart through the dynamic aspect of the sequences. Clinical acquisitions consist of sparse 2D images instead of 3D volumes, taken at landmark points of the ECG to cover the whole heartbeat. A stack of short axis images and a small number of long axis views are generally acquired. Efforts have been made to accelerate acquisitions at the acquisition stage as well as at post-processing. A major part of current research in medical image processing focuses on deep learning approaches driven by large datasets. However, most of those methods leave out the dynamic aspect of temporal data and treat frames of cine MRI sequences individually. We propose a super resolution network based on the U-net and long short-term memory layers to exploit the temporal aspect of the dynamic cardiac cine MRI data. When given a sequence of low resolution long axis images, our method is able to render a high resolution sequence. Results on synthetic data simulating a stack of short axis images show quantitative and qualitative improvements over traditional interpolation methods or the equivalent machine learning method using a single frame, including the ability of the network to recover important image features such as the apex.

Keywords: Super-resolution · Cardiac cine MRI · Deep learning

1 Introduction

Cardiac cine MRI allows functional and structural analysis of the heart. Due to its exceptional soft tissue contrast, reproducibility and safety considerations it is commonly taken as the gold standard for cardiac imaging. To capture the whole heartbeat in a sequence of images, scans are produced at landmark times synchronised with ECG readings. To minimise the imaging times, clinical acquisitions consist of anisotropic 2D slices instead of a 3D volume. A stack of parallel short axis (SA) slices and a small number of orthogonal long axis (LA) slices are generally acquired for each frame of the sequence. The number of slices in the SA stack is dependent on the size of the heart but generally ranges between 8 and 12, and the number of LA slices is also variable. Standardised protocols

D. Stoyanov et al. (Eds.): RAMBO 2018/BIA 2018/TIA 2018, LNCS 11040, pp. 23–31, 2018.
https://doi.org/10.1007/978-3-030-00946-5_3

such as the UK biobank protocol include three LA views: the vertical long axis (VLA, also called 2-chamber view), the horizontal long axis (HLA, also called 4-chamber view), and the left ventricular outflow tract (LVOT) view [1, 2]. Some of the main issues associated with cine MRI are the slice misalignment occurring due to patient motion and breath hold variations between acquisitions, intensity differences between slices due to flow artefacts and magnetic field inhomogeneities, and sometimes contrast agents, as well the sparsity of the data occasionally resulting in a lack of coverage of the left ventricle by the SA stack [3]. The dynamic aspect of cardiac MRI is used to evaluate cardiovascular function metrics such as the ejection fraction and the stroke volume, to quantify wall motion and thickness and identify scar tissue in follow-up scans from patients who have suffered a myocardial infarct.

The MRI pulse sequence most commonly used in cardiac cine MRI for left ventricular structural and functional analysis is the b-SFFP sequence. This is due to its excellent signal-to-noise ratio per unit time and T2/T1 contrast and the fact that it does not suffer from excessive signal loss from motion [4]. There also exists a 3D version of the b-SFFP sequence, which allows isotropic acquisitions but in turn has worse contrast between blood and the myocardium and is therefore not commonly used in clinical practice.

MRI acquisitions may be accelerated at the acquisition stage, by undersampling k-space and reconstructing images with incomplete data, which is referred to as compressed sensing. Most compressed sensing approaches work on an individual image basis. One of the few that uses temporal context is [5] where a dynamic 2D+t dictionary is learnt and used to recover missing k-space data.

The limitations caused by the relatively long time required for MRI acquisition have also led to interest in the development of super resolution methods at the post-processing end of the imaging pipeline. A large part of the literature uses non-machine learning approaches. Most of these methods involve least squares error regularisation and assume overlap between numerous slices [6]. Few approaches to super resolution of medical images, more specifically cardiac cine MRI, actually make use of the temporal aspect. In work by Odille *et al.*, a parallel SA stack and two additional stacks taken at orthogonal orientations are used to produce a 3D reconstruction of the heart using regularised least squares, after applying a motion compensating algorithm using the data from the whole cine sequence [7].

Recently, machine learning methods have dominated the research in the biomedical image analysis field. With the increasing availability of computing power, large labelled datasets and open source libraries, deep learning has quickly become the benchmark for many tasks such as image classification and segmentation. The first application of deep learning to image super-resolution consisted of a simple network with three layers, inspired by the idea behind dictionary learning applications to super resolution. The first layer has a small filter size similar to a LR dictionary extracting a small LR image patch, the third layer a larger filter size similar to a HR dictionary upsampling to a bigger higher resolution patch, and the middle layer introduces a non linear mapping between the two [8]. A small number of training images underlines the simplicity of the approach, which shows pleasing results on natural images, and has become a benchmark in deep learning super resolution.

Some of the best results in image segmentation have been produced by the U-net architecture introduced by Ronneberger et al. [9]. The U-net is a convolutional neural network, similar to an autoencoder but including skip connections between input and output layers. The skip connections allow high frequency as well as low frequency information to be processed and make it suitable for super resolution, for which it has been applied to 3D microscopy in two recent studies. The first of them uses a U-net to generate a residual image containing the high frequency information to be added to the LR input [10]. The second compares a U-net to a Super-Resolution Convolutional Neural Network (SRCNN) [8] in 3D to upsample synthetically downsampled microscopy images, showing that both architectures can be used for the task at hand with the U-net consistently outperforming SRCNN [11].

Deep learning has also been applied to super resolution of cardiac MRI in [12], where a single image and a multi-image network are trained to predict residuals which are added to the LR image and give it high frequency information. The data used in that study comes from synthetically down-sampled 3D b-SFFP acquisitions that do not require realignment to account for breathing between acquisitions or patient motion. The same group recently extended the network to an anatomically constrained neural network that resembles a U-net and is able to do super resolution and segmentation aided by the addition of shape priors [13]. In contrast, our work aims to improve standard dynamic 2D data acquired in clinical practice, using the dynamic information in the time sequence to improve the reconstruction. We present a network learning a one-to-one mapping between low resolution (LR) and high resolution (HR) 2D image sequences to generate additional HR LA views from a dynamic SA stack.

Recurrent neural networks (RNN) and especially long short term memory (LSTM) are starting to be applied in medical image analysis. Recurrence can be applied in a spatial sense, by considering adjacent slices in a 3D image. In a study on prostate MRI for cancer segmentation, adjacent 2D slices were fed into a U-net fitted with recurrent layers at every convolution [14]. RNNs have been applied to cardiac cine MRI first by Poudel et al. [15], at the lowest resolution level of a U-net to take advantage of low frequency features in consecutive frames of the cardiac cycle. LSTMs have been applied to enhance performance of myocardium segmentations in cardiac cine MRI sequences [16]. In that study, similar to [15], recurrent layers are present in the lower resolution levels of the network architecture.

Up to our knowledge, recurrent networks have not been used for cardiac cine MRI sequence reconstruction. In this paper we propose a method using temporal recurrence to recover HR LA slices from LR acquisitions. Our results show that introducing recurrence improves the quality of the reconstruction, as compared to equivalent single-frame approaches.

2   Materials and Methods

Our method uses an architecture inspired by the U-net, with added recurrent layers, sharing some characteristics with those used in [14–16] for segmentation. While [14] used recurrence on all levels of a U-net, [16] only on the two lower resolution levels, and [15] only on the lowest resolution level, we included recurrence layers on the first two layers, corresponding to the highest resolutions. We limited the number of levels to the first two for two reasons: to save memory and because unlike with segmentation work where the lower frequency features are more important, we are particularly interested in the high frequency information which is needed to convert LR into HR images.

Figure 1 shows the network architecture. The network we propose is inspired by the U-net with a contractive part and skip connections sensitive to low and high frequency details, respectively. At the first and second levels, we introduced LSTM convolution layers. There are a total of five levels in the network each initiated by a 2×2 Max pooling layer. The input data has a size of $128 \times 128 \times 10$, the lowest level therefore operates on samples of size $8 \times 8 \times 10$ where only the very low frequency features are present. We chose to put the recurrent layers on the top levels since we want to enhance the high frequency features of the images and they are mostly present in the first and second levels. Going down to the

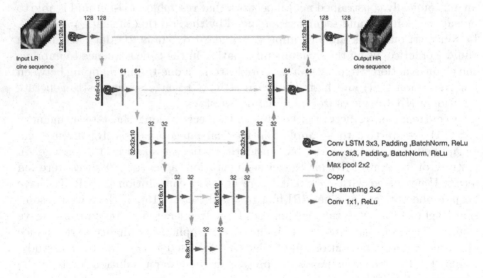

Fig. 1. Network architecture. A network inspired by the U-net with four LSTM modules at the top of the network aiming to enhance high frequency features by taking into account the dynamic aspect of the cine sequence on the original image size and after the first max pooling operation which decreases the image size by a factor of two. Filter numbers are indicated on the diagram on top of the blue bars after every convolution. Arrows represent the different operations. Height, width, and time sizes are shown for every level. (Color figure online)

third level, the data is now $32 \times 32 \times 10$ which we deemed to be less relevant to the high frequency content. We also trained a U-net with the same architecture where all the convolution layers are conventional convolutions with filters of size 3×3, to compare performance between a context sensitive and a static network. Training was performed using an Adam optimiser to minimise mean squared error over 90 epochs, with a learning rate of $4.5.10^{-5}$. The network was written in Python using the Keras library (https://keras.io) running on Tensorflow backend, and training was performed on a Nvidia GeForce GTX 1080 Ti 256 RAM GPU.

2.1 Data

LA views from the Kaggle Data Science Bowl Cardiac Challenge Data [17] were used in training. The dataset consists of cine MRI sequences of over five hundred patients. Every data set has 30 frames, however the number of SA and LA slices differ, as a standardised imaging protocol was not used. VLA and HLA acquisitions were present for most of the patients but a non negligible part of the data had only one or no LA views. The patients have a large spread of age and size which is advantageous to preserve the generalisation properties of the method.

After discarding unusable data (e.g. the ones affected by very strong artefacts or wrongly labeled as LA) by visual inspection, all remaining images were resampled to isotropic resolution of $1.4 \, \text{mm} \times 1.4 \, \text{mm}$, rotated to the same upright orientation where the base is towards the top of the image and the apex towards the bottom, and down-sampled in the baso-apical direction to match the slice thickness of standard SA slices of $10 \, \text{mm}$. In this way, we generated images similar to those that would be reconstructed from the SA stack. Every sequence was also normalised such that all image intensities lie in the range between 0 and 1. We did not differentiate between HLA and VLA views, both were included together in the training, validation and testing datasets. In this way, we aimed to demonstrate the ability of the method to recover images with different appearance (e.g. in terms of the number of chambers), with the eventual goal of using the network to produce slices in any arbitrary orthogonal orientation from SA stacks.

After splitting the sequences of 30 frames into shorter sequences of 10 frames each (to reduce the time needed for training), 3342 LR-HR sequence pairs of 10 frames per sequence were available. 3000 sequences were used for training, 171 set aside for validation, and 171 for testing, ensuring that none of the split sequences were spanning over the training and the validation or testing set. For the static network, all the frames in a sequence were used, which increased the training, validation, and testing data by a factor of 30.

3 Results

Results on the first 5 frames of a HLA sequence are shown in Fig. 2. A representative result on 5 non-adjacent frames of a VLA sequence can be seen in Fig. 3, with the cardiac contraction more easily visible due to the frames spanning a longer time. Both figures display a sequence from the unseen testing dataset using cubic interpolation in the first row, the result of using static frames only in the second row, the result of the proposed network in the third row, and the ground truth on the bottom row. Each frame has been magnified around the apex, one of the features that is most prone to being missed by the SA stack acquisition. The proposed network manages to recover the apex across the sequence, with much better definition than previously used standard U-Nets.

In addition to qualitative improvements, the peak signal-to-noise ratio (PSNR) and structural similarity (SSIM) of the dynamic network output outperform the static network and interpolation. More quantitative results are shown in Table 1, which contains the average values for PSNR and SSIM of the whole testing data set and shows that the dynamic network output is superior to the static network as well as interpolation.

Table 1. Quantitative evaluation (PSNR and SSIM) of interpolated, single frame U-net, and the proposed network results on the whole testing data set which has not been seen by the networks in training.

	Interpolated	U-net	LSTM
PSNR	23.17 dB	25.23 dB	26.57 dB
SSIM	0.72	0.77	0.81

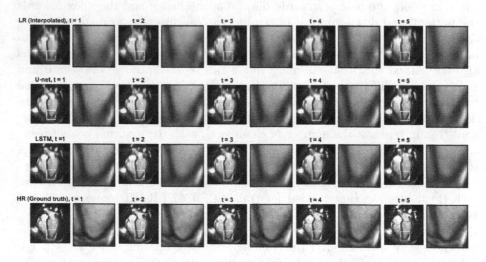

Fig. 2. Result on the first 5 frames of a HLA view cine sequence. The top row shows the LR interpolated input, the second row shows the result given by the static U-net, the third the result given by network including LSTM layers, and the bottom row shows the HR ground truth. This proposed enhanced 4-chamber sequence has a PSNR of 25.28 dB and a SSIM of 0.82 while the static U-net gives a PSNR of 23.83 dB and a SSIM of 0.79 and the interpolated sequence a PSNR of 22.15 dB and a SSIM of 0.73.

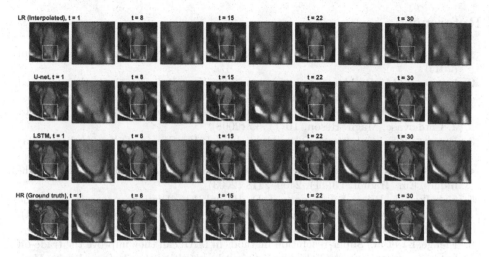

Fig. 3. Result on the 1st, 8th, 15th, 22nd, and 30th frames of a VLA view cine sequence. The top row shows the LR interpolated input, the second row shows the result given by the static U-net, the third the result given by network including LSTM layers, and the bottom row shows the HR ground truth. This proposed enhanced 2-chamber sequence has a PSNR of 27.55 dB and a SSIM of 0.83 while the static U-net gives a PSNR of 25.69 dB and a SSIM of 0.78 and the interpolated sequence a PSNR of 22.23 dB and a SSIM of 0.71.

4   Discussion and Conclusion

We have showed that there is an advantage to using the temporal context for super resolution of cardiac cine MRI sequences, in comparison to the more common approach of reconstructing individual frames. Our proposed architecture, which includes LSTM layers on the upper layers of a U-net, gives qualitatively and quantitatively superior results to an equivalent U-net architecture with no recurrence.

In order to concentrate on the effects of recurrence on reconstructions, we chose experiments that avoid common acquisition artifacts such as misalignment between slices and intensity mismatches. Future work will look into the reconstruction from clinical SA stacks suffering from these artifacts, as well as reconstruction of arbitrarily oriented slices, eventually aiming to reconstruct complete 3D datasets.

Acknowledgments. NMB acknowledges the support of the RCUK Digital Economy Programme grant number EP/G036861/1 (Oxford Centre for Doctoral Training in Healthcare Innovation).

References

1. Petersen, S.E., et al.: UK Biobank's cardiovascular magnetic resonance protocol (2015)
2. Kramer, C.M., Barkhausen, J., Flamm, S.D., Kim, R.J., Nagel, E.: Standardized cardiovascular magnetic resonance imaging (CMR) protocols, society for cardiovascular magnetic resonance: board of trustees task force on standardized protocols. J. Cardiovasc. Magn. Reson. **10**(1), 35 (2008)
3. Ferreira, P.F., Gatehouse, P.D., Mohiaddin, R.H., Firmin, D.N.: Cardiovascular magnetic resonance artefacts. J. Cardiovasc. Magn. Reson. **15**(1), 41 (2013)
4. Scheffler, K., Lehnhardt, S.: Principles and applications of balanced SSFP techniques. Eur. Radiol. **13**(11), 2409–2418 (2003)
5. Caballero, J., Price, A.N., Rueckert, D., Hajnal, J.V.: Dictionary learning and time sparsity for dynamic MR data reconstruction. IEEE Trans. Med. Imaging **33**(4), 979–994 (2014)
6. Plenge, E., et al.: Super-resolution methods in MRI: can they improve the trade-off between resolution, signal-to-noise ratio, and acquisition time? Magn. Reson. Med. **68**(6), 1983–1993 (2012)
7. Odille, F., Bustin, A., Chen, B., Vuissoz, P.-A., Felblinger, J.: Motion-corrected, super-resolution reconstruction for high-resolution 3D cardiac cine MRI. In: Navab, N., Hornegger, J., Wells, W.M., Frangi, A.F. (eds.) MICCAI 2015. LNCS, vol. 9351, pp. 435–442. Springer, Cham (2015). https://doi.org/10.1007/978-3-319-24574-4_52
8. Dong, C., Loy, C.C., He, K., Tang, X.: Learning a deep convolutional network for image super-resolution. In: Fleet, D., Pajdla, T., Schiele, B., Tuytelaars, T. (eds.) ECCV 2014. LNCS, vol. 8692, pp. 184–199. Springer, Cham (2014). https://doi.org/10.1007/978-3-319-10593-2_13
9. Ronneberger, O., Fischer, P., Brox, T.: U-Net: convolutional networks for biomedical image segmentation. In: Navab, N., Hornegger, J., Wells, W.M., Frangi, A.F. (eds.) MICCAI 2015. LNCS, vol. 9351, pp. 234–241. Springer, Cham (2015). https://doi.org/10.1007/978-3-319-24574-4_28
10. Weigert, M., Royer, L., Jug, F., Myers, G.: Isotropic reconstruction of 3D fluorescence microscopy images using convolutional neural networks. In: Descoteaux, M., Maier-Hein, L., Franz, A., Jannin, P., Collins, D.L., Duchesne, S. (eds.) MICCAI 2017. LNCS, vol. 10434, pp. 126–134. Springer, Cham (2017). https://doi.org/10.1007/978-3-319-66185-8_15
11. Heinrich, L., Bogovic, J.A., Saalfeld, S.: Deep learning for isotropic super-resolution from non-isotropic 3D electron microscopy. In: Descoteaux, M., Maier-Hein, L., Franz, A., Jannin, P., Collins, D.L., Duchesne, S. (eds.) MICCAI 2017. LNCS, vol. 10434, pp. 135–143. Springer, Cham (2017). https://doi.org/10.1007/978-3-319-66185-8_16
12. Oktay, O., et al.: Multi-input cardiac image super-resolution using convolutional neural networks. In: Ourselin, S., Joskowicz, L., Sabuncu, M.R., Unal, G., Wells, W. (eds.) MICCAI 2016. LNCS, vol. 9902, pp. 246–254. Springer, Cham (2016). https://doi.org/10.1007/978-3-319-46726-9_29
13. Oktay, O., et al.: Anatomically constrained neural networks (ACNNs): application to cardiac image enhancement and segmentation. IEEE Trans. Med. Imaging **37**(2), 384–395 (2018)

14. Zhu, Q., Du, B., Turkbey, B., Choyke, P., Yan, P.: Exploiting interslice correlation for MRI prostate image segmentation, from recursive neural networks aspect. Complexity **2018**, 10 (2018). https://doi.org/10.1155/2018/4185279. Article ID 4185279
15. Poudel, R.P.K., Lamata, P., Montana, G.: Recurrent fully convolutional neural networks for multi-slice MRI cardiac segmentation. In: Zuluaga, M.A., Bhatia, K., Kainz, B., Moghari, M.H., Pace, D.F. (eds.) RAMBO/HVSMR - 2016. LNCS, vol. 10129, pp. 83–94. Springer, Cham (2017). https://doi.org/10.1007/978-3-319-52280-7_8
16. Zhang, D., et al.: A multi-level convolutional LSTM model for the segmentation of left ventricle myocardium in infarcted porcine cine MR images. In: 2018 IEEE 15th International Symposium on Biomedical Imaging (ISBI 2018), pp. 470–473. IEEE (2018)
17. Kaggle data science bowl cardiac challenge data (2015). https://www.kaggle.com/c/second-annual-data-science-bowl/data

Automated CNN-Based Reconstruction of Short-Axis Cardiac MR Sequence from Real-Time Image Data

Eric Kerfoot[✉], Esther Puyol Anton, Bram Ruijsink, James Clough,
Andrew P. King, and Julia A. Schnabel

Division of Imaging Sciences and Biomedical Engineering,
King's College London, London, UK
eric.kerfoot@kcl.ac.uk

Abstract. We present a methodology for reconstructing full-cycle respiratory and cardiac gated short-axis cine MR sequences from real-time MR data. For patients who are too ill or otherwise incapable of consistent breath holds, real-time MR sequences are the preferred means of acquiring cardiac images, but suffer from inferior image quality compared to standard short-axis sequences and lack cardiac ECG gating. To construct a sequence from real-time images which, as close as possible, replicates the characteristics of short-axis series, the phase of the cardiac cycle must be estimated for each image and the left ventricle identified, to be used as a landmark for slice re-alignment. Our method employs CNN-based deep learning to segment the left ventricle in the real-time sequence, which is then used to estimate the pool volume and thus the position of each image in the cardiac cycle. We then use manifold learning to account for the respiratory cycle so as to select images of the best quality at expiration. From these images a selection is made to automatically reconstruct a single cardiac cycle, and the images and segmentations are then aligned. The aligned pool segmentations can then be used to calculate volume over time and thus volume-based biomarkers.

Keywords: Automatic segmentation · Real time cardiac imaging
Image-based motion correction

1 Introduction

Short axis cine (SAX) is the primary cardiac magnetic resonance imaging (cMRI) protocol for assessing cardiac function, but relies on electrocardiogram (ECG) gating and breath holds during acquisition. The protocol requires the subject to lie still, restricting it to acquisitions at rest, and to perform breath holds, which not all patients can do due to pathology or age. Free breathing non-gated real-time cine (RT) is an alternative protocol which has recently been proposed as a solution to the above problem [10, 11]. This method acquires images over multiple cardiac cycles at the same locations in the left ventricle (LV) as SAX, both

D. Stoyanov et al. (Eds.): RAMBO 2018/BIA 2018/TIA 2018, LNCS 11040, pp. 32–41, 2018.
https://doi.org/10.1007/978-3-030-00946-5_4

eliminating the need for patient cooperation during breath holds and allowing imaging during movement and distorted ECG signals, eg. during exercise. A less demanding scanning sequence such as RT greatly expands the number of patients who can be scanned, and using RT to assess cardiac function during exercise has its own diagnostic potential [3]. Developing a methodology for improving the quality of RT imaging would therefore provide a new and effective tool for clinicians.

However the RT series suffers from poor image quality, in terms of greater noise and artefacts, compared to SAX sequences, as well as patient motion from respiration and minor body shifts. The images of this series are thus neither aligned in space nor in time as each plane starts acquisition at arbitrary points in the cardiac cycle. This significantly hinders clinical applicability, as through-plane motion of the heart results in significant variability in quantified volumes. In order to approach clinically acceptable standards, these issues need to be compensated for, and to calculate biomarkers with comparable accuracy to conventional cine, a motion corrected ECG gated cine image series should be reconstructed. Specifically images must be retained at end-expiration only to eliminate geometric and position variation, and these must be aligned so that the LV region in each image is correctly aligned in space.

In this paper we propose a workflow for accomplishing this reconstruction using convolutional neural networks (CNN) for automatic segmentation of the LV, manifold learning for estimating respiratory cycles, and an image processing pipeline which uses the information from these two sources to create a single-cycle image series. Our workflow uses automatically generated segmentations alone for determining cardiac cycle position for images. This contrasts with approaches in [1,13] which estimate the R-R interval using the image frequency domain and then determine which images are end-diastole based on semi-automated segmentation, and other techniques including [5] which use stable ECG signals for reconstruction. Furthermore our method does not require complex k-space reconstruction techniques [4] which are not widely available in clinical practice. Analysis techniques used to assess SAX series can then be applied to this reconstructed series to calculate biomarkers.

Our novel contribution is a workflow which wholly automates the process of reconstructing a single-cycle image series from the input RT series, eliminating both the need for manual segmentation and inter-observer variability. This contrasts with previous work which involved manual input in the reconstruction pipeline [13]. The next sections will describe the steps in the workflow in detail, present results of applying the workflow to volunteer images, and then discuss the further work necessary to refine the technique.

2   Methodology

The automated workflow shown in Fig. 1 transforms a RT series spanning multiple cardiac cycles, containing images neither aligned in space nor corrected for respiration, into a single-cycle series corrected for spatial alignment and containing only end-expiration images. The input image series is a 4-dimensional image

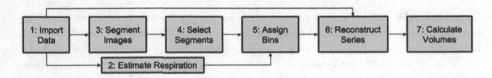

Fig. 1. Outline of the image processing workflow

volume storing 3D image volumes capturing cardiac geometry over time (3D+t). The output image is also 4D, but contains only a single cardiac cycle, removing the respiratory variability and correctly aligning the sequence to reconstruct an image similar to the standard SAX sequence. The steps in this workflow are outlined here in brief and expanded in the following subsections:

1. Data Import: Image data is imported from the Dicom files and converted to Nifti format using Eidolon [8]. This is the most convenient and reliable tool for this step although any Nifti file from other sources is acceptable.
2. Estimate Respiration: Manifold learning is used to estimate the position of each image in the respiratory cycle, and images not at end-expiration are rejected.
3. Segment Images: A neural network trained to segment the myocardium of the left ventricle is applied to each image, providing a myocardial mask.
4. Select Segments: Each mask is assessed for correctness and quality to remove malformed segmentations outside the LV region.
5. Assign Bins: All images not rejected in the previous steps are assigned to a position in the cardiac cycle. Firstly, images at end-diastole are identified by measuring the pool volumes of their myocardial masks. Other images are then assigned to bins representing phases of the cardiac cycle using the time differences between the identified end-diastole images at the start and end of that cardiac cycle.
6. Reconstruct Series: A reconstructed series is created by selecting an image from each cycle position for every slice position.
7. Calculate Volumes: The reconstruction is also applied to the myocardial mask associated with each image to produce a single-cycle segment series which can be used to calculate volume properties.

2.1 Deep Learning Segmentation

Our technique relies on a convolutional neural network trained to segment LV myocardial tissue in real-time images. The network architecture (Fig. 2) is based on U-Net [12,16] using residual units [7] and is implemented in Tensorflow. Each numbered section of the encoding phase of the network is implemented using the residual unit definition on the left, where the number indicates the output number of filters. Upsampling in the decoding phase is done with a transpose convolution followed by a single set of batchnorm-prelu-conv2D operations.

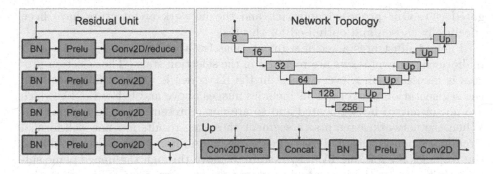

Fig. 2. Topology of the segmentation network.

Residual units use Parametric Rectified Linear Unit (PReLU) [6] for activation and are defined with 4 series of batchnorm-prelu-convolution operations. Downsampling in the encoding phase of the network is done using striding on the first convolution of the residual unit.

The training data for the network consists of RT series images from 10 volunteers segmented manually by a clinician resulting in a dataset of 3153 greyscale image/mask pairs. Figure 3 shows a selection of augmented image/mask pairs taken from the training dataset. During training, data augmentation [9,15] is applied to the images to ensure the model does not overfit to the dataset. Specifically, a random selection of rotation, transposition, flip, shift, and zoom operations are applied to each image/mask pair of a batch. Segmenting RT imaging is particularly challenging as RT image quality is inferior to conventional

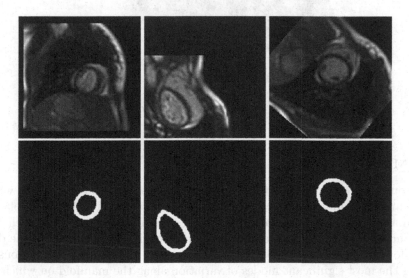

Fig. 3. Example augmented image/mask pairs from the training dataset.

gated cine. Our proposed approach and the network architecture have been specifically chosen and optimised for this task.

Figure 4 illustrates a set of segmentations for a real-time image series after malformed segmentations are removed in the selection stage. The selection process is necessary since every image in the RT series is used for inference with the segmentation network. This includes images above and below the LV which are not meant to be segmented and so are not represented in the training set. When the network attempts to segment these the results are not well-formed circular segmentations, and must be identified and filtered out. Secondly, during the respiration cycle the LV may deform or move through the image plane sufficiently to distort the image and produce poor segmentations. The expectation is that the RT image will capture enough cardiac cycles that there will be a well-segmented representative somewhere to reconstruct a single cycle.

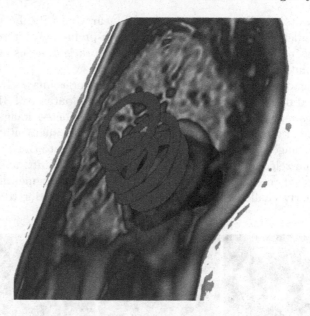

Fig. 4. Example automatically generated segmentation

2.2   Manifold Learning

To account for respiratory motion we select the frames at end-expiration, which is the current standard for assessment for cardiac volumes. Here we use Laplacian Eigenmaps (LE) [2] to automatically estimate the respiratory state in each slice in the image stack. LE is a manifold learning technique which embeds the data into a low-dimensional space while preserving local neighbourhood relations by finding the most significant modes of variation along the manifold on which the original data lies. When applied to a sequence of cine cardiac images, we find that this variation consistently corresponds to the respiratory cycle.

Using each image's coordinates in the low-dimensional embedding we assign a true or false value stating whether each image is within some specified margin of the end-respiration state. MR images, rather than myocardial masks, are used at this step as regions outside the heart also contain information about the respiratory state and help in this categorisation.

2.3   Image Processing

In addition to Eidolon and Tensorflow, our workflow uses Python with the Numpy, Scipy, and Nibabel libraries for array types, scientific functions, and Nifti loading respectively. Our workflow is implemented as a Jupyter notebook which guides the user through the process of applying the operations. This is available as open source on our repository at https://github.com/ericspod/RealtimeReconWorkflow.

Select Segments. In this stage each 2D image is analysed individually to filter out bad segmentations. Due to image quality and subject motion not all images present usable cardiac geometry and thus cannot be correctly segmented. A segmentation is rejected if it does not have exactly one cavity (i.e. the LV chamber), if it contains fewer than 100 pixels, or if the surface area of a convex hull enclosing the segmentation is at least 15% larger than the area of the segmentation including pool. This ensures that only a segmentation representing a relatively smooth annulus is accepted. The value of 100 pixels for minimal size has been found in our analysis to be a rational rejection criteria for images of 256×256 pixels, and similarly the 15% size criteria has been found to reject highly irregular segmentations.

Assign Bins. At this stage images at end-expiration have been selected using manifold learning, these are then assigned to a position in the cardiac cycle based on the segmentation areas. Each image with a segmentation is assigned the surface area of their segmentation's pools. Images with areas larger than its non-zero neighbours are assumed to be as ED, and so an identifiable cardiac cycle is a list of contiguous images in time, which all have surface areas, from one of these maximal images up to the but not including the next. These individual cycles must be a certain length to be accepted, if so each image in the cycle is assigned a value representing their position in the cycle from 0 to 1.

The cycles thus defined will vary in length and so the values assigned to each image do not all fall easily into obvious bins. A histogram is computed for the percentages to determine what the bins should be such that no bin is empty, which then allows a bin number to be assigned to each image. Each bin represents a frame of a single cardiac cycle, where bin 0 is the ED frame. Bins contain many images, however with the filtering done for segmentation quality and respiration they should all represent the same geometry at the same moment in the cardiac cycle.

Reconstruct Series. With bins assigned to each image (excepting those rejected for poor segmentation or respiratory motion), reconstructing a short-axis like image becomes a process of selecting an image from each bin for each image plane. The number of bins has been chosen to ensure that each bin is represented by at least one image from each image plane, however typically there will be many images to choose from at each plane per bin. Our current strategy is to select, for particular plane and bin, the image whose segmentation's pool has a surface area closest to the mean of all those in its bin. The time offset between frames is taken from the original images and if this value correctly represents the per-image time since ED this will be preserved in the final output image.

Having selected the images for each slice at each timestep, the same process is applied to the segmentations to produce a second segmentation series. The average of the image centroids from this series is calculated, then each image in the segment series and its corresponding image in the reconstructed SAX-like image are shifted in the XY plane to be centred at this position.

This produces an image and a segmentation series which accounts for patient movement during scanning which is not respiratory in origin, although aligning all images does produce non-physiological results since the left ventricle is not entirely conical but flatter on the septal side. For the purposes of various 2D assessment criteria, for example estimating ejection fraction, this does not impact results but does aid in observing wall motion abnormalities.

Calculate Volumes. Pool volumes are calculated by summing up the number of pixels in the pools of the segmentations. Volumes are then summed in the depth dimension then multiplied by the voxel volume of the original image to give a total per timestep volume.

3   Results

We scanned seven participants using the real-time protocol twice with a rest interval between scans at St. Thomas' Hospital, London, UK, using a 1.5T Philips Ingenia MR scanner (Philips, Best, Netherlands). All participants were healthy volunteers with ages ranging from 20 to 32, 4 males and 3 females. Due to the length of the scan sequence a much larger dataset of 100 frames was acquired for each subject. These frames are significantly dissimilar even within one patient due to breathing and exercise motion. Therefore these datasets represent a larger training dataset than the number of participants would seem to imply. We did not consider clinical patient participants for this study since their morphological details will not vary significantly from healthy volunteers as observed in the used RT sequences.

Figure 5 shows an example of reconstructed CINE-like sequence and segmentations at end-diastole for all the slices. We can see that the slices are correctly aligned and segmentations allow for accurate assessment of volumes.

For a further validation, we compared the volumes obtained with the proposed reconstruction pipeline cine with a previously validated, non-gated real-time imaging protocol (non-gated RT) that uses manual selection of respiratory

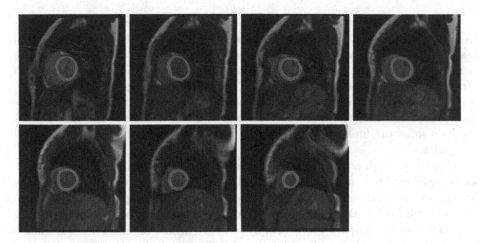

Fig. 5. Example reconstructed CINE-like image series for all slices at ED.

Table 1. Median and inter-quartile range (iqr) of EDV and ESV for the proposed method and the non-gated MRI method, and differences.

	EDV (mL)	ESV (mL)
Proposed	117.0 (iqr: 31.75)	37.0 (iqr: 14.31)
Non-gated MRI	113.6 (iqr: 32.73)	46.1 (iqr: 17.02)
Difference	−3.07 (iqr: 12.00)	0.85 (iqr: 12.48)

state [10]. Table 1 summarises the ED volume (EDV) and end-systolic volume (ESV) for the two methods.

The results obtained with the proposed automatic pipeline correlated well with the manual results from the non-gated MRI sequence. Visual inspection of this sort is standard clinical practice and thus our results are comparable to assessments considered sufficiently accurate for diagnostic purposes. From a clinical perspective, the differences between results are within expected ranges between inter-observer measurements in the reference standard [10,13], and so are diagnostically valid.

4   Conclusion and Future Work

We have in this paper demonstrated a workflow for reconstructing a single-cycle image series from a real-time series. This is in multiple ways an extension of previous work on reconstruction of respiratory and cardiac gated cine SAX [13], whose method relied on manual input to determine the location of the heart. Furthermore, the previous method for estimating temporal and spatial motions of the images were obtained from changes in image contrast, resulting in sub-optimal alignment and blurring of the images due to inaccurate motion estimation.

Other pipelines have been proposed for cine reconstruction from ungated, free-breathing MR. However, these methods often rely on complex, self-tailored k-space acquisition and reconstruction schemes [4]. Whereas these techniques benefit from utilising raw data instead of reconstructed RT images for reconstruction of gated cine MR, such frameworks have limited clinical applicability, as they are not available in most clinical MR facilities. Our technique is available as standalone Python software or integrated into Eidolon, a free cardiac MR analysis software, and can therefore be implemented using a standard personal computer.

Due to the high acceleration factors needed for RT imaging, image quality is lower compared to conventional cine. Although this did not result in a significant impact on measurements of the most frequently obtained parameters (cardiac volumes and function), specific details and features of boundaries are less distinct and can possibly impact more comprehensive cardiac assessment. Our future research goals include investigating the use of autoencoders [14] as a method of improving image quality.

Our process of assigning images to cardiac phase bins relies the assignment of an ED image using the local maximal pool volume. This is not strictly true and so there is some approximation in how images are assigned to cardiac cycle position. This does not optimally utilise the RT information, as the independency of acquisition and cardiac frequency likely results in different offsets of images from 'true' ED between the different cycles acquired per slice. Exploitation of this knowledge will make it possible to create smaller (and thus more) bins and therefore increase temporal resolution of the reconstructed images.

With this work, we have shown a feasible technique for a complete automatic pipeline for the reconstruction of cardiac and respiratory gated cine MR from RT imaging and subsequent quantification of key parameters of cardiac function. When extended to include the full heart, including the basal part of the ventricle and the atria, this technique can be of great benefit in imaging of subjects that are unable to hold their breath or lie still, such as children or severely ill patients. Furthermore, as demonstrated our work allows imaging during diagnostic scans employing physical exercise.

Acknowledgements. This research was partly supported by the National Institute for Health Research (NIHR) Biomedical Research Centre (BRC) at Guy's and St Thomas' NHS Foundation Trust. Views expressed are those of the authors and not necessarily of the NHS, the NIHR, or the Dept. of Health.

References

1. van Amerom, J., et al.: Fetal cardiac cine imaging using highly accelerated dynamic MRI with retrospective motion correction and outlier rejection. Magn. Reson. Med. **79**, 327–338 (2017)
2. Belkin, M., Niyogi, P.: Laplacian eigenmaps for dimensionality reduction and data representation. Neural Comput. **15**(6), 1373–1396 (2003)

3. Cahalin, L.P., et al.: A meta-analysis of the prognostic significance of cardiopulmonary exercise testing in patients with heart failure. Heart Fail. Rev. **18**(1), 79–94 (2013)
4. Feng, L., Axel, L., Chandarana, H., Block, K.T., Sodickson, D.K., Otazo, R.: XD-GRASP: Golden-angle radial MRI with reconstruction of extra motion-state dimensions using compressed sensing. Magn. Reson. Med. **75**(2), 775–788 (2016)
5. Hansen, M., Sørensen, T., Arai, A., Kellman, P.: Retrospective reconstruction of high temporal resolution cine images from real-time MRI using iterative motion correction. Magn. Reson. Med. **68**(3), 741–750 (2012)
6. He, K., Zhang, X., Ren, S., Sun, J.: Delving deep into rectifiers: Surpassing human-level performance on imagenet classification. CoRR abs/1502.01852 (2015)
7. He, K., Zhang, X., Ren, S., Sun, J.: Identity mappings in deep residual networks. CoRR abs/1603.05027 (2016)
8. Kerfoot, E., et al.: Eidolon: visualization and computational framework for multi-modal biomedical data analysis. In: Zheng, G., Liao, H., Jannin, P., Cattin, P., Lee, S.-L. (eds.) MIAR 2016. LNCS, vol. 9805, pp. 425–437. Springer, Cham (2016). https://doi.org/10.1007/978-3-319-43775-0_39
9. Krizhevsky, A., Sutskever, I., Hinton, G.E.: Imagenet classification with deep convolutional neural networks. In: Proceedings of the 25th International Conference on Neural Information Processing Systems, vol. 1, pp. 1097–1105. NIPS 2012, Curran Associates Inc., USA (2012)
10. La Gerche, A., et al.: Cardiac MRI: a new gold standard for ventricular volume quantification during high-intensity exercise. Circ. Cardiovasc. Imaging **6**(2), 329–338 (2013)
11. Lurz, P., et al.: Feasibility and reproducibility of biventricular volumetric assessment of cardiac function during exercise using real-time radial k-t SENSE magnetic resonance imaging. J. Magn. Reson. Imaging **29**(5), 1062–1070 (2009)
12. Ronneberger, O., Fischer, P., Brox, T.: U-net: Convolutional networks for biomedical image segmentation. CoRR abs/1505.04597 (2015)
13. Ruijsink, B.: Semi-automatic cardiac and respiratory gated MRI for cardiac assessment during exercise. In: Cardoso, M.J. (ed.) CMMI/SWITCH/RAMBO - 2017. LNCS, vol. 10555, pp. 86–95. Springer, Cham (2017). https://doi.org/10.1007/978-3-319-67564-0_9
14. Rumelhart, D.E., Hinton, G.E., Williams, R.J.: Parallel distributed processing: Explorations in the microstructure of cognition, vol. 1. chap. Learning Internal Representations by Error Propagation, pp. 318–362. MIT Press, Cambridge (1986)
15. Simard, P.Y., Steinkraus, D., Platt, J.: Best practices for convolutional neural networks applied to visual document analysis. Institute of Electrical and Electronics Engineers, Inc. August 2003
16. Zhang, Z., Liu, Q., Wang, Y.: Road extraction by deep residual u-net. CoRR abs/1711.10684 (2017)

An Unbiased Groupwise Registration Algorithm for Correcting Motion in Dynamic Contrast-Enhanced Magnetic Resonance Images

Mia Mojica and Mehran Ebrahimi[(⊠)]

Faculty of Science, University of Ontario Institute of Technology,
2000 Simcoe Street North, Oshawa, ON L1H 7K4, Canada
{mia.mojica,mehran.ebrahimi}@uoit.ca
http://www.ImagingLab.ca/

Abstract. A simple and computationally efficient algorithm for performing unbiased groupwise registration to correct motion in a dataset of contrast-enhanced magnetic resonance (DCE-MR) images is presented. All the DCE-MR images in the sequence are registered simultaneously and updates to the reference are computed using an averaging technique that takes into account all the transformations aligning each image to the current reference. The method is validated both subjectively and quantitatively using an abdominal DCE-MRI dataset. When combined with the normalized gradient field dissimilarity measure, it produced promising results and showed significant improvements compared to those obtained from an existing motion correction approach.

Keywords: DCE-MRI registration · Multilevel elastic registration
Normalized gradient field · Groupwise registration

1 Introduction

Over the last years, dynamic contrast-enhanced magnetic resonance imaging (DCE-MRI) has been a useful clinical technique in the characterization of tumor biology. It involves the acquisition of a sequence of images acquired pre- and post-injection of a bolus of a contrast agent. The uptake of the contrast agent from this sequence of images can be quantified via a concentration vs. time curve, which in turn allows us to characterize vascular permeability [13].

DCE-MRI continues to be a crucial component in identifying appropriate patient treatment response. However, motion present in the dataset has to first be compensated to accurately convert signal intensity changes to contrast agent concentrations [7]. Image registration has been demonstrated to be effective in obtaining a motionless dataset from a sequence of DCE-MR images [1,2,6,8].

Some registration methods for DCE images include reducing motion in the dataset through a floating image reference scheme combined with principal component analysis, as presented in [7]. In their paper, an intensity correction term

© Springer Nature Switzerland AG 2018
D. Stoyanov et al. (Eds.): RAMBO 2018/BIA 2018/TIA 2018, LNCS 11040, pp. 42–52, 2018.
https://doi.org/10.1007/978-3-030-00946-5_5

was added to the similarity measure for pairwise registration. In [12], the registration problem was divided into sub-problems using auxiliary images computed from the conditional probability distribution of image pairs. These auxiliary images were registered to the original images using the sum of squared differences.

We introduce a groupwise registration approach combined with an NGF-based pairwise step for correcting motion and subsequently validate the proposed scheme on a set of abdominal dynamic contrast-enhanced MR images. The groupwise framework used in this paper assumes equal weight for all pairwise transformations to come up with an update to the reference image. It effectively reduces naturally occurring motion induced by the respiration process and is able to align images in spite of the changes in contrast.

2 Pairwise Registration

Constructing a motion-corrected dataset through groupwise registration entails aligning the subjects to the same reference geometry. In this paper, we used a combination of affine and elastic (also referred to as "non-parametric registration" in [9]) to initialize each groupwise iteration.

2.1 Mathematical Model

Given a template and a reference image $\mathcal{T}, \mathcal{R} : \Omega \subset \mathbb{R}^2 \to \mathbb{R}$, we wish to find a transformation $y : \Omega \to \mathbb{R}^2$ such that a transformed version $\mathcal{T}[y]$ of the template image $\mathcal{T}$ is similar to the reference $\mathcal{R}$. This is equivalent to the optimization problem

$$\min_y \mathcal{J}[y] = \mathcal{D}[\mathcal{T}[y], \mathcal{R}] + \alpha \mathcal{S}[y]. \tag{1}$$

The term $\mathcal{D}$ in the joint functional $\mathcal{J}$ is called a distance measure and it quantifies the similarity between the transformed template and the reference image. The second term $\mathcal{S}$ is the regularization term, which makes the registration problem well-posed.

In our implementations, we have tested the following distance measures:

a. Normalized Gradient Field (NGF)

$$\mathcal{D}^{\mathrm{NGF}}[\mathcal{T}, \mathcal{R}] = \mathrm{NGF}[\mathcal{T}, \mathcal{R}] = \int_\Omega 1 - \left(\mathrm{NGF}[\mathcal{T}(x)]^T \, \mathrm{NGF}[\mathcal{R}(x)]\right)^2 dx \tag{2}$$

where $\mathrm{NGF}[\mathcal{T}]$ denotes the normalized gradient field of $\mathcal{T}$, defined by

$$\mathrm{NGF}[\mathcal{T}] = \mathrm{NGF}[\mathcal{T}, \eta] = \frac{\nabla \mathcal{T}}{\sqrt{|\nabla \mathcal{T}|^2 + \eta^2}}$$

and η is an edge parameter. The NGF is suited for aligning images where intensity changes appear at corresponding positions. These intensity changes are given by the image gradient $\nabla \mathcal{T}$.

b. Sum of Squared Differences with Intensity Correction (SSDIC)

In [7], intensity correction was used in combination with the SSD to partially account for intensity changes between image volumes. Instead of solving for a reasonable transformation aligning $\mathcal{T}$ and $\mathcal{R}$, we find one that matches the "intensity-corrected" template T^c to the reference, where

$$T^c = \mathcal{T} + c, \quad c = (\mathcal{R} - \mathcal{T}) * \mathrm{N}(0, \sigma),$$

and $\mathrm{N}(0, \sigma)$ is a Gaussian kernel with a mean and standard deviation of 0 and σ, respectively. The template image is transformed using the optimal deformation aligning the intensity-corrected template to the reference image.

The above distance measures are approximated using a midpoint quadrature rule on a cell-centered grid with uniform mesh spacing.

2.2   Multilevel Affine and Elastic Registration

The discretized form of the registration problem in (1) is solved from the coarsest to the finest level. We perform an affine registration at the coarsest level and use the resulting optimal transformation to initialize y^{ref} in the regularization term $\mathcal{S}[y]$, which is given by the elastic potential of the transformation y [9]:

$$\mathcal{S}[y] = \text{Elastic Potential} \left[y - y^{\mathrm{ref}} \right].$$

The starting guess for the optimal transformation at every succeeding level is taken to be the prolongated version of the solution y^h from the preceding level.

3   Groupwise Registration

Groupwise registration has been used in a wide range of applications, including normalizing structural and functional MR data [3]. In [5], the performance of a groupwise registration method with a principal component analysis-based metric for correcting motion in DCE-MR images of the liver was evaluated.

Here, we adopt the method used in [4,11] to correct motion in a sequence of DCE-MR images and coupled it with the pairwise registration step discussed in the previous section.

Each groupwise iteration is initialized by mapping every image in the dataset to the current reference image. The reference image is then updated using an averaging technique that takes into account all the transformations obtained from the pairwise registration step. The update to the reference is given by

$$\mathcal{R}_{\mathrm{mean}}^{n+1}(\mathrm{x}^h) = \frac{1}{N} \sum_{i=1}^{N} \mathcal{T}_i \left(y_i^n \circ [y_{\mathrm{mean}}^n]^{-1}(\mathrm{x}^h) \right), \tag{3}$$

where

- N refers to the size of the dataset,

- $\mathbf{x}^h$ is the original grid,
- $\mathcal{T}_i$ are the DCE-MR images ($i = 1, 2, \ldots, N$),
- y_i^n is the mapping that aligns the ith image in the sequence to the nth reference image,
- y_{mean}^n is the mean of the transformations y_i^n at the nth iteration, and
- $y_i^n \circ [y_{\text{mean}}^n]^{-1}$ is the composition of y_i^n with the inverse of y_{mean}^n.

Performing the update process described in (3) leads to an average geometry $\mathcal{R}_{\text{mean}}$ and a collection of transformations aligning the subjects to $\mathcal{R}_{\text{mean}}$.

In our implementations, we used the following approximation for the inverse of the average transformation field y_{mean}^n:

$$\left[y_{\text{mean}}^n(\mathbf{x}^h)\right]^{-1} \approx -y_{\text{mean}}^n(\mathbf{x}^h) + 2\mathbf{x}^h. \tag{4}$$

A detailed outline of the groupwise registration framework is given in our previous work [10].

4 Experiments and Results

A sequence of abdominal MR images was used for validation. The scans were acquired with a T1-weighted FSPGR sequence. Spatial resolution was 1.88 mm by 1.88 mm by 8 mm in the S/I, L/R, and A/P directions respectively. Temporal resolution was approximately 3.7 seconds per volume [7].

We applied the proposed groupwise algorithm to visually assess how well it eliminates real and complex patient motion. For quantitative validation, the groupwise scheme was applied to a dataset with simulated motion. The resulting sequence of registered images is then compared against the ground truth (the motionless dataset). For experiments that made use of the SSDIC metric, the standard deviation was chosen heuristically to be $\sigma = 2.7$.

4.1 Real Patient Motion

Every groupwise iteration was initialized by a pairwise alignment of the subjects to the current reference geometry. In Fig. 1, we demonstrate how using different distance measures can affect the overall efficiency of the proposed method. Figures 1(f) and (i) show the optimal transformations that register Fig. 1(b) to (a) obtained using the NGF and SSDIC. Figures 1(d) and (g) show the transformed versions of the template image. Observe that the NGF and SSDIC were able to align corresponding features correctly, with only slight misregistrations near the borders from using SSDIC. We also quantified the efficiency of the distance measure by computing the difference between the transformed template and the reference image. Ideally, if registration were done properly, this difference should only exhibit the regions with contrast differences. This was the case with the NGF and the SSDIC, as demonstrated in Figs. 1(e) and (h).

Next, we present results obtained from separate experiments using two significantly different initial reference images (one before and one after the contrast

Table 1. Mean Squared Error of the SI curves as a measure of the accuracy of the registration methods.

α	ROI 1				ROI 2			
	PW-NGF	GW-NGF	PW-SSDIC	GW-SSDIC	PW-NGF	GW-NGF	PW-SSDIC	GW-SSDIC
100	1.68E-03	1.36E-04	2.01E-03	2.20E-03	4.91E-04	1.79E-04	1.61E-02	1.57E-02
200	1.20E-03	2.18E-04	6.40E-04	6.81E-04	5.34E-04	1.86E-04	4.81E-03	4.84E-03
600	2.12E-04	6.34E-05	7.10E-04	7.68E-04	3.30E-04	8.02E-05	1.10E-03	9.77E-04

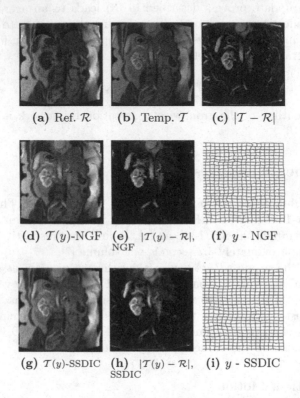

(a) Ref. $\mathcal{R}$ (b) Temp. $\mathcal{T}$ (c) $|\mathcal{T} - \mathcal{R}|$

(d) $\mathcal{T}(y)$-NGF   (e) $|\mathcal{T}(y) - \mathcal{R}|$, NGF   (f) y - NGF

(g) $\mathcal{T}(y)$-SSDIC   (h) $|\mathcal{T}(y) - \mathcal{R}|$, SSDIC   (i) y - SSDIC

Fig. 1. Results of Pairwise Registration of DCE-MR images. (a) reference, (b) template image, (c) difference image between the template and reference, (d) and (g) are the transformed templates, (e) and (h) are the difference images between the transformed template and the reference image, (f) and (i) are the optimal transformations aligning the template to the reference image using different distance measures.

agent had been absorbed) in order to demonstrate that the proposed method for correcting motion in DCE-MR datasets is indeed unbiased regardless of the chosen initial reference. Figures 2(a) and (d) show the two initial reference images used. Next to the reference images are the final mean images computed using the NGF and SSDIC, respectively. Notice that the groupwise scheme converged to the same final average image when the same distance measure was used.

Table 2. Standard Deviation of the SI curves as means of quantifying the amount of remaining motion in the sequence of registered images.

	ROI 1				ROI 2			
α	PW-NGF	GW-NGF	PW-SSDIC	GW-SSDIC	PW-NGF	GW-NGF	PW-SSDIC	GW-SSDIC
100	2.71E-02	2.48E-02	2.82E-02	2.88E-02	1.79E-02	1.43E-02	5.12E-02	5.27E-02
200	2.29E-02	2.27E-02	2.69E-02	2.95E-02	2.32E-02	2.15E-02	5.00E-02	5.03E-02
600	2.48E-02	2.43E-02	2.78E-02	2.88E-02	3.47E-02	3.46E-02	4.77E-02	4.75E-02

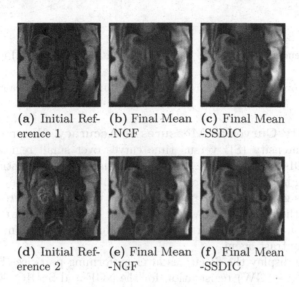

(a) Initial Ref-   (b) Final Mean   (c) Final Mean
erence 1   -NGF   -SSDIC

(d) Initial Ref-   (e) Final Mean   (f) Final Mean
erence 2   -NGF   -SSDIC

Fig. 2. Unbiased groupwise registration. The computation of the final mean image is independent of the initial reference.

For instance, the final mean images Fig. 2(b) and (e) are the same in spite of "evolving" from different initial references.

In Fig. 3, we show the rate of convergence of the groupwise scheme by plotting the average change in pixel values between successive iterates for the reference image against the iteration number. After around seven iterations, the average change in intensity values dropped from approximately 0.08 to 0.005, where the intensity values of the images in the dataset lie in the interval [0,1].

4.2   Simulated Motion

Simulated motion was added to a motionless dataset similar to [7]. Non-rigid diaphragm motion during respiration combined with rigid rotations at point x during time t was modelled by

$$\Delta SI(x,t) = \Delta SI_{\max} \sin\left(\frac{\pi x}{x_{\max}}\right)\left|\sin\left(\frac{\pi t}{t_b}\right)\right|.$$

In the above equation, $\Delta SI_{\max}$ is the maximum SI displacement, $x_{\max}$ is the maximum LR extent of the patient, and t_b is the duration of a full breath.

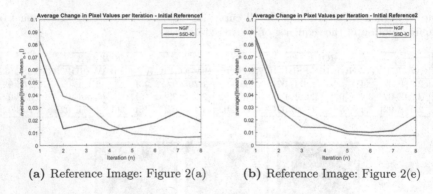

(a) Reference Image: Figure 2(a)   **(b)** Reference Image: Figure 2(e)

Fig. 3. Convergence of the groupwise algorithm to a stable mean image.

Signal Intensity Curves as Measures of Accuracy. We present statistics on the signal intensity (SI) versus time curves over small regions of interest (ROIs). The ROIs considered are regions with relatively large motion shifts that are also affected by the administration of the contrast agent. They are shown in Fig. 4. SI curves give us an idea of how well the registration corrects motion in the dataset. Without motion, these curves would be smooth. However, naturally occurring motion present in our dataset introduced changes unrelated to the uptake of the contrast agent.

In Fig. 5, we display the SI curves after performing pairwise (PW) registration and groupwise (GW) registration for the NGF and SSDIC. All 4 methods were able to mitigate the effects of diaphragm motion and contrast change as demonstrated by smaller peaks in their SI curves compared to that from the simulated data. However, it is important to note the persistence of high fluctuations after using the SSDIC with either a pairwise or groupwise approach. This signifies misregistration in the specified region of interest. On the other hand, we obtained relatively smoother curves for the same ROIs after combining groupwise registration with NGF. See Figs. 5(b), (d).

We measured the mean-squared error for each curve to quantify how close our final registered images are to the ground truth. Out of all the methods we implemented, GW-NGF had the smallest mean-squared error. In some cases, it

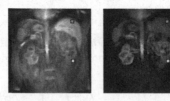

Fig. 4. Regions of interest considered in the sequence of DCE-MR data with simulated motion. Green = ROI1; Red = ROI2 (Color figure online)

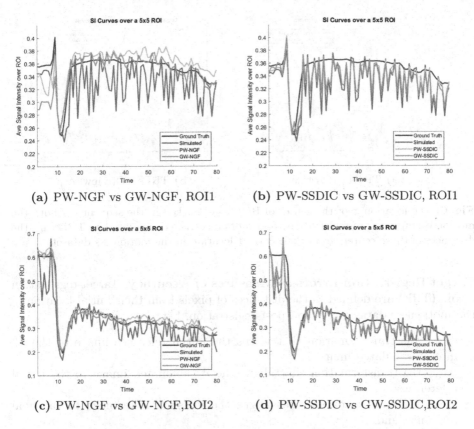

(a) PW-NGF vs GW-NGF, ROI1   **(b)** PW-SSDIC vs GW-SSDIC, ROI1

(c) PW-NGF vs GW-NGF,ROI2   **(d)** PW-SSDIC vs GW-SSDIC,ROI2

Fig. 5. The signal intensity vs. time curves pre- and post-pairwise and groupwise registration for different ROIs.

even resulted to a ten-fold improvement in the MSE compared with the other methods.

The standard deviation was also calculated to quantify the amount of motion in the registered images. Again, the GW-NGF yielded the best results, implying that there were smaller fluctuations in the SI curves and less misregistrations in the ROIs considered. On the other hand, using the SSDIC with the groupwise scheme was either a hit or miss. Notice from the convergence of the method visualized in Fig. 3 that the final average change in pixel values fluctuated close to the initial average change in intensity values. This could suggest that the final reference image might be similar to the initial reference and that some of the motion correction made in the previous iterations were cancelled out.

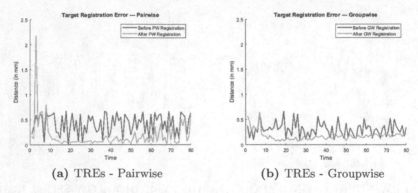

(a) TREs - Pairwise   (b) TREs - Groupwise

Fig. 6. The location x of the center of ROI1 was tracked in the sequence of both the motion-corrupted (pre-registration) and motion-corrected images. The TREs are the distances of these centers from their correct location in the motionless dataset.

Target Registration Errors as Measures of Accuracy. Target registration errors (TRE) are defined as the distances of pixels from their initial location in the motionless dataset pre- and post-registration. Let

- ϕ_i be the transformation that warps the initial reference image to the ith motion-simulated image I_i,
- y_{PW_i} the transformation that aligns the ith simulated image to the initial reference,
- y_{GW_i} the transformation that aligns the ith simulated image to the final reference, and
- ψ the transformation aligning the final groupwise mean to the initial reference image.

Then the pairwise TREs before and after registration, respectively, are given by

$$|x - \phi_i(x)| \text{ and } |x - \phi_i(y_{\text{PW}_i}(x))|.$$

On the other hand, the groupwise TREs are given by

$$|x - \psi(\phi_i(x))| \text{ and } |x - \psi(\phi_i(y_{\text{GW}_i}(x)))|.$$

Shown in Fig. 6 are the TREs for both PW-NGF and GW-NGF. Observe that the TRE post-GW registration had a smaller average compared to the usual pairwise approach. These are consistent with the results we obtained by analyzing the average signal intensity values over the same ROI in the previous section.

5   Conclusions

In this paper, we presented a computationally efficient and unbiased groupwise registration approach for correcting motion in a sequence of dynamic contrast-enhanced images. We also demonstrated how different distance measures affect the performance of a multilevel elastic registration algorithm for registering contrast-enhanced images and found that both the NGF and SSDIC are able to account for contrast changes between the template and reference images. Finally, we conclude that the groupwise approach combined with the NGF yielded the smoothest SI curves and the smallest TREs, implying that this method eliminates motion more accurately than methods that simply register against an arbitrarily chosen image from the dataset.

Acknowledgments. This work was supported in part by an NSERC Discovery grant and Deborah Saucier Early Researcher Award for Mehran Ebrahimi. Mia Mojica is supported by an Ontario Trillium Scholarship (OTS). The authors would like to acknowledge Dr. Anne Martel of Sunnybrook Research Institute, Toronto, Ontario, Canada for great discussions and for providing the DCE-MRI data.

References

1. Ebrahimi, M., Lausch, A., Martel, A.L.: A Gauss-newton approach to joint image registration and intensity correction. Comput. Methods Programs Biomed. **112**(3), 398–406 (2013)
2. Ebrahimi, M., Martel, A.L.: A general PDE-framework for registration of contrast enhanced images. In: Yang, G.-Z., Hawkes, D., Rueckert, D., Noble, A., Taylor, C. (eds.) MICCAI 2009. LNCS, vol. 5761, pp. 811–819. Springer, Heidelberg (2009). https://doi.org/10.1007/978-3-642-04268-3_100
3. Geng, X., Christensen, G.E., Gu, H., Ross, T.J., Yang, Y.: Implicit reference-based group-wise image registration and its application to structural and functional MRI. Neuroimage **47**(4), 1341–1351 (2009)
4. Helm, P.A.: A novel technique for quantifying variability of cardiac anatomy: application to the dyssynchronous failing heart. Ph.D thesis, The Johns Hopkins University 164 (2005)
5. Jansen, M., Kuijf, H., Veldhuis, W., Wessels, F., Van Leeuwen, M., Pluim, J.: Evaluation of motion correction for clinical dynamic contrast enhanced MRI of the liver. Phys. Med. Biol. **62**(19), 7556 (2017)
6. Kim, M., Wu, G., Shen, D.: Groupwise registration of breast DCE-MR images for accurate tumor measurement. In: 2011 IEEE International Symposium on Biomedical Imaging: From Nano to Macro, pp. 598–601. IEEE (2011)
7. Lausch, A., Ebrahimi, M., Martel, A.: Image registration for abdominal dynamic contrast-enhanced magnetic resonance images. In: 2011 IEEE International Symposium on Biomedical Imaging: From Nano to Macro, pp. 561–565. IEEE (2011)
8. Martel, A., Froh, M., Brock, K., Plewes, D., Barber, D.: Evaluating an optical-flow-based registration algorithm for contrast-enhanced magnetic resonance imaging of the breast. Phys. Med. Biol. **52**(13), 3803 (2007)
9. Modersitzki, J.: FAIR: Flexible Algorithms for Image Registration, vol. 6. SIAM (2009)
10. Mojica, M., Pop, M., Sermesant, M., Ebrahimi, M.: Multilevel non-parametric groupwise registration in Cardiac MRI: application to explanted porcine hearts. In: Pop, M. (ed.) STACOM 2017. LNCS, vol. 10663, pp. 60–69. Springer, Cham (2018). https://doi.org/10.1007/978-3-319-75541-0_7

11. Peyrat, J.M., et al.: A computational framework for the statistical analysis of cardiac diffusion tensors: application to a small database of canine hearts. IEEE Trans. Med. imaging **26**(11), 1500–1514 (2007)
12. Sun, Y., Yan, C.H., Ong, S.-H., Tan, E.T., Wang, S.-C.: Intensity-based volumetric registration of contrast-enhanced MR breast images. In: Larsen, R., Nielsen, M., Sporring, J. (eds.) MICCAI 2006. LNCS, vol. 4190, pp. 671–678. Springer, Heidelberg (2006). https://doi.org/10.1007/11866565_82
13. Tofts, P.: T1-weighted DCE imaging concepts: Modelling, acquisition and analysis. MAGNETOM Flash **3**, 30–39 (2010)

Fourth International Workshop on Breast Image Analysis, BIA 2018

Siamese Network for Dual-View Mammography Mass Matching

Shaked Perek$^{(\boxtimes)}$, Alon Hazan, Ella Barkan, and Ayelet Akselrod-Ballin

IBM Research, Haifa, Israel
{shaked.perek,alon.hazan,ella,ayeletb}@il.ibm.com

Abstract. In a standard mammography screening procedure, two X-ray images are acquired per breast from two views. In this paper, we introduce a patch based, deep learning network for lesion matching in dual-view mammography using a Siamese network. Our method is evaluated on several datasets, among them the large freely available digital database for screening mammography (DDSM). We perform a comprehensive set of experiment, focusing on the mass correspondence problem. We analyze the effect of transfer learning between different types of dataset, compare the network based matching to classic template matching and evaluate the contribution of the matching network to the detection task. Experimental results show the promise in improving detection accuracy by our approach.

Keywords: Biomedical imaging · Deep learning · Mammography

1 Introduction

Mammography (MG), the primary imaging modality for breast cancer screening, typically utilizes a standard dual-view procedure. Two X-ray projection views are acquired for each breast, a craniocaudal (CC) and a mediolateral oblique (MLO) view. Examining the correspondence of a suspected finding in two separate compression views, enables the radiologist to better classify an abnormality. Studies have shown that using a two-view analysis helps radiologists reduce false positive masses caused by overlapping tissues that resemble a mass, and ultimately helps achieve a higher detection rate [17]. Although Computer Aided Diagnosis (CAD) algorithms were developed to assist radiologists, their usefulness has been debated. This is partially due to the many false positives they produce, especially for masses and architectural distortions. We propose a novel approach for identifying the correspondences between masses detected in different views, to further improve the detection and classification of MG algorithms.

Previous work on MG classification employed hand-crafted features, such as texture, size, histogram matching, distance from the nipple, and more. The extracted features were then classified together using various techniques to assess the similarity between image pairs. [11] demonstrated the positive effect of dual-view analysis, which detects suspicious mass in one view and its counterpart

© Springer Nature Switzerland AG 2018
D. Stoyanov et al. (Eds.): RAMBO 2018/BIA 2018/TIA 2018, LNCS 11040, pp. 55–63, 2018.
https://doi.org/10.1007/978-3-030-00946-5_6

in the other view. Based on geometric location, this analysis fuses both sets of features and classifies them with linear discriminant analysis. [1] used dual view analysis to improve single-view detection and classification performance by combining the dual-view score with the single-view score. Features were obtained manually using candidate location, shape, and image characteristics.

Deep learning approaches have already shown impressive results in MG detection and classification. [3] presents a micro-calcification (MC) classification that uses a dual-view approach based on two neural networks; this is followed by a single neuron layer that produces the decision based on the concatenated features from both full image views. [15] presents a multiscale convolutional neural networks (CNN) for malignancy classification of full images and sub-image patches integrated with a random forest gating network. Dhungelz et al. [5] proposed a multi-view deep residual network (Resnet) to automatically classify MG as normal/benign/malignant. The network consists of six input images, CC and MLO together with binary masks of masses and MC. The output of each Resnet is concatenated, followed by a fully connected layer that determines the class. Similarly, [6] proposed a two-stage network approach that operates on the four full images: CC and MLO of the left and right breasts. The second stage concatenates the four view-specific representations to a second softmax layer, producing the output distribution.

Most multi-view deep learning approaches to MG are applied on unregistered full images and concatenates the features obtained by the network on each view separately. In contrast, we propose a Siamese approach that focuses on matching localized patch pairs of masses from dual views. Siamese networks are neural networks that contain at least two sub-networks, with identical configuration, parameters, and weights. During training, updates to either path are shared between the two paths. To address the correspondence problem, previous works used the **Siamese network** [10] to simultaneously train inputs together. [4] uses this type of network for a face verification task, in which each new face image was compared with a previously known face image. [16] demonstrate the advantage of Siamese networks by detecting spinal cord mass in different resolutions. Sharing parameters leads to fewer parameters allowing training with smaller datasets. The subnetworks representation is related, and thus better suited for the comparison task.

Our work entails three key contributions: (1) A novel deep learning dual view algorithm for mass detection and localization in breast MG based on Siamese networks, which have not been used before to solve lesion correspondence in MG. (2) A careful set of experiments using several datasets to study the contribution of the network components, also showing that the network is better than the classic template matching approach. (3) Evaluation on the DDSM database.

2   Methods

For this study, our input took unregistered CC/MLO MG images and matched between lesions appearance in both views. Below, we describe the network matching architecture, the experimental methodology including fine-tuning and comparison to template matching and how the matching architecture is integrated into an automatic detection pipeline.

2.1 Matching Architecture

Our approach extends the work presented by Han et al. [8]. The authors developed MatchNet, a CNN approach for patch-based matching between two images. The network consists of two sub-networks. The first is a **feature network**, a Siamese neural network, in which a pair of patches, extracted from the CC and MLO views are inserted and processed through one of two networks. Both paths consist of interchanging layers of convolutions and pooling, which are connected via shared weights. The second is the **metric network**, which concatenates the two features, contains three fully connected layers and uses a softmax for feature comparison. Dropout layers were added after layers FC1 and FC2 with value of 0.5. The network is jointly trained with a cross entropy loss. Figure 1(c), presents the modified network, including the network's ensemble approach.

The mammography datasets employed for this study were created by defining a positive image pair label, as the detections annotated by a radiologist in each view, while a negative pair label is defined by matching false detection with annotated detections in the other view.

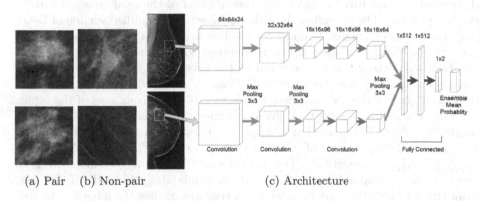

(a) Pair   (b) Non-pair   (c) Architecture

Fig. 1. The dual-view matching architecture. Columns (a, b) are illustration of ROI input patches from two views, CC and MLO. (a) Matching pair of images (b) Non matching images. (c) Patch pairs from CC and MLO views are inserted to the network. The feature network, consists of interchanging layers of convolutions and pooling, share parameters between paths. The metric network has fully connected layers with dropout, produce the final decision by networks ensemble.

2.2 Fine Tuning the Network

Fine-tuning and transfer learning have shown to improve performance results despite of specific application domains [14, 18]. To adapt MatchNet to the task of matching detections from different MG views, we first evaluated fine-tuning. We fine-tuned by training the layers of the metric network, i.e. the three fully connected layers and the last convolution layer from the feature network. We used three different datasets, as described in the Experiment and Results section, including: Photo tourism (natural image pairs)[12], Digital Database for Screening Mammography (DDSM) [9] and In-house dataset. We used the trained weights of one dataset domain to fine tune the other datasets.

2.3   Template Matching

Template matching, which extracts sub-image patches and computes a similarity measure that reflects the template and image patch correspondence, has been used extensively in computer vision [2]. We compare our deep learning network to template matching with normalized cross correlation. Intuitively, we assume that the similarity of image patches of a mass in one view with the same mass in the other view under deformations, will be higher than the similarity with a different mass or region of the breast [7].

2.4   Dual-View Automatic Lesion Detection

We integrated two components, a **matching architecture** and a single-view **detection algorithm** to exploit the contribution of the dual-view network to the full pipeline. The detection algorithm is based on a modified version of U-net [13], which was originally designed for the biomedical image processing field. In the original U-net, the output size is identical to the input size. However, for our task segmentation is not required at the pixel level, since the boundary of tumors and healthy tissue is ill-defined. Thus, we modified the U-net output, so that each pixel of the output, corresponds to a 16×16 pixels area of the input.

The system flow is such that, given a dual-view pair of images as input, the single-view detection algorithm is applied separately on the CC, MLO image I_{cc}, I_{MLO} and outputs a set of candidate patches, $P_{CC} = \{p_{CC}^1, ...p_{CC}^N\}, P_{MLO} = \{p_{MLO}^1, ...p_{MLO}^M\}$ respectively. The objective of the matching architecture is to identify the correspondences. If both patch candidates, CC and MLO views, from the detection flow, are identified as a true lesion, then the label for the pair will be true and accordingly considered a positive match. We assign labels to each pair based on the Dice Coefficient threshold δ, between two masks, defined by a detection contour and ground truth lesion contour respectively. For our experiments, we used $\delta = 0.1$ as the threshold. Any contour with a larger score is said to be a true lesion.

3   Experiments and Results

3.1   Data Description

We carried out the experiments on three datasets: (a) The Photo Tourism dataset [12], consists of three image datasets: Trevi fountain, Notre Dame and Yosemite.

Which is similar to the dataset used in the MatchNet paper [8]. It consists of 1024×1024 bitmap images, containing a 16×16 array of image patches. Each image patch has 64×64 pixels and has several matching images that differ in contrast, brightness and translation. (b) The Digital Database for Screening Mammography (DDSM) [9], contains 2620 cases of four-view MG screenings. It includes radiologist ground truth annotations for normal, benign and malignant image. 1935 images contain tumors. (c) The In-house dataset includes benign and malignant tumor ground truth annotations, from both CC/MLO MG views for either left, right or both breasts. It contains 791 tumor pairs. Figure 1(a, b) shows some tumor pairs from In-house dataset used as positive examples for the network versus negative examples. We randomly split the data into training (80%) and testing (20%) subsets of patients. The partitioning was patient-wise to prevent training and testing on images of the same patient.

3.2   Patch Preprocessing and Augmentations

We extracted ROI patches from the full MG images of 4000×6000 pixels by cropping a bounding box around each detection contour. Each such bounding box was enlarged by 10% in each dimension to include useful information around the lesion border. The extracted patches were then resized to 64×64 to generate the input to the network. We normalized all the datasets by subtracting the mean of each image and dividing by the standard deviation of each patch, avoiding the proposed MatchNet normalization [12].

Augmentation was utilized throughout the training stage on all three datasets, such that each patch was flipped left and right and rotated by $90°$, $180°$, $270°$. Each augmented patch was matched with all the others augmented patches. Medical datasets are generally unbalanced. Namely, the number of positive pairs are significantly smaller than the negative pairs. Thus, we train two networks, each network has a balanced input of positive pairs and randomly selected negative pairs. In the testing stage, we evaluate each test image through all networks, and achieve a final score using a mean probability.

We trained with a learning rate of 0.0001, Adam optimizer and batch size of 512. Experiments were performed on a Titan X Pascal GPU. Training time for DDSM models took 4 h. Testing time with model ensemble took 6 s.

3.3   Fine Tuning the Network

We studied the contribution of fine-tuning on the results in three experiments. Full training on Photo tourism and fine tuning with (i) In-house (ii) DDSM (iii) Full training on DDSM and fine tuning with In-house. (i+ii) were done using Notredam dataset. The results for these tests are presented in Fig. 2, where the upper and lower subfigures correspond to the In-house and DDSM dataset respectively. The comparison of the In-house and DDSM full training results (AUC 0.969, 0.92) with the fine tuning results (AUC 0.973, 0.91) did not show a clear advantage over the fine tuning process. This can be explained by two factors: the domain transfer effect, namely despite the Notredam large dataset

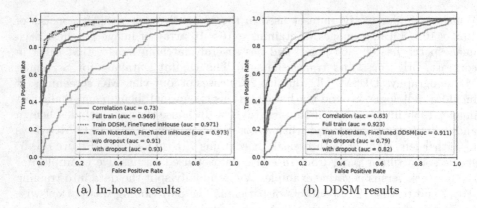

(a) In-house results   (b) DDSM results

Fig. 2. Fine tuning ROC results. The figures demonstrate the different experiment performed to evaluate the ability of the matching architecture to classify MG pairs and non pairs. (a) In-house dataset shows no advantage for fine tuning. (b) DDSM dataset shows best result by full train (cyan). (Color figure online)

of image pairs, natural images are different than medical images. Second, the Noterdam dataset pairs are much more similar to each other than the different views pairs from the breast images, which go through deformation.

Fine tuning the DDSM with the In-house dataset in (iii), obtained (AUC 0.971) compared to full training of (AUC 0.969). DDSM is a large MG dataset, however it is acquired with a different imaging technique from the In-house data (full field digital mammography) and this might explain the similar results. The ROC plot also shows the improvement in AUC by adding dropout in Fig. 2.

3.4   Template Matching

The cross-correlation score was transformed from the range of $[-1, 1]$ to $[0, 1]$ to represent the score as probabilities. The correlation presented in Fig. 2 obtained significantly lower results of AUC 0.73, 0.63 on In-house, DDSM respectively.

3.5   Dual-View Automatic Lesion Detection

To evaluate the contribution of the matching architecture to the full detection pipeline, we applied the single-view detection algorithms on the CC, MLO image pairs followed by the matching architecture on the DDSM dataset. In some cases, detections will appear only for one view and not in the other. These cases cannot be evaluated using the matching architecture. Thus, two possibilities arise, exclude all detections without a pair or include them. Figure 3(a) shows the classification of the set of patches into positive and negative matches, generates an AUROC of 0.864, 0.81 depending on whether the small set of detections with no-pairs were included or excluded. We conclude that it is reasonable to include these detection as some tumors may be identified only in a single view.

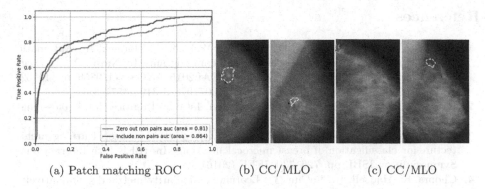

(a) Patch matching ROC   (b) CC/MLO   (c) CC/MLO

Fig. 3. Results of automatic lesion detection pipeline. (a) Green curve includes detections with no-pair in second view, orange curve excludes those detection. Detection examples on DDSM dataset (b, c). Red contours denote automatically detected pairs that correspond to GT while, the cyan contours are false positive automatic detections that were reduced by the dual-view algorithm. (Color figure online)

Additionally, Fig. 3(a) shows that proposed approach can reduce the false positive detection rate while keeping a high sensitivity. For MG pairs matching, we can keep a sensitivity of 0.99 and specificity of 0.19. Namely, by keeping the standalone detections we are able to reduce the false positives by almost 20%. Fig. 3(b, c), illustrates the full pipeline prediction on MG images. Probabilities of the false detections pairs (in cyan) are omitted in the final detection output. This is similar to the approach used by human radiologists, first detecting suspicious findings and then analyzing them by comparing the dual-view appearance.

4   Discussion

Finding correspondence between patches from different views of the same breast is a challenging task. Each image from MLO/CC views undergoes nonlinear deformations which can make the lesions very different from each other. On the other hand, being able to detect the lesion in both views can help the radiologists reach more accurate findings. In this work, we propose a dual-view Siamese based network, in which the architecture learns a patch representation and similarity for lesion matching. We demonstrate the advantage of a learned distance metric implemented in the network and its value in addition to a single view detection. This work can also be extended to 3D mammography by applying 3D patches. Future work will extend this work to other types of findings such as calcifications and will utilize mass location information to better eliminate false positives.

References

1. Amit, G., Hashoul, S., Kisilev, P., Ophir, B., Walach, E., Zlotnick, A.: Automatic dual-view mass detection in full-field digital mammograms. In: Navab, N., Hornegger, J., Wells, W.M., Frangi, A.F. (eds.) MICCAI 2015. LNCS, vol. 9350, pp. 44–52. Springer, Cham (2015). https://doi.org/10.1007/978-3-319-24571-3_6
2. Ballard, D.H., Brown, C.M.: Computer Vision, 1st edn. Prentice Hall Professional Technical Reference, New York (1982)
3. Bekker, A.J., Greenspan, H., Goldberger, J.: A multi-view deep learning architecture for classification of breast microcalcifications. In: IEEE 13th International Symposium on ISBI, pp. 726–730. IEEE (2016)
4. Chopra, S., Hadsell, R., LeCun, Y.: Learning a similarity metric discriminatively, with application to face verification. In: IEEE Computer Society Conference on CVPR, vol. 1, pp. 539–546. IEEE (2005)
5. Dhungel, N., Carneiro, G., Bradley, A.P.: Fully automated classification of mammograms using deep residual neural networks. In: ISBI, pp. 310–314. IEEE (2017)
6. Geras, K.J., Wolfson, S., Shen, Y., Kim, S., Moy, L., Cho, K.: High-resolution breast cancer screening with multi-view deep convolutional neural networks. arXiv preprint arXiv:1703.07047 (2017)
7. Giger, M.L., Karssemeijer, N., Schnabel, J.A.: Breast image analysis for risk assessment, detection, diagnosis, and treatment of cancer. Annu. Rev. Biomed. Eng. **15**, 327–357 (2013)
8. Han, X., Leung, T., Jia, Y., Sukthankar, R., Berg, A.C.: MatchNet: unifying feature and metric learning for patch-based matching. In: CVPR. IEEE (2015)
9. Heath, M., Bowyer, K., Kopans, D., Moore, R., Kegelmeyer, P.: The digital database for screening mammography. In: Digital Mammography, pp. 431–434 (2000)
10. Koch, G., Zemel, R., Salakhutdinov, R.: Siamese neural networks for one-shot image recognition. In: ICML Deep Learning Workshop, vol. 2 (2015)
11. Paquerault, S., Petrick, N., Chan, H.P., Sahiner, B., Helvie, M.A.: Improvement of computerized mass detection on mammograms: fusion of two-view information. Med. Phys. **29**(2), 238–247 (2002)
12. http://phototour.cs.washington.edu/patches/default.htm (2007)
13. Ronneberger, O., Fischer, P., Brox, T.: U-Net: convolutional networks for biomedical image segmentation. In: Navab, N., Hornegger, J., Wells, W.M., Frangi, A.F. (eds.) MICCAI 2015. LNCS, vol. 9351, pp. 234–241. Springer, Cham (2015). https://doi.org/10.1007/978-3-319-24574-4_28
14. Tajbakhsh, N., Shin, J.Y., Gurudu, S.R., Hurst, R.T., Kendall, C.B., Gotway, M.B., Liang, J.: Convolutional neural networks for medical image analysis: full training or fine tuning? IEEE TMI **35**(5), 1299–1312 (2016)
15. Teare, P., Fishman, M., Benzaquen, O., Toledano, E., Elnekave, E.: Malignancy detection on mammography using dual deep convolutional neural networks and genetically discovered false color input enhancement. J. Digit. Imaging **30**(4), 499–505 (2017)
16. Wang, J., Fang, Z., Lang, N., Yuan, H., Su, M.Y., Baldi, P.: A multi-resolution approach for spinal metastasis detection using deep siamese neural networks. Comput. Biol. Med. **84**, 137–146 (2017)

17. Warren, R.M., Duffy, S., Bashir, S.: The value of the second view in screening mammography. Br. J. Radiol. **69**(818), 105–108 (1996)
18. Yosinski, J., Clune, J., Bengio, Y., Lipson, H.: How transferable are features in deep neural networks? In: Advances in Neural Information Processing Systems, pp. 3320–3328 (2014)

Large-Scale Mammography CAD
with Deformable Conv-Nets

Stephen Morrell[1]([✉]), Zbigniew Wojna[1], Can Son Khoo[1],
Sebastien Ourselin[2], and Juan Eugenio Iglesias[1]

[1] Medical Physics and Biomedical Engineering,
University College London, London, UK
stephen.morrell@gmail.com
[2] School of Biomedical Engineering and Imaging Sciences,
King's College London, London, UK

Abstract. State-of-the-art deep learning methods for image processing are evolving into increasingly complex meta-architectures with a growing number of modules. Among them, region-based fully convolutional networks (R-FCN) and deformable convolutional nets (DCN) can improve CAD for mammography: R-FCN optimizes for speed and low consumption of memory, which is crucial for processing the high resolutions of to $50\,\mu$m used by radiologists. Deformable convolution and pooling can model a wide range of mammographic findings of different morphology and scales, thanks to their versatility. In this study, we present a neural net architecture based on R-FCN/DCN, that we have adapted from the natural image domain to suit mammograms—particularly their larger image size—without compromising resolution. We trained the network on a large, recently released dataset (Optimam) including 6,500 cancerous mammograms. By combining our modern architecture with such a rich dataset, we achieved an area under the ROC curve of 0.879 for breast-wise detection in the DREAMS challenge (130,000 withheld images), which surpassed all other submissions in the competitive phase.

1 Introduction

Breast cancer is the most commonly diagnosed cancer and the second leading cause of cancer death in U.S. women [1]. Timely and accurate diagnosis is of paramount importance since prognosis is improved by early detection and treatment, notably before metastasis has occurred. Screening asymptomatic women with mammography reduces disease specific mortality by between 20% and 40% [1] but incorrect diagnosis remains problematic. Radiologists achieve an area under the ROC curve (AUC) between 0.84 and 0.88 [2], depending on expertise and use of computer aided detection (CAD).

CAD for mammography was first approved 20 years ago but some studies showed it to be ineffective [3] or counterproductive [2] because of over-reliance. Early CAD methods used simple handcrafted features and produced many false positive detections [2]. The best of these "classical", feature-engineered methods,

D. Stoyanov et al. (Eds.): RAMBO 2018/BIA 2018/TIA 2018, LNCS 11040, pp. 64–72, 2018.
https://doi.org/10.1007/978-3-030-00946-5_7

represented by e.g., [4,5], plateaued at 90% sensitivity for masses at one false positive per image [5], and at 84% area of overlap in segmentation [4].

Deep learning (DL) has enhanced image recognition tasks, building on GPUs, larger data sets and new algorithms. Convolutional neural nets (CNNs) have been applied to mammography, outperforming classical methods. For example, Dhungel et al. [6] used CNNs to achieve state of the art results in mass classification. In a recent study, Kooi et al. [7] proposed a two-stage system in which a random forest classifier first generated proposals for suspicious image patches, and a CNN then classified such patches into malignant or normal groups. Kooi's system was trained on a large private dataset of 40,506 images (6,729 cases) of which 634 were cancerous, and achieved an AUC of 0.941 in patch classification— representing significant improvement beyond prior work.

Despite the adoption of CNNs and increasing size of datasets, mammographic analysis still lags work on natural images in dataset size and algorithm comparability. Databases like ImageNet [8] and MS COCO [9] include millions of instances. Moreover, these public datasets enable independent verification of algorithmic performance with private test sets. Very recently, the Optimam [10] and Group Health datasets have begun to approach ImageNet and MS Coco sizes. Group Health was made available under the DREAMS Digital Mammography Challenge [11] (henceforth "the Challenge"), which used a verified hidden test set to benchmark comparisons between methods. The Challenge had 1,300 participants, and was supported by the FDA and IBM among others.

Moreover, CNN architectures now include a plethora of new techniques for detection, classification and segmentation [12–14]. It has also been shown that integration of these tasks in unified architectures – rather than pipelining networks – not only enables more efficient end-to-end training, but also achieves higher performance than when tasks are performed independently (e.g., [14]). This is due to sharing of features that use richer locality information in the labels – segmentations or bounding boxes.

Here we present our submission to the second phase ("collaborative") of the Challenge. Our contribution includes the selection of architectures from the natural image domain, adaptation to mammography to balance the trade-off between high resolution and network size (computational tractability) for fine feature detection, e.g., microcalcifications, data augmentation and score aggregation. In particular, the presented system is – to the best of our knowledge – the highest resolution DL mammography object detection system ever trained.

2   Methods

2.1   Network Architecture

Even though our objective is classifying whole images, we chose a detection architecture to exploit the rich bounding box information in our training dataset (Optimam), and also to increase the interpreteability of the results, which is useful for clinicians. Our choice of meta-architecture is Region-based Fully Convolutional Networks (R-FCN) [15], which are more memory-efficient than the popular

Faster Region-based Convolutional Neural Nets (F-RCNN) [16]. R-FCNs were enhanced with Deformable Convolutional Networks (DCN) [12], which dynamically model spatial transformations for convolutions and Regions of Interest (ROI) Pooling, depending on the data's current features:

$$y(\boldsymbol{p}_0) = \sum_{\boldsymbol{p}_n \in \mathcal{R}} \boldsymbol{w}(\boldsymbol{p}_n) \cdot \boldsymbol{x}(\boldsymbol{p}_0 + \boldsymbol{p}_n + \Delta\boldsymbol{p}_n),$$

where y is the filter response at a location $\boldsymbol{p}_0$; $\mathcal{R}$ is a neighborhood around $\boldsymbol{p}_0$; and $\boldsymbol{w}$ and $\Delta\boldsymbol{p}_n$ are learnable sets of weights and offsets, respectively. The versatility of adaptive convolution and pooling enables DCNs to model a wider spectrum of shapes and scales, which is appropriate in mammography – where features of interest can be of very different sizes (from barely perceptible microcalcifications to large masses) and forms (foci, asymmetries, architèctural distortions).

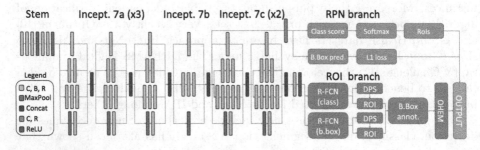

Fig. 1. Network architecture used in this study. C, B and R stand for convolution, batch norm and ReLU layers; RPN for region proposal network; DPS (ROI) for deformable position sensitive ROI; and OHEM [17] for online hard example mining.

A diagram of our architecture is shown in Fig. 1. It starts with a detection backbone, followed by two parallel branches: a region proposal network (RPN) branch, and a region of interest (ROI) branch – as per the R-FCN meta-architecture. The RPN branch [16] proposes candidate ROIs, which are applied on the score maps from the Inception 7b module. The ROI branch uses deformable position sensitive (DPS) score maps to generate class probabilities. Analogously to deformable convolutions, deformable ROI pooling modules include a similar parallel branch (Fig. 4 in [12]), in order to compute the offsets. Deformable pooling can directly replace its plain equivalent and can be trained with back propagation.

2.2   Adaptations

Backbone: Our backbone is descended from Inception v3 [18] from which we selected the first 7 layers (the "stem") and modules 7A, 7B and 7C. Choosing Inception, for which pre-trained weights from natural images were published, allowed transfer learning which showed beneficial for mammographic image analysis [19]. We included early layers on the assumption these are more consistent between domains. We chose consecutive layers to preserve co-adaption of weighs where possible. We compared to other recent architectures [20–22] in a pilot dataset but results were weaker; we did not pursue them.

Resolution-Related Trade-Offs: Current GPU memory constraints preclude full size mammographic images in deep CNNs – yet radiologists regularly zoom in to the highest level of detail. In particular, malignant microcalcifications may only be discerned at $\sim$50 μm resolution (approximately $4,000 \times 5,000$ pixels). Leading CNNs are designed for maximal GPU memory usage when fed natural images, which have two orders of magnitude fewer pixels, so the CNNs must be trimmed judiciously for mammography. This results in a trade-off between backbone choice, module selection, image downsampling, batch size, and number of channels in the different layers. We selected Inception v3 for its superior trade-off between parameter parsimoniousness and accuracy in natural images [23]. Its successor, Inception ResNet v2, was used in [12] but would have restricted images to $1,300 \times 1,300$ pixels. We included fewer repeats of modules 7A, 7B and 7C: three, one and two repeats, respectively; pilot experiments showed fewer layers to be sufficient for mammograms, whose content is less heterogeneous than natural images. We reduced batch size to one image per GPU. The channels are co-adapted in the pretrained weights and we ultimately retained them all. These choices, combined with meta-architecture and framework choices, enabled input size of $2,545 \times 2,545$ pixels (i.e. minimum downsample factor of 0.42), the highest resolution used for mammography classification to the best of our knowledge.

Data Augmentation: Training is more effective if additional augmented data are included. Each training image was rotated through 360° in 90° increments and flipped horizontally, thus included eight times per epoch. We opted for the benefit of using rotated images despite induced "anatomical" noise, i.e., implausible anatomy. We also used the same four rotations and flipping at inference. We did not use random noise or random crops (which are standard in the natural image domain), to avoid omitting lesions at the image edge.

Aggregation of Multiple Views: Screening exams usually consist of two views (cranio-caudal, CC, and medio-lateral oblique, MLO) of each breast, giving four images per exam. For each of these images we generated 8 predictions, when including augmentations. Each subjects's probability of malignancy lesion was calculated by computing the mean over views and augmentations for each laterality, and then taking the maximum over the two sides; other combination rules were explored but yielded inferior results (see results in Sect. 3.3).

3   Experiments and Results

3.1   Data

Two datasets were released in 2016/17, which were substantially larger than prior digital mammography datasets. These are the Optimam [10] dataset, which we used in training, and Group Health (GH), used in testing. The ground truths were determined by biopsy. Using standardised data makes comparisons objective and reproducible, e.g., as for ImageNet in the natural image domain. We believe these new benchmarks will allow attribution to future architectures.

Group Health images are a representative sample of 640,000 screening mammogram images, approximately 0.5% cancerous, provided in the Challenge. All machines were Hologic and maximum image size was $3,300 \times 4,100$ pixels. The GH data were not downloadable, excepting a small pilot set of 500 images for prototyping. The data are kept on IBM's cloud and are not accessible directly. Challenge participants could only upload models, run inference on the cloud, and receive a score. While this hampers testing experiments, it preserves patient confidentiality and ensures veracity of results. We used two subsets of GH in our study: 1. GH-13K, a subset of approximately 13,000 images with cancer prevalence inflated artificially by a factor of four; and 2. GH-Validation, a representative subset with 130,000 images, which was used for final testing and ranking and which the organisers intend to keep open for future testing, providing a hitherto absent way to benchmark performance.

Optimam consists of 78,000 selected digital screening and symptomatic mammograms including approximately 7,500 findings with bounding boxes of which 6,500 were cancerous. It included preprocessed and magnification images. Mammography machines were mainly Hologic and GE, and maximum image size was $4,000 \times 5,000$ pixels. Most teams in phase 2 of the Challenge used Optimam.

3.2 Experimental Setup

We trained our network on all Optimam images with findings. We trained our architecture on three different classes: negative, benign and malignant findings. For subsequent analyses, we used the score of the malignant class as prediction score. Pixel intensities were normalised across different manufacturers and devices using the corresponding lookup tables. We chose MXNet http://mxnet. incubator.apache.org/, for its memory-efficiency which surpasses most frameworks including TensorFlow. In terms of parameters, we used the same values as in the original publications describing the different DL modules, with two main differences: 1. We changed the scale of the input images, as explained in Sect. 2.2; and 2. In order to reflect the much lower risk of overlap and occlusion observed in mammography compared with natural images, we reduced the RPN positive overlap parameter from 0.7 to 0.5, and the proposal NMS threshold from 0.7 to 0.1. Training took 48 h on two NVIDIA TitanX GPUs.

We chose AUC on breast or patient classification as measure of diagnostic accuracy. AUC is used frequently to estimate the diagnostic performance of both CAD and radiologists. Compared with metrics like specificity at sensitivity or partial AUC, which are usually applied at high sensitivity levels and may be used to evaluate screening radiologists, AUC measures diagnostic accuracy across all probability thresholds, so is a comprehensive metric. Use cases for DL algorithms may range form automated flagging of some positive cases for immediate follow up – where high precision at high confidence thresholds is key – to safely excluding normal mammograms – where high negative predictive value at low confidence thresholds prevails.

We conducted three sets of experiments. First, we tested a number of design choices on the pilot set, then second on the GH-13K dataset, changing one or two key variables at a time while holding others constant. We tested backbone choices, scales, train and test augmentation and aggregation. Each evaluation on GH-13K took a day on the IBM cloud. Finally, we submitted our final model for testing on GH-Validation, which took approximately 8 days.

3.3 Results

Table 1 summarises results from our GH-13K experiments. Experiments 1–5 explored combinations of backbones and scales. In terms of backbone, empirical results showed that Inception was superior to ResNet [24] (1 vs. 2 and 5). In terms of scales, the main conclusion was that performance peaked when train and test inference was run at the higher scale (2, 8); however, accuracy dropped when testing size exceeded training (3, 4). Experiments 6–8 assessed the impact of augmentation (6), as well as answering the question of how to aggregate augmentation scores (7). In general, these experiments showed that: (a) augmentation at inference does help; and (b) within a single breast, taking the mean over views and augmented images outperformed the alternative of

Table 1. Summary of GH-13K results. Legend for consistent variables: R - ResNet backbone; M - mean probability over augmentations and views, maximum over laterality; I - Inception backbone; N - No augmentation at inference. The scale is in pixels.

Exp. #	Changed variable	AUC before	AUC after	Consistent variables
1	Train and Test Scale: 2145 to 2545	0.8352	0.8227	R, M, N
2	Train and Test Scale: 2145 to 2545	0.8595	0.8667	M, I
3	Increased test image size: 2500 to 2900	0.8173	0.8143	I
4	Increased test image size: 2900 to 3300	0.8143	0.8039	I
5	Changed backbone: Resnet to Inception	0.8352	0.8584	M, N
6	Added augmentation at inference	0.8584	0.8667	M, I
7	Max over breast's images changed to mean	0.8591	0.8667	I
8	As for 8 above and inference scale: 2,454 to 2,545	0.8511	0.8667	I
9	Adapted Inception ResNet v2. Image size of $1,600 \times 1,600$	N/A	0.7366	M, I, N

taking the maximum (we still use the maximum across lateralities). Row 9 shows a test AUC of 0.74 on GH-Validation from the competitive phase of the Challenge using a classification net (an adapted Inception ResNet v2), TensorFlow with the largest possible resolution under that setup ($1,600 \times 1,600$, much smaller than our current model, thus leading to a 0.15 decrease in AUC).

Based on these results, we submitted our final architecture described in Sect. 2 for testing on the large GH-Validation dataset. In the first sub-challenge, which records the AUC by breast purely on imaging and blinded to demographic information, we achieved $AUC = 0.879$ (standard deviation: 0.00914), see Fig. 2(e), which is 0.005 above the top AUC in the competitive phase of the Challenge. It was also the highest single-model AUC in the collaborative phase, 0.014 below an ensemble of detection models, and higher than all patch-based models. The second sub-challenge is on subject-wise AUC, with access to both images and demographics. Despite ignoring demographics, our architecture gave $AUC = 0.868$, behind only the top score in the competitive phase (a patch-based curriculum-trained model) by 0.006. Twenty-five method descriptions from this phase are available at synapse.org, but details of the collaborative phase, including performance of patch-based models trained on Optimam, is embargoed pending publication by the Challenge. Figure 2 shows sample outputs from GH.

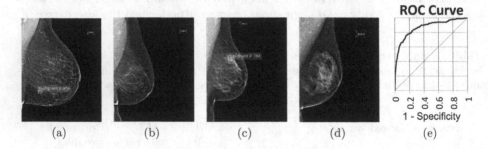

(a)   (b)   (c)   (d)   (e)

Fig. 2. (a) True positive prediction ($p = 0.90$ probability of malignancy) of an inconspicuous lesion on a left MLO of a 73 year old woman. (b) True negative (malignancy: $p = 0.06$) for left MLO view of a 66 year old woman. (c) False positive ($p = 0.78$) on left MLO of a 43 year old woman, due to hyper-intense region. (d) False negative ($p = 0.03$) for left CC view of a 61 year old woman. (e) ROC by breast, AUC = 0.879.

4   Discussion and Conclusion

We have presented a two-stage detection network trained on strongly labelled data which achieved 0.879 AUC by breast on a large unseen representative screening test set, operating at high resolution. Important questions remain, e.g., the impact of deformable modules, ameliorating batch size = 1 in batch normalisation, image rotation, the use of architectures that handle multiple scales (FPNs), single pass models, comparison to the different setup in [7] and clinical applicability. Exploring these directions, along with integrating demographic features into the architecture, will be in a future journal extension. As mammographic training databases grow and the rapid progress in DL for machine vision continues, we hope this will provide a first benchmark in mammogram classification on an public yet hidden test set.

References

1. American Cancer Society: What are the key statistics about breast cancer?
2. Lehman, C., Wellman, R., Buist, D., Kerlikowske, K., Tosteson, A., Miglioretti, D.: Diagnostic accuracy of digital screening mammography with and without computer-aided detection. JAMA Intern. Med. **175**, 1828 (2015)
3. Gross, C.P., et al.: The cost of breast cancer screening in the medicare population. JAMA Intern. Med. **173**(3), 220 (2013)
4. Jiang, M., Zhang, S., Zheng, Y., Metaxas, D.N.: Mammographic mass segmentation with online learned shape and appearance priors. In: Ourselin, S., Joskowicz, L., Sabuncu, M.R., Unal, G., Wells, W. (eds.) MICCAI 2016. LNCS, vol. 9901, pp. 35–43. Springer, Cham (2016). https://doi.org/10.1007/978-3-319-46723-8_5
5. Karssemeijer, N., te Brake, G.M.: Detection of stellate distortions in mammograms. IEEE Trans. Med. Imaging **15**(5), 611–619 (1996)
6. Dhungel, N., Carneiro, G., Bradley, A.P.: The automated learning of deep features for breast mass classification from mammograms. In: Ourselin, S., Joskowicz, L., Sabuncu, M.R., Unal, G., Wells, W. (eds.) MICCAI 2016. LNCS, vol. 9901, pp. 106–114. Springer, Cham (2016). https://doi.org/10.1007/978-3-319-46723-8_13
7. Kooi, T., Litjens, G., Ginneken, B.V., Gubern-mérida, A., Sánchez, C.I., Mann, R., Heeten, A.D., Karssemeijer, N.: Large scale deep learning for computer aided detection of mammographic lesions. Med. Image Anal. **35**, 303–312 (2017)
8. Russakovsky, O., et al.: ImageNet large scale visual recognition challenge. IJCV **115**(3), 211–252 (2015)
9. Lin, T.-Y., et al.: Microsoft COCO: common objects in context. In: Fleet, D., Pajdla, T., Schiele, B., Tuytelaars, T. (eds.) ECCV 2014. LNCS, vol. 8693, pp. 740–755. Springer, Cham (2014). https://doi.org/10.1007/978-3-319-10602-1_48
10. Royal Surrey County Hospital: The Optimam Mammography Image Database
11. Sage Bionetworks: The Digital Mammography DREAM Challenge (2016)
12. Dai, J., et al.: Deformable convolutional networks. In: CVPR, pp. 764–773 (2017)
13. Lin, T.Y., Dollár, P., Girshick, R., He, K., Hariharan, B., Belongie, S.: Feature pyramid networks for object detection. In: CVPR, vol. 1, p. 4 (2017)
14. He, K., Gkioxari, G., Dollár, P., Girshick, R.: Mask R-CNN. In: 2017 IEEE International Conference on Computer Vision (ICCV), pp. 2980–2988. IEEE (2017)
15. Dai, J., Li, Y., He, K., Sun, J.: R-FCN: object Detection via Region-based Fully Convolutional Networks, May 2016
16. Ren, S., He, K., Girshick, R., Sun, J.: Faster R-CNN: towards real-time object detection with region proposal networks. In: Advances in Neural Information Processing Systems, pp. 91–99 (2015)
17. Shrivastava, A., Gupta, A., Girshick, R.: Training region-based object detectors with online hard example mining. In: Proceedings of the IEEE Conference on Computer Vision and Pattern Recognition, pp. 761–769 (2015)
18. Szegedy, C., Vanhoucke, V., Shlens, J., Wojna, Z.: Rethinking the Inception Architecture for Computer Vision. (2015)

19. Carneiro, G., Nascimento, J., Bradley, A.P.: Unregistered multiview mammogram analysis with pre-trained deep learning models. In: Navab, N., Hornegger, J., Wells, W.M., Frangi, A.F. (eds.) MICCAI 2015. LNCS, vol. 9351, pp. 652–660. Springer, Cham (2015). https://doi.org/10.1007/978-3-319-24574-4_78
20. Hu, J., Shen, L., Sun, G.: Squeeze-and-Excitation Networks (2017)
21. Huang, G., Liu, Z., van der Maaten, L., Weinberger, K.Q.: Densely Connected Convolutional Networks, 1–12. arXiv preprint (2016)
22. Xie, S., Girshick, R., Dollár, P., Tu, Z., He, K.: Aggregated Residual Transformations for Deep Neural Networks (2016)
23. Canziani, A., Paszke, A., Culurciello, E.: An analysis of deep neural network models for practical applications, 7p. Arxiv (2016)
24. He, K., Zhang, X., Ren, S., Sun, J.: Deep residual learning for image recognition. In: CVPR, pp. 770–778 (2016)

Domain Adaptation for Deviating Acquisition Protocols in CNN-Based Lesion Classification on Diffusion-Weighted MR Images

Jennifer Kamphenkel[1(✉)], Paul F. Jäger[1], Sebastian Bickelhaupt[2],
Frederik Bernd Laun[2,3], Wolfgang Lederer[4], Heidi Daniel[5],
Tristan Anselm Kuder[6], Stefan Delorme[2], Heinz-Peter Schlemmer[2],
Franziska König[2], and Klaus H. Maier-Hein[1]

[1] Division of Medical Image Computing, German Cancer
Research Center (DKFZ), Heidelberg, Germany
j.kamphenkel@dkfz.de
[2] Department of Radiology, DKFZ, Heidelberg, Germany
[3] Institute of Radiology, University Hospital Erlangen, Erlangen, Germany
[4] Radiological Practice at the ATOS Clinic, Heidelberg, Germany
[5] Radiology Center Mannheim (RZM), Mannheim, Germany
[6] Medical Physics in Radiology, DKFZ, Heidelberg, Germany

Abstract. End-to-end deep learning improves breast cancer classification on diffusion-weighted MR images (DWI) using a convolutional neural network (CNN) architecture. A limitation of CNN as opposed to previous model-based approaches is the dependence on specific DWI input channels used during training. However, in the context of large-scale application, methods agnostic towards heterogeneous inputs are desirable, due to the high deviation of scanning protocols between clinical sites. We propose model-based domain adaptation to overcome input dependencies and avoid re-training of networks at clinical sites by restoring training inputs from altered input channels given during deployment. We demonstrate the method's significant increase in classification performance and superiority over implicit domain adaptation provided by training-schemes operating on model-parameters instead of raw DWI images.

Keywords: Convolutional neural networks
Diffusion-weighted MR imaging · Deep learning · Lesion classification
Domain adaptation

1 Introduction

As mammography suffers from high amounts of false positive findings, a promising image modality for breast cancer classification is DWI, which aims at

---

J. Kamphenkel, P. F. Jäger—Contributed equally.

© Springer Nature Switzerland AG 2018
D. Stoyanov et al. (Eds.): RAMBO 2018/BIA 2018/TIA 2018, LNCS 11040, pp. 73–80, 2018.
https://doi.org/10.1007/978-3-030-00946-5_8

reducing the number of biopsies through reliable early diagnosis [1]. The model-based state of the art for DWI signal exploitation is diffusion kurtosis imaging (DKI), where diffusion properties are estimated in suspicious tissue to distinguish between malignant and benign tumor cells [2,3]. An end-to-end q-space deep learning approach (E2E) has recently been shown to outperform DKI-based approaches by optimally exploiting input correlations using CNNs [4,5]. However, a limitation of E2E is the inherent input dependence of CNNs [6], which in this case are trained on specific diffusion-weighted images acquired at certain *b-values*, i.e. strengths and timings of gradient fields. This limitation is crucial for large-scale clinical application, since DWI scanning protocols deviate between sites and standardization is not expected in the near future. Furthermore, due to limited training data, it is desirable to ship trained models across clinical sites for inference on unseen images acquired with arbitrary local protocols. This procedure implies heterogeneities between training data and local inference data, e.g. in the form of *shifted* or *missing* b-values.

Generative models such as generative adversarial networks [7,8] and variational autoencoders [9,10] have recently succeeded at domain transformations. Such models could potentially be used to transform altered test-time inputs to original input channels used during training, yet do not eliminate input dependencies. Similar to other domain adaptation methods such as fine-tuning of models on new input or common representation learning of inputs [11], they themselves need to be trained on specific input alteration modes. As model fits such as DKI come with an inherent robustness towards input variations, input independence could potentially be achieved by operating on the fit parameters instead of raw DWI inputs. However, this robustness is proportional to the number of observed values, which, as will be shown, is not sufficient in typical DWI acquisition setups.

In this paper, we propose model-based domain adaptation, where the original training channels are derived from DKI using the altered inputs at test time. This method does not require training and hence can be deployed in any clinical setting without prior assumptions about protocol deviations. We show that this method significantly reduces input dependencies by optimally exploiting input correlations (E2E) based on estimations from the DKI model. We further demonstrate the superiority of our approach over training networks on DKI parameters (fit-to-end, F2E).

2   Methods

2.1   DWI Data Set

This study is performed on a data set of 221 patients and is equal to the data set used for E2E training [4,5]. For each patient, images of four b-values 0, 100, 750 and 1500 s mm^{-2} with a slice thickness of 3 mm were acquired using two different 1.5 T MR scanners. The in-plane resolution of one scanner had to be upsampled by a factor 2 to match the other scanners resolution of 1.25 mm. Prior to DWI scanning, all patients were diagnosed with BI-RADS [12] ≥ 4

from mammography screenings. A core-needle biopsy was performed to secure diagnosis, which resulted in 121 malignant and 100 benign lesions. The biopsy result served as the classification ground truth. Lesions were manually segmented as regions of interest (ROI) by expert radiologist without knowledge about the biopsy results. As 23 images do not contain any visible lesion, those subjects were predicted as benign. Figure 1 shows an example set of diffusion-weighted images for one patient.

Fig. 1. Sample slice of diffusion-weighted images of one patient at distinct b-values and the segmentation of the lesion on b = 1500 s mm^{-2} (right).

2.2 Diffusion Kurtosis Imaging

DKI is the the state of the art model for DWI signal exploitation in lesion classification. To derive diagnostically conclusive tissue parameters, DKI estimates the apparent diffusion coefficient (ADC) and additionally the apparent kurtosis coefficient (AKC) which quantifies deviations from free Gaussian diffusion induced by diffusion restrictions and diffusion heterogeneity [13]. These parameters are estimated by fitting the DKI model to measured signal intensities $S(b)$ in each voxel:

$$S(b) = (\theta^2 + S_0 \ exp(-b \ ADC + \frac{1}{6} \ b^2 \ ADC^2 \ AKC)^2)^{0.5} \qquad (1)$$

where S_0 is the signal intensity for b0 (b = 0), the b-value is the strength of diffusion weighting [14]. Furthermore, the model accounts for a background signal level induced by fat signal contamination in the lesion using the mean signal intensity θ of an additionally segmented fat area for each patient. In DKI, ADC and AKC are used most commonly to determine the malignancy of a suspicious lesion by averaging the coefficients over an ROI to obtain global coefficients [2]. Notably, we updated the DKI fit of [5] by not omitting $S(0)$ and added fat calibration to increase DKI fitting performance according to [14].

2.3 End-to-End Q-Space Deep Learning

E2E has recently been proposed as a successful model-free approach to classifying suspicious breast lesions [4,5]. Classification is performed by feeding the raw signal intensities of the segmented ROI into a CNN. Using 1×1 convolutions, deep diffusion coefficients are learned mimicking DKI parameters by correlating signal intensities of each pixel across DWI input channels. Subsequently, the network extracts features related to texture and geometry, which are globally pooled and fed through a softmax layer to obtain probabilities of malignancy.

2.4   Model-Based Domain Adaptation

To overcome dependence on specific b-values and enable clinical applicability of lesion classification regardless of scanning protocols, we propose to perform model-based domain adaptation (MBDA). During inference, the DKI model is fit to the signal intensities of all available (potentially altered) b-values. In order to restore the original set of b-values seen during training, the fitted model is used to derive estimates of the signal intensities $S(b)$ at the missing b-values (see Formula 1). Subsequently, the restored set of inputs is fed into the trained model to obtain classification scores (see Fig. 2 top).

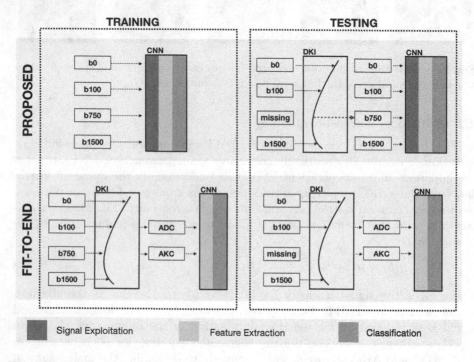

Fig. 2. Concept of our proposed method for the *missing scenario* (top). The missing b-value is derived from a DKI-model and used as CNN input. The fit-to-end architecture trained on ADC and AKC is used for comparison (bottom).

Experimental Setup. Two scenarios of heterogeneous inputs were studied: *shifted scenario*, where one measured b-value in the inference data is provided at a different (shifted) value w.r.t. the training data, and *missing scenario*, where one measured b-value in the inference data is missing w.r.t. the training data. Both scenarios were imitated by training and testing on respective subsets of the four b-values provided by the utilized data set. Note, that scenarios comprising alterations of multiple inputs were not studied due to the limited number of b-values provided. Furthermore, no alterations were applied to b0 as in practice all protocols include at least one b-value equal or close to zero [13–15].

An upper bound performance for MBDA is given by training and testing on the same subset of b-values (*matched input*). A lower bound performance for MBDA is given by testing on the altered inputs without domain adaptation (*altered input*). To compare our approach against the implicit domain adaptation of DKI, we train on DKI fit parameters ADC and AKC by feeding the parameter maps directly into the feature extraction and classification modules of the CNN (F2E). During testing, ADC and AKC are fitted using the altered inputs (see Fig. 2 bottom). For inference subsets containing only two b-values, which causes the DKI model to be under-constrained, we set $AKC = 0$.

The network details and training setup are equal to the setup reported in [5]. The signal exploitation module is omitted for F2E training. The networks are trained using 5-fold cross validation with 60% training-, 20% validation- and 20% test data and selected based on the lowest validation error.

Evaluation. Evaluation is conducted by comparing the area under the receiver operator curves (AUC). Significance tests were performed using DeLong's method and corrected for multiple testing using the Holm-Bonferroni-Method (initial $\alpha = 0.05$).

3 Results

Results are shown in Table 1. The observed moderate decrease of performance caused by a general absence of inputs (*matched input*) indicates a general redundancy of information across b-values of the input images. For instance, subsets of three b-values seem to roughly contain the same information as the original four b-values with respect to overall performance. However, strong input dependence is observed in both E2E and F2E (*altered input*, i.e. no domain adaptation) with an average decrease of 19.2% and 10.6%. MBDA is able to significantly increase this lower bound performance in the shifted scenario (12.4%) and missing scenario (16.8%) (see Fig. 3). Comparing F2E to E2E, F2E *altered input* performs on average slightly better than E2E *altered input*, i.e. 7.1% for shifted scenario and 4.4% for missing scenario, indicating a positive effect of implicit domain adaptation. E2E with MDBA considerably outperforms F2E by 5.3% for shifted scenario and 12.4% for missing scenario. Notably, extrapolation to large b-values is a poorly constrained problem, which causes performance drops across all explored methods. As expected, F2E only works when constraining the DKI model (setting $AKC = 0$) during CNN training.

Table 1. Results comparing all explored methods. All numbers report AUC except for p-values. x marks the available b-values. o marks the derived b-value. * marks observed significance.

a) Shifted Scenario.

Training b-values				E2E Matched Input	F2E Matched Input	Testing b-values				E2E Altered Input	F2E Altered Input	MBDA	p-value E2E;MBDA	p-value E2E;F2E
b0	b100	b750	b1500			b0	b100	b750	b1500					
x	x	x		0.893±0.04	0.819±0.05	x	x	o	x	0.741±0.06	0.768±0.05	**0.848±0.05**	0.0005*	0.011
						x	o	x	x	0.831±0.05	0.845±0.05	**0.893±0.04**	0.0052*	0.0622
x	x		x	0.882±0.04	0.855±0.05	x	x	x	o	0.799±0.06	**0.817±0.06**	0.751±0.07	0.1426	0.1132
						x	o	x	x	0.831±0.05	0.845±0.05	**0.880±0.04**	0.0019*	0.816
x		x	x	0.886±0.04	0.892±0.04	x	x	x	o	0.725±0.07	**0.845±0.05**	0.766±0.07	0.3199	0.0416
						x	x	o	x	0.737±0.07	0.844±0.05	**0.871±0.05**	6.96e-5*	0.422
x	x			0.777±0.06	0.674±0.072	x	o	x		0.680±0.07	0.679±0.07	**0.794±0.06**	0.00014*	0.0018*
						x	o		x	0.666±0.07	0.679±0.07	**0.791±0.06**	0.0002*	0.0015*
x		x		0.889±0.04	0.871±0.05	x	x	o		0.723±0.07	0.608±0.08	**0.796±0.06**	0.0467	4.08e-6*
						x		o	x	0.752±0.06	0.833±0.06	**0.869±0.05**	0.0009*	0.1426
x			x	0.882±0.04	0.877±0.05	x	x		o	0.729±0.07	0.589±0.08	**0.757±0.06**	0.4864	0.0002*
						x		x	o	0.817±0.06	0.825±0.06	**0.866±0.05**	0.0643	0.1485

b) Missing Scenario.

As for subsets of two available b-value images DKI is manually constrained by setting $AKC = 0$, performances for both training with and without the constraint are reported (DKI/ADC)

Training b-values				E2E Matched Input	F2E Matched Input (DKI/ADC)	Testing b-values				E2E Altered Input	F2E Altered Input	MBDA	p-value E2E;MBDA	p-value E2E;F2E (DKI/ADC)
b0	b100	b750	b1500			b0	b100	b750	b1500					
x	x	x	x	0.898±0.05	0.896±0.05	x	x	x	o	0.678±0.07	0.655±0.07	**0.745±0.07**	0.1463	0.0449*
						x	x	o	x	0.604±0.08	0.667±0.07	**0.882±0.04**	1.4e-12*	8.76e-8*
						x	o	x	x	0.823±0.53	0.678±0.07	**0.901±0.04**	0.00028*	1.04e-8*
x	x	x		0.893±0.04	0.819±0.05/ 0.859±0.05	x	x	o		0.513±0.08	0.522±0.08/ 0.617±0.07	**0.780±0.06**	2.1e-7*	1.18e-8*/ 0.00014*
						x	o	x		0.817±0.05	0.514±0.08/ 0.857±0.08	**0.891±0.04**	0.00026*	2.2e-16*/ 0.1041
x	x		x	0.882±0.04	0.855±0.05/ 0.860±0.05	x	x		o	0.512±0.08	0.612±0.08/ 0.652±0.074	**0.755±0.06**	6.92e-6*	0.00067*/ 0.0125*
						x	o		x	0.818±0.05	0.647±0.08/ 0.875±0.05	**0.879±0.04**	0.0003*	3.63e-9*/ 0.8804
x		x	x	0.886±0.04	0.892±0.04/ 0.860±0.05	x		x	o	0.657±0.07	0.646±0.07/ 0.836±0.05	**0.878±0.04**	5.14e-9*	8.72e-10*/ 0.1036
						x		o	x	0.649±0.07	0.699±0.07/ **0.868±0.05**	**0.868±0.04**	3.24e-7*	2.66e-6*/ 0.997

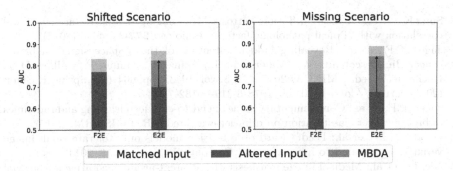

Fig. 3. Mean AUC derived from Table 1. Matched input represents the upper bound with matching b-value subsets during training and inference. Altered Input represents the lower bound by testing on the altered subset without domain adaptation. E2E with MBDA significantly improves the robustness towards heterogeneous inputs compared to F2E with altered inputs (implicit domain adaptation) in both scenarios.

4 Discussion

The results of this study suggest that model-based domain adaptation is an effective approach to overcome input dependencies and avoid re-training at clinical sites during large-scale application of DWI lesion classification. MBDA significantly increases the performance for both missing and shifted input scenarios by combining optimal exploitation of input correlations of raw DWI with DKI-based signal estimation to restore information lost due to altered input. In other words, MBDA is a "minimal invasive" method, which leaves unaltered input untouched, while the implicit domain adaptation performed by training and testing on fit parameters generates entirely new fit parameters given altered input, discarding unaltered correspondences. The latter works in theory, given a sufficient number of b-value images, but suffers from fitting instabilities in a typical DWI setup. In addition, strong assumptions have to be made on the amount of b-value images available during clinical inference prior to CNN training (as manually constraining the model by setting $AKC = 0$ might be required), which contradicts the desire for input independence. Future research includes studying multiple input alterations on data sets providing a larger number of b-values, application on unsegmented breast DWI, investigating the generalization of deep learning models trained on large DWI data sets and exploring the applicability to further entities.

References

1. Lauby-Secretan, B.: Breast-cancer screening-viewpoint of the IARC working group. New Engl. J. Med. **372**(24), 2353–2358 (2015)
2. Wu, D.: Characterization of breast tumors using diffusion kurtosis imaging (DKI). PloS One **9**(11), e113240 (2014)

3. Sun, K.: Breast cancer: diffusion kurtosis MR imaging diagnostic accuracy and correlation with clinical-pathologic factors. Radiology **277**(1), 4655 (2015)
4. Jäger, P.F., et al.: Revealing hidden potentials of the q-Space signal in breast cancer. In: Descoteaux, M., Maier-Hein, L., Franz, A., Jannin, P., Collins, D.L., Duchesne, S. (eds.) MICCAI 2017. LNCS, vol. 10433, pp. 664–671. Springer, Cham (2017). https://doi.org/10.1007/978-3-319-66182-7_76
5. Jäger, P.F., et al.: Complementary value of end-to-end deep learning and radiomics in breast cancer classification on diffusion-weighted MR. In: ISMRM (2017)
6. Ghodrati, M., et al.: Feedforward object-vision models only tolerate small image variations compared to human. Front. Comput. Neurosci. **8**, 74 (2014)
7. Nie, D., et al.: Medical image synthesis with context-aware generative adversarial networks. In: MICCAI, pp. 417–425 (2017)
8. Isola, P., et al.: Image-to-image translation with conditional adversarial networks. In: IEEE Conference on CVPR, p. 5967 (2017)
9. Rezende, D., Jimenez, S.M., Wierstra, D.: Stochastic backpropagation and approximate inference in deep generative models. ICML **32**(2), 1278–1286 (2014)
10. Kingma, D., Welling, M.: Auto-encoding variational bayes. In: ICLR (2014)
11. Havaei, M., et al.: HeMIS: Hetero-modal image segmentation. In: MICCAI, pp. 469–477 (2016)
12. Balleyguier, A.C., et al.: BI-RADS^{TM} classification in mammography. Eur. J. Radiol. **61**(2), 192–194 (2007)
13. Jensen, J.H., et al.: Diffusional kurtosis imaging: the quantification of nongaussian water diffusion by means of magnetic resonance imaging. Magn. Reson. Med. **53**(6), 1432–1440 (2005)
14. Bickelhaupt, S., et al.: Radiomics based on adapted diffusion kurtosis imaging helps to clarify most mammographic findings suspicious for cancer. Radiology **287**(3), 761–770 (2018)
15. Roethke, M.C., et al.: Evaluation of diffusion kurtosis imaging versus standard diffusion imaging for detection and grading of peripheral zone prostate cancer. Invest. Radiol. **50**(8), 483–489 (2015)

Improved Breast Mass Segmentation in Mammograms with Conditional Residual U-Net

Heyi Li[1(✉)], Dongdong Chen[1], William H. Nailon[2], Mike E. Davies[1], and David Laurenson[1]

[1] Institute for Digital Communications, University of Edinburgh, Edinburgh, UK
{heyi.li,d.chen,mike.davies,dave.laurenson}@ed.ac.uk
[2] Oncology Physics Department, Edinburgh Cancer Centre, Western General Hospital, Edinburgh, UK
bill.nailon@luht.scot.nhs.uk

Abstract. We explore the use of deep learning for breast mass segmentation in mammograms. By integrating the merits of residual learning and probabilistic graphical modelling with standard U-Net, we propose a new deep network, Conditional Residual U-Net (CRU-Net), to improve the U-Net segmentation performance. Benefiting from the advantage of probabilistic graphical modelling in the pixel-level labelling, and the structure insights of a deep residual network in the feature extraction, the CRU-Net provides excellent mass segmentation performance. Evaluations based on INbreast and DDSM-BCRP datasets demonstrate that the CRU-Net achieves the best mass segmentation performance compared to the state-of-art methodologies. Moreover, neither tedious pre-processing nor post-processing techniques are not required in our algorithm.

Keywords: Mammogram mass segmentation · Structured prediction
Deep residual learning

1 Introduction

Breast cancer is the most frequently diagnosed cancer among women across the globe. Among all types of breast abnormalities, breast masses are the most common but also the most challenging to detect and segment, due to variations in their size and shape and low signal-to-noise ratio [6]. An irregular or spiculated margin is the most important feature in indicating a cancer. The more irregular the shape of a mass, the more likely the lesion is malignant [12]. Oliver *et al.* demonstrated in their review paper that mass segmentation provides detailed morphological features with precise outlines of masses, and plays a crucial role in a subsequent cancerous classification task [12].

The main roadblock faced by mass segmentation algorithms is the insufficient volume of contour delineated data, which directly leads to inadequate

© Springer Nature Switzerland AG 2018
D. Stoyanov et al. (Eds.): RAMBO 2018/BIA 2018/TIA 2018, LNCS 11040, pp. 81–89, 2018.
https://doi.org/10.1007/978-3-030-00946-5_9

accuracy [4]. The U-Net [13], as a Convolutional Neural Network (CNN) based segmentation algorithm, is shown to perform well with limited training data by interlacing multi-resolution information. However, the CNN segmentation algorithms including the U-Net are limited by the weak consistency of predicted pixel labels over homogeneous regions. To improve the labelling consistency and completeness, probabilistic graphical models [5] have been applied for mass segmentation, including Structured Support Vector Machine (SSVM) [7] and Conditional Random Field (CRF) [6] as a post-processing technique. To train the CRF integrated network in an end-to-end way, the CRF with the mean-field inference is realised as a recurrent neural network [14]. This is applied on mass segmentation [15], and achieved the state-of-art mass segmentation performance. Another limitation of CNN segmentation algorithms is that as the depth of the CNNs increase for better performing deep features, they may suffer from the gradient vanishing and exploding problems, which are likely to hinder the convergence [8]. Deep residual learning is shown to address this issue by mapping layers with residuals explicitly instead of mapping the deep network directly [8].

In this work, the CRU-Net is proposed to precisely segment breast masses with small-sample-sized mammographic datasets. Our main contributions include: (1) the first neural network based segmentation algorithm that considers both pixel-level labelling consistency and efficient training via integrating the U-Net with CRF and deep residual learning; (2) the first deep learning mass segmentation algorithm, which does not require any pre-processing or post-processing techniques; (3) the CRU-Net achieves the best mass segmentation performance on the two most commonly used mammographic datasets when compared to other related methodologies.

2   Methodology

The proposed algorithm CRU-Net is schematically shown in Fig. 1. The inputs are mammogram regions of interest (ROIs) that contain masses and the outputs

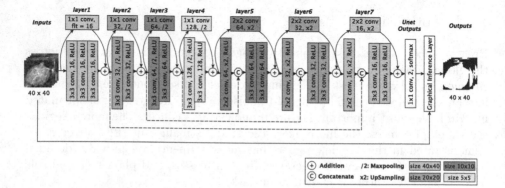

Fig. 1. Proposed CRU-Net Structure

are the predicted binary images. In this section, a detailed description of applied methods is introduced: our U-Net with residual learning, followed by the pixel-level labelling with graphical inference.

2.1 U-Net with Residual Learning

The U-Net is shown to perform well with a limited volume of training data for segmentation problems in medical imaging [13], which suits our situation. However, the gradient vanishing and explosion problem, which hinders the convergence, is not considered in the U-Net. We integrate residual learning into the U-Net to precisely segment breast masses over a small sample size training data. Assuming $x : \Omega \to \mathbb{R}$ (Ω represents the image lattice) as an ROI and $y : \Omega \to \{0,1\}$ as the corresponding binary labelling image (0 denotes background pixels and 1 for the mass pixels), the training set can be represented by $\mathcal{D} = \{(x^{(n)}, y^{(n)})\}_{n \in \{1,...,N\}}$.

The U-Net comprises of a contractive downsampling and expansive upsampling path with skip connections between the two parts, which makes use of standard convolutional layers. The output of mth layer with input $x^{(n)}$ at pixel (i,j) is formulated as follows:

$$y_{i,j}^{(n,m)} = h_{ks}(\{x_{s_i+\delta_i, s_j+\delta_j}\}_{0 \leq \delta_i, \delta_j \leq k})$$ (1)

where k represents for kernel size, s for stride or maxpooling factor, and h_{ks} is the layer operator including convolution, maxpooling and the ReLU activation function.

Then we integrate the residual learning into the U-Net, which solves the applied U-Net network mapping $\mathcal{H}(x)$ with:

$$\mathcal{F}(x) := \mathcal{H}(x) - W * x$$ (2)

thus casting the original mapping into $\mathcal{F}(x) + W * x$, where W is a convolution kernel and linearly projects x to match $\mathcal{F}(x)$'s dimensions as Fig. 1. As the U-Net layers resize the image, residuals are linearly projected either with 1×1 kernel convolutional layer along with maxpooling or upsampling and 2×2 convolution to match dimensions. The detailed residual connections of layer 2 and layer 6 are described in Fig. 2. These layers are shown as examples as all residual layers have analogous structure. In the final stage, a 1×1 convolutional layer with softmax activation creates a pixel-wise probabilistic map of two classes (background and masses). The residual U-Net loss energy for each output during training is defined with categorical cross-entropy. Mathematically,

$$f = -\sum_{i,j} \log P(y_{i,j}^{(n)} \mid x^{(n)}; \theta)$$ (3)

where P is the residual U-Net output probability distribution at position (i,j) given the input ROI $x^{(n)}$ and parameters θ.

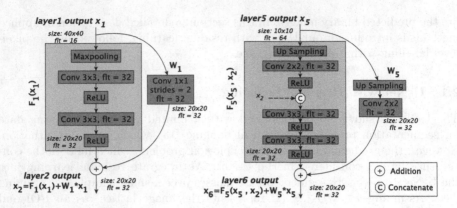

Fig. 2. Residual Learning illustration for layer2 and layer6. Other layers are equivalent to this example but with different parameters.

Note that the standard U-Net is designed for images of size 572×572. Here we modify the standard U-Net to adapt mammographic ROIs (40×40) with zero-padding for downsampling and upsampling. Residual short-cut additions are calculated in each layer. After that, feature maps are concatenated as: layer 1 with layer 7, layer 2 with layer 6, layer 3 with layer 5 as shown in Fig. 1. Both original ROIs and U-Net Outputs are then fed into the graphical inference layer.

2.2 Graphical Inference

Graphical models are recently applied on mammograms for mass segmentation. Among them, CRF incorporates the label consistency with similar pixels and provide sharp boundary and fine-grained segmentation. Mean field iterations are applied as the inference method to realise the CRF as a stack of RNN layers [14,15]. The cost function for CRF (g) can be defined as follows:

$$g = A(\boldsymbol{x}^{(n)}) - \exp\Big(\sum_{i,j \in V} P\big(y_{i,j}^{(n)}\big) + \sum_{p,q \in E} \phi(y_p^{(n)}, y_q^{(n)} \mid \boldsymbol{x}^{(n)}) \Big) \qquad (4)$$

where A is the partition function, P is the unary function which is calculated on the residual U-Net output, and ϕ is the pair-wise potential function which is defined with the label compatibility $\mu(y_p^{(n)}, y_q^{(n)})$ for position p and q [14], Gaussian kernels k_G^1, k_G^2 and corresponding weights $\omega_G^{(1)}$, $\omega_G^{(2)}$ [10] as $\phi(y_p^{(n)}, y_q^{(n)} \mid \boldsymbol{x}^{(n)}) = \mu(y_p^{(n)}, y_q^{(n)})\big(\omega_G^{(1)} k_G^{(1)}(\boldsymbol{x}^{(n)}) + \omega_G^{(2)} k_G^{(2)}(\boldsymbol{x}^{(n)})\big)$ [6,15].

Finally, by integrating (3) and (4) the total loss energy in the CRU-Net for each input $\boldsymbol{x}^{(n)}$ is defined as:

$$\ell = (1 - \lambda)f + \lambda \cdot g(f, \boldsymbol{x}^{(n)}) \qquad (5)$$

where $\lambda \in [0, 1]$ is a trade-off factor, which is empirically chosen as 0.67. And the whole CRU-Net is trained by backpropagation.

3 Experiments

3.1 Datasets

The proposed method is evaluated on two publicly available datasets INbreast [11] and DDSM-BCRP [9]. INBreast is a full-field digital mammographic dataset (70 μ m pixel resolution), which is annotated by a specialist with lesion type and detailed contours for each mass. 116 accurately annotated masses are contained with mass size ranging from $15\,mm^2$ to $3689\,mm^2$. The DDSM-BCRP [9] database is selected from the Digital Database for Screening Mammography (DDSM) database, which contains digitized film screen mammograms (43.5 microns resolution) with corresponding pixel-wise ground truth provided by radiologists.

To compare the proposed methods with other related algorithms, we use the same dataset division and ROIs extraction as [6,7,15], in which ROIs are manually located and extracted with rectangular bounding boxes and then resized into 40 × 40 pixels using bicubic interpolation [6]. In work [6,7,15], extracted ROIs are pre-processed with the Ball and Bruce technique [1], which our algorithms do not require. The INbreast dataset is divided into 58 training and 58 test ROIs; The DDSM-BCRP is divided into 87 training and 87 test ROIs [6]. The training data is augmented by horizontal flip, vertical flip, and both horizontal and vertical flip.

3.2 Experiment Configurations

In this paper, each component of the CRU-Net is experimented, including $\lambda = 0, 1, 0.67$ and the CRU-Net without residual learning (CRU-Net, No R). In the CRU-Net, convolutions are first computed with kernel size 3 × 3, which are then followed by a skip to compute the residual as shown in Fig. 1. The feature maps in each downsampling layer are of size 16, 32, 64, and 128 respectively, while the ROIs spatial dimensions are 40 × 40, 20 × 20, 10 × 10 and 5 × 5. To avoid over-fitting, dropout layers are involved with 50% dropout rate. The resolution of two datasets are different, with the DDSM's much higher than the INbreast's. To address this, the convolutional kernel size for DDSM is chosen as 7 × 7 by experimental grid search. All other hyper parameters are identical. The whole CRU-Net is optimized by the Stochastic Gradient Descent algorithm with the Adam update rule.

3.3 Performance and Discussion

All state-of-art methods and the CRU-Net' performances are shown in the Table 1, where [15] are reproduced, results of [2,3,6,7] are from their papers. Table 1 shows that our proposed algorithm performs better than other published algorithms on both data sets. In INbreast, the best Dice Index (DI) 93.66% is obtained with CRU-Net, No R ($\lambda = 0.67$) and a similar DI 93.32% is achieved by its residual learning; while in DDSM-BCRP, all state-of-art algorithm performs similarly and the best DI 91.43% is obtained by CRU-Net ($\lambda = 0$). The CRU-Net performs worse on DDSM-BCRP than INbreast, which is because of its worse data quality. To better understand the dice coefficients distribution in test sets,

Table 1. Mass segmentation performance (DI, %) of the CRU-Net and several state-of-art methods on test sets. λ is the trade off loss factor as (5).

Methodology	INbreast	DDSM-BCRP	Residual	Preprocess	Postprocess
Cardoso *et al.* [3]	88	-	-	-	-
Beller *et al.* [2]	-	70	-	-	-
Dhungel *et al.* [7]	88	87	×	✓	✓
Dhungel *et al.* [6]	90	90	×	✓	✓
Zhu *et al.* [15]	89.36 ± 0.37	90.62 ± 0.16	×	✓	×
U-Net	92.99 ± 0.23	90.08 ± 0.62	×	×	×
CRU-Net ($\lambda = 0$)	92.72 ± 0.09	$\mathbf{91.43 \pm 0.02}$	✓	×	×
CRU-Net ($\lambda = 1$)	92.60 ± 0.24	91.41 ± 0.02	✓	×	×
CRU-Net, No R ($\lambda = 0.67$)	$\mathbf{93.66 \pm 0.10}$	91.14 ± 0.09	×	×	×
CRU-Net ($\lambda = 0.67$)	93.32 ± 0.12	90.95 ± 0.26	✓	×	×

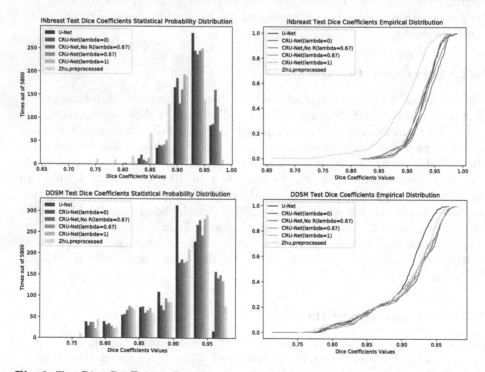

Fig. 3. Test Dice Coefficients Distribution of INbreast Dataset. The first row shows the distribution of INbreast dataset and the second row shows DDSM's. The left figures depict the histogram of test dice coefficients and the rights show the sampled cumulative distribution.

Fig. 3 shows the histogram of dice coefficients and sampled cumulative distribution of two datasets. In those figures we can observe that the CRU-Net achieves a higher proportion of cases with DI > 95%. In addition, all algorithms follow a similar distribution, but Zhu's algorithm has a bigger tail than others on the INbreast data. To visually compare the performances, example contours from the CRU-Net ($\lambda = 0.67$) and Zhu's algorithms are shown in Fig. 4. It depicts that while achieving a similar DI value to Zhu's method, the CRU-Net obtains a less noisy boundary. To examine the tail in Zhu's DIs histogram (DI ≤ 81%), Fig. 5 compares the contours of the hard cases, which suggests that the proposed CRU-Net provides better contours for irregular shape masses with less noisy boundaries.

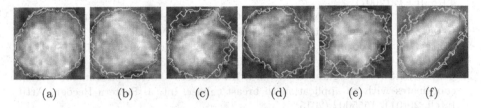

| | | | | | |
| (a) | (b) | (c) | (d) | (e) | (f) |

Fig. 4. Visualized comparison of segmentation results (DI > 81%) between CRU-Net and Zhu's work. Red lines denote the radiologist's contour, blue lines are the CRU-Net's results ($\lambda = 0.67$), and green lines denote Zhu's method results. (Color figure online)

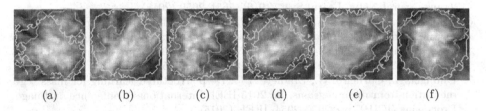

| | | | | | |
| (a) | (b) | (c) | (d) | (e) | (f) |

Fig. 5. Visualized comparison of segmentation results between CRU-Net ($\lambda = 0.67$) method and Zhu's work on the 5 hardest cases, when Zhu's DI ≤ 81%. Red lines denote the radiologist's contour, blue lines are the CRU-Net's results, and green lines are from Zhu's method. From (a) to (f), Zhu's DIs are: 70.16%, 73.47%, 76.11%, 72.95%, 80.36% and 79.98%. The CRU-Net's corresponding DIs are: 87.51%, 92.43%, 88.52%, 95.01%, 93.50% and 91.33%. (Color figure online)

4   Conclusions

In summary, we propose the CRU-Net to improve the standard U-Net segmentation performance via incorporating the advantages of probabilistic graphic models and deep residual learning. The CRU-Net algorithm does not require any tedious preprocessing or postprocessing techniques. It outperforms published state-of-art methods on INbreast and DDSM-BCRP with best DIs as 93.66% and 91.14% respectively. In addition, it achieves higher segmentation accuracy when the applied database is of higher quality. The CRU-Net provides similar contour shapes (even for hard cases) to the radiologist with less noisy boundary, which plays a vital role in subsequent cancerous diagnosis.

References

1. Ball, J.E., Bruce, L.M.: Digital mammographic computer aided diagnosis (CAD) using adaptive level set segmentation. In: 29th Annual International Conference of the IEEE Engineering in Medicine and Biology Society, EMBS 2007, pp. 4973–4978. IEEE (2007)
2. Beller, M., Stotzka, R., Müller, T.O., Gemmeke, H.: An example-based system to support the segmentation of stellate lesions. In: Meinzer, H.P., Handels, H., Horsch, A., Tolxdorff, T. (eds.) Bildverarbeitung für die Medizin 2005. Springer, Heidelberg (2005). https://doi.org/10.1007/3-540-26431-0_97
3. Cardoso, J.S., Domingues, I., Oliveira, H.P.: Closed shortest path in the original coordinates with an application to breast cancer. Int. J. Pattern Recogn. Artif. Intell. **29**(01), 1555002 (2015)
4. Carneiro, G., Zheng, Y., Xing, F., Yang, L.: Review of deep learning methods in mammography, cardiovascular, and microscopy image analysis. In: Lu, L., Zheng, Y., Carneiro, G., Yang, L. (eds.) Deep Learning and Convolutional Neural Networks for Medical Image Computing. ACVPR, pp. 11–32. Springer, Cham (2017). https://doi.org/10.1007/978-3-319-42999-1_2
5. Chen, D., Lv, J., Yi, Z.: Graph regularized restricted Boltzmann machine. IEEE Trans. Neural Netw. Learn. Syst. **29**(6), 2651–2659 (2018)
6. Dhungel, N., Carneiro, G., Bradley, A.P.: Deep learning and structured prediction for the segmentation of mass in Mammograms. In: Navab, N., Hornegger, J., Wells, W.M., Frangi, A.F. (eds.) MICCAI 2015. LNCS, vol. 9349, pp. 605–612. Springer, Cham (2015). https://doi.org/10.1007/978-3-319-24553-9_74
7. Dhungel, N., Carneiro, G., Bradley, A.P.: Deep structured learning for mass segmentation from mammograms. In: 2015 IEEE International Conference on Image Processing (ICIP), pp. 2950–2954. IEEE (2015)
8. He, K., Zhang, X., Ren, S., Sun, J.: Deep residual learning for image recognition. In: Proceedings of the IEEE Conference on Computer Vision and Pattern Recognition, pp. 770–778 (2016)
9. Heath, M., Bowyer, K., Kopans, D., Moore, R., Kegelmeyer, P.: The digital database for screening mammography. In: Digital Mammography, pp. 431–434 (2000)
10. Krähenbühl, P., Koltun, V.: Efficient inference in fully connected CRFs with Gaussian edge potentials. In: Advances in Neural Information Processing Systems, pp. 109–117 (2011)
11. Moreira, I.C., Amaral, I., Domingues, I., Cardoso, A., Cardoso, M.J., Cardoso, J.S.: INbreast: toward a full-field digital mammographic database. Acad. Radiol. **19**(2), 236–248 (2012)
12. Oliver, A., Freixenet, J., Marti, J., Perez, E., Pont, J., Denton, E.R., Zwiggelaar, R.: A review of automatic mass detection and segmentation in mammographic images. Med. Image Anal. **14**(2), 87–110 (2010)

13. Ronneberger, O., Fischer, P., Brox, T.: U-Net: convolutional networks for biomedical image segmentation. In: Navab, N., Hornegger, J., Wells, W.M., Frangi, A.F. (eds.) MICCAI 2015. LNCS, vol. 9351, pp. 234–241. Springer, Cham (2015). https://doi.org/10.1007/978-3-319-24574-4_28
14. Zheng, S., et al.: Conditional random fields as recurrent neural networks. In: Proceedings of the IEEE International Conference on Computer Vision, pp. 1529–1537 (2015)
15. Zhu, W., Xiang, X., Tran, T.D., Hager, G.D., Xie, X.: Adversarial deep structured nets for mass segmentation from Mammograms. arXiv preprint arXiv:1710.09288 (2017)

Improving Breast Cancer Detection
Using Symmetry Information
with Deep Learning

Yeman Brhane Hagos[1,3,4,5]([✉]), Albert Gubern Mérida[1], and Jonas Teuwen[1,2]

[1] Department of Radiology and Nuclear Medicine,
Radboud University Medical Center, Nijmegen, The Netherlands
Yeman.Hagos@radboudumc.nl
[2] Delft University of Technology, Delft, The Netherlands
[3] University of Burgundy, Dijon, France
[4] University of Cassino and Southern Lazio, Cassino, Italy
[5] University of Girona, Girona, Spain

Abstract. Convolutional Neural Networks (CNN) have had a huge success in many areas of computer vision and medical image analysis. However, there is still an immense potential for performance improvement in mammogram breast cancer detection Computer-Aided Detection (CAD) systems by integrating all the information that radiologist utilizes, such as symmetry and temporal data. In this work, we proposed a patch based multi-input CNN that learns symmetrical difference to detect breast masses. The network was trained on a large-scale dataset of 28294 mammogram images. The performance was compared to a baseline architecture without symmetry context using Area Under the ROC Curve (AUC) and Competition Performance Metric (CPM). At candidate level, AUC value of 0.933 with 95% confidence interval of [0.920, 0.954] was obtained when symmetry information is incorporated in comparison with baseline architecture which yielded AUC value of 0.929 with [0.919, 0.947] confidence interval. By incorporating symmetrical information, although there was no a significant candidate level performance again ($p = 0.111$), we have found a compelling result at exam level with CPM value of 0.733 ($p = 0.001$). We believe that including temporal data, and adding benign class to the dataset could improve the detection performance.

Keywords: Breast cancer · Digital mammography
Convolutional neural networks · Symmetry · Deep learning
Mass detection

1 Introduction

Breast cancer is the second most common cause of cancer death in women after lung cancer in the United States, which covers around 30% of cancers diagnosed and the chance of women dying from breast cancer is 2.6% [1].

© Springer Nature Switzerland AG 2018
D. Stoyanov et al. (Eds.): RAMBO 2018/BIA 2018/TIA 2018, LNCS 11040, pp. 90–97, 2018.
https://doi.org/10.1007/978-3-030-00946-5_10

Mammography is the main imaging modality used to detect breast abnormalities at an early stage. Breast masses are most dense and appear in grey to white pixel intensity with oval or irregular shape [2]. Normally, irregular shaped masses are suspicious [2,3]. Breast cancer screening has shown a reduction in mortality rate of between 40% and 45% for women who were undergoing mammogram screening regularly [4]. However, mammogram screening has drawbacks due to False Positive (FP) recalls, such as FP biopsy and cost associated with the unnecessary follow up [5]. Therefore, it is necessary to increase sensitivity for early stage detection and increase specificity to reduce FP detection.

Nowadays, with a massive amount of data and computational power, Deep Learning (DL) has shown a remarkable success in natural language processing [6] and object detection and recognition [7]. This has opened an interest in applying DL in medical image processing and analysis. However, care should be taken as the way we as humans interpret natural images and medical images are different in some cases. Eventually, the performance of DL method will be compared with the radiologist and thus, the CNN should preferably be given all the information that radiologist utilize. For instance, during the reading of screening mammograms, radiologists use priors, multiple views and look for asymmetries between the two breasts.

DL has been explored for Digital Mammogram (DM) image analysis. Some of them work directly on the whole image [3,5], and others focused on patch based [8]. [5] proposed a multi-view single stage CNN breast mammogram classification that works at original resolution. To address memory issue, aggressive convolution and pooling layers with stride greater than one were proposed. It is stated also that this approach suffers from loss of spatial information. In the work by [8], incorporating symmetry and temporal context improves detection of malignant soft tissue lesion, in which random forest classifier was used for mass detection and CNN for classification.

In this study, we conducted an investigation to analyze the performance gain of integrating symmetry information into a CNN to detect malignant lesions on a large scale mammography database. First, a database of 7196 exams which contains 28294 images was collected from different sites in the Netherlands. Previous work by [9] was employed to detect suspicious candidates locations. Then, patches centered on the points were extracted to train a two input CNN to reduce FP candidates. Left and right breast images were considered as contra-later images to each other, and a patch in a primary image and an exact reflection or mirror on the contra-lateral were considered as a pair of inputs to the network.

2   Materials and Methods

2.1   Dataset

The mammogram images used were collected from General Electric, Siemens, and Hologic from women attending for diagnostic purpose between 2000 and 2016. The images are anonymized and approved by the regional ethics board after summary review, with a waiver of a full review and informed consent [10].

The database contains 7196 exams. For most of the exams, Medio Lateral
Oblique (MLO) and Cranio-Caudal (CC) views of both breasts are provided,
resulting in 28294 DM images in totals. All images with malignant lesions were
histopathologically confirmed, while normal exams were selected if they had at
least two years of negative follow-up. From 7196 DM exams, 2883 exams (42%)
contained a total of 3023 biopsy-verified malignant lesions. The exact distribution of the dataset is shown in Table 1. In the whole dataset, 1315 exams does
not have either left or right breast images of MLO and/or CC views.

Training, validation and test data split was done at patient level to evaluate
the generalization of the model developed. Data was randomly split into training
(50%), validation (10%) and testing (40%) while making sure exams from each
vendors present in each partition proportionally.

Table 1. Distribution of DM dataset used including their vendor.

	General Electric	Siemens	Hologic
Number of studies	2248	1518	3430
Normal images	7771	5842	12288
Images with malignant lesions	1292	255	1476

2.2   Candidate Selection

Previous work by [9] was employed to detect suspicious mass candidates. Figure 1
shows sample MLO view DM images of left and right breast. Likelihood of a pixel
to be part of a mass was computed using local lines and distribution of gradient

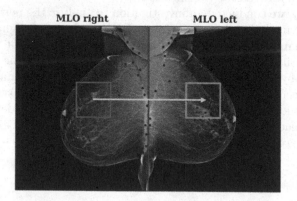

Fig. 1. An illustrative example showing center location of suspected masses in a sample MLO views of right and left breast mammogram images, and patches used to train
symmetry CNN model. The green box represents a patch centered on a positive candidate on MLO view of right breast DM image, and its corresponding symmetry patch at
the same location on the contra-lateral image is displayed in blue. (Color figure online)

Table 2. Number of suspicious candidates. The numbers after + indicate candidates from exams without left or right breast images. Positive refers to candidates inside malignant mass and negative candidates are outside a mass.

Candidates	Training	Validation	Test
Negative	$337366 + 2359$	$61833 + 1093$	$250293 + 6154$
Positive	$2217 + 58$	$927 + 30$	$727 + 67$

orientation features. Then, a global threshold was applied to the likelihood image to generate regions that are considered as suspicious. The red and green points correspond to suspected candidate center locations of mass. The green point is a true mass and others are false positive candidates. Table 2 details the number of suspicious candidates from training, validation and test data.

3   Patch Extraction and Augmentation

To extract patches, the contra-lateral images were flipped horizontally to place both images in the same space. Maximum size of the mass in our dataset was about 5 cm, and a patch size of 300×300 pixels (6 cm $\times$ 6 cm) was considered to provide enough context to discriminate soft tissue lesions. We reduced the number of training negative candidates by ensuring a sufficient distance (at least 2 cm) from a lesion and an inter-negative candidate distance of 1.4 cm. This resulted in 253476 (74.6%) negatives patches.

As an augmentation scheme, initially positive patches were flipped and Gaussian blurred with standard deviation between $[0.2, 3]$. Then, with probability of 0.5 one of the three augmentations were applied to both negative and positive patches: scaling, translation around the center and rotation. The parameters for these augmentations were uniformly selected from $[0.88, 1.25]$, $[-25, 25]$ and $[-30°, 30°]$, respectively.

4   Network Architecture and Training

In addition to incorporating symmetry information, a single input baseline architecture was trained. The baseline architecture is a variant of VGG architecture [11] as shown in Fig. 2a and it consists of feature extraction and classification parts. The feature extraction section has a series of seven convolutional layers with $\{16, 32, 32, 64, 64, 128, 128\}$ filters each followed by a max pooling layer. Convolution was performed with a stride of $(1, 1)$ and valid padding. The classification part is composed of three dense layers with $\{300, 300, 2\}$ neurons and with dropout (rate = 0.5) regularization after the first dense layer. ReLU activation was chosen for all layers but softmax for the last. Global Average Pooling (GAP) [12] was applied after the last convolutional layer while the other layers are followed by 3×3 max pooling. The advantage of GAP over flattening is

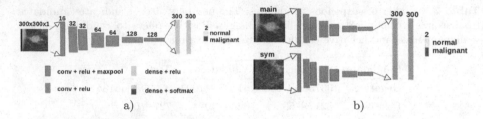

Fig. 2. CNN architectures: (a) Baseline architecture (b) Symmetry model architecture

it minimizes overfitting by reducing the number of parameters. The symmetry model has two inputs, the primary patch and a contra-lateral patch as shown in Fig. 2b. The parallel streams were transfer learned from the baseline architecture in Fig. 2a without weight sharing. The features from the parallel stream were concatenated and fed to the classifier. The classification part is similar to the baseline model. For exams without a contra-lateral image, zero matrices were used as a symmetry image.

Weights of both networks were initialized using Glorot weight initialization and optimized using Stochastic Gradient Decent (SGD) with time-based learning rate scheduler with an initial learning rate (ILR) of 10^{-2} for baseline architecture and 10^{-3} for the symmetry model, decay rate (ILR/200), and momentum (0.9). Mini-batch size of 64 was used and for each epoch, all positives samples were presented twice and an equal number of randomly sampled negatives, ensuring balance in each batch. Model with highest AUC on validation was selected as the best model. Furthermore, we monitored AUC for early stopping with patience of 20 epochs.

5   Result

All the experiments were conducted in Keras [13], and results presented are on a separately held 40% of the data. Candidate level quantitative evaluation was done using AUC and Free Receiver Operating Characteristic (FROC) along with CPM [14] for image and exam level performance analysis. Moreover, a 95% confidence interval and p-values of AUC and CPM were computed using bootstrapping [15], using 1000 bootstraps.

Table 3 reveals AUC values of the candidate selection, baseline and symmetry models. AUC value of 0.896 with 95% confidence interval of [0.879, 0.913] was obtained by the model used for candidate selection. The baseline architecture that processes a single Region of Interest (ROI) image yielded an AUC value of 0.929 with 95% confidence interval [0.916, 0.942], which is significantly better than the candidate selection stage performance ($p = 0.004$). Incorporating symmetry information improved the AUC to 0.933 with [0.919, 0.947] 95% confidence interval, although it was not significant ($p = 0.111$) in comparison with baseline architecture. For symmetry model, a zero matrix was used as a substitute when contra-lateral image is missing and a separate evaluation is presented

Table 3. AUC comparison of candidate selection, baseline and symmetry network. Symmetry* represents evaluation of symmetry model on candidates with missing contra-lateral patch.

	Candidate selection	Baseline	Symmetry	Symmetry*
AUC	0.896	0.929	0.933	0.866

in Table 3. The separate evaluation resulted in an AUC value of 0.866 with 95% significance interval of [0.788, 0.930]. A symmetry model was trained without augmentation and the best model resulted in AUC value of 0.91. This shows the proposed augmentation has significantly improved detection AUC. Figure 3 present image and exam based FROC comparison of the three models. In our test set, the symmetry model showed a better performance ($p = 0.001$) compared to the baseline architecture at both image and exam level. At an image level, CPM value of 0.716, 0.718, and 0.744 with 95% confidence interval of [0.682, 0.750], [0.679, 0.756], and [0.723, 0.794] was obtained for candidate selection, baseline and symmetry model, respectively. Moreover, during exam level evaluation sensitivity of the model that incorporates symmetry context was found to be better than the other model throughout the whole False Positive Rate (FPR) range, resulting in CPM value and confidence interval of 0.733 [0.721, 0.823] compared to 0.682 [0.671, 0.746] and 0.702 [0.687, 0.772] for candidate selection and baseline model, respectively.

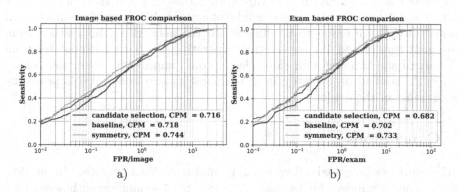

Fig. 3. FROC comparison of candidate selection, baseline and symmetry models; (a) Image based FROC. (b) Exam based FROC.

6 Discussion

The proposed patch augmentation method showed an improvement in the generalization of the CNN model and thus, the performance of the classifier. Symmetry model trained without patch augmentation yielded AUC value of 0.91 on

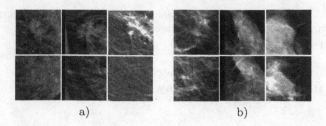

a)   b)

Fig. 4. Sample patches with an improved prediction using symmetry model: (a) Positive patches that were misclassified by baseline architecture and correctly classified by symmetry model. (b) Negative patches that were misclassified by baseline architecture and correctly classified by symmetry model. The top and bottom row images are primary and contra-lateral pairs, respectively.

a test set, in comparison to 0.933 when augmentation was applied. Moreover, incorporating symmetry information helps in learning distinctive features when there is a low-intensity contrast between mass and the background as shown in Fig. 4a. For the malignant candidates in Fig. 4a, without symmetry context malignancy probability was found to be below 0.2, however, integrating symmetrical information increased the malignancy prediction to a value greater than 0.7. Moreover, the negative patches in Fig. 4b were predicted as malignant masses by the baseline model (probability greater than 0.9), however, after including symmetrical context, their malignancy probability was found less than 0.1.

One of the main limitations of this work is that only soft tissue lesions were studied and detecting calcification will be of added value. Secondly, some benign abnormalities were found to be difficult for the network to differentiate from malignant candidates. We expect that separating the benign candidates from the normal and training with three classes could improve the detection performance. As studied in [8], integrating temporal context could also improve the performance of the model.

7   Conclusions

In this work, we proposed a deep learning approach that integrates symmetrical information to improve breast mass detection from mammogram images. Previous work by Karssemeijer et al. [9] was used to detect suspicious candidates. The FP candidates were reduced by learning symmetrical differences between primary and contra-lateral patches. AUC was employed as a performance measure at candidate level, whilst CPM was computed for image and exam level evaluation. We have found that our proposed approach reduces FP predictions compared to baseline architecture. An AUC value 0.933 ($p = 0.111$) with 95% confidence interval of [0.919, 0.947] was obtained at candidate level and 0.733 ($p = 0.001$) CPM with 95% confidence interval of [0.721, 0.823] was achieved with our symmetry model.

Training with a dataset which includes more time points could possibly improve reliability and detection accuracy [8], and will be part of our future work.

References

1. Rakhlin, A., Shvets, A., Iglovikov, V., Kalinin, A.A.: Deep convolutional neural networks for breast cancer histology image analysis. In: Campilho, A., Karray, F., ter Haar Romeny, B. (eds.) ICIAR 2018. LNCS, vol. 10882, pp. 737–744. Springer, Cham (2018). https://doi.org/10.1007/978-3-319-93000-8_83
2. Oliver, A., et al.: A review of automatic mass detection and segmentation in mammographic images. Med. Image Anal. **14**(2), 87–110 (2010)
3. Dhungel, N., Carneiro, G., Bradley, A.P.: Fully automated classification of mammograms using deep residual neural networks. In: 2017 IEEE 14th International Symposium on Biomedical Imaging (ISBI 2017), pp. 310–314. IEEE (2017)
4. Feig, S.A.: Effect of service screening mammography on population mortality from breast carcinoma. Cancer Interdiscip. Int. J. Am. Cancer Soc. **95**(3), 451–457 (2002)
5. Geras, K.J., Wolfson, S., Shen, Y., Kim, S., Moy, L., Cho, K.: High-resolution breast cancer screening with multi-view deep convolutional neural networks. arXiv preprint arXiv:1703.07047 (2017)
6. Bahdanau, D., Cho, K., Bengio, Y.: Neural machine translation by jointly learning to align and translate. arXiv preprint arXiv:1409.0473 (2014)
7. Wang, X., et al.: Deep learning in object recognition, detection, and segmentation. Found. Trends® Sig. Process. **8**(4), 217–382 (2016)
8. Kooi, T., et al.: Large scale deep learning for computer aided detection of mammographic lesions. Med. Image Anal. **35**, 303–312 (2017)
9. Karssemeijer, N.: Local orientation distribution as a function of spatial scale for detection of masses in mammograms. In: Kuba, A., Šáamal, M., Todd-Pokropek, A. (eds.) IPMI 1999. LNCS, vol. 1613, pp. 280–293. Springer, Heidelberg (1999). https://doi.org/10.1007/3-540-48714-X_21
10. de Moor, T., Rodriguez-Ruiz, A., Mann, R., Teuwen, J.: Automated soft tissue lesion detection and segmentation in digital mammography using a U-Net deep learning network. arXiv preprint arXiv:1802.06865 (2018)
11. Simonyan, K., Zisserman, A.: Very deep convolutional networks for large-scale image recognition. arXiv preprint arXiv:1409.1556 (2014)
12. Lin, M., Chen, Q., Yan, S.: Network in network. arXiv preprint arXiv:1312.4400 (2013)
13. Chollet, F., et al.: Keras (2015). (2017)
14. Setio, A.A.A., et al.: Validation, comparison, and combination of algorithms for automatic detection of pulmonary nodules in computed tomography images: the LUNA16 challenge. Med. Image Anal. **42**, 1–13 (2017)
15. Efron, B., Tibshirani, R.J.: An Introduction to the Bootstrap. CRC Press, Boca Raton (1994)

Conditional Infilling GANs for Data Augmentation in Mammogram Classification

Eric Wu[1,2](✉), Kevin Wu[1,2](✉), David Cox[1], and William Lotter[1,2]

[1] Harvard University, Cambridge, MA, USA
ericwu09@gmail.com
[2] DeepHealth, Inc., Boston, MA, USA

Abstract. Deep learning approaches to breast cancer detection in mammograms have recently shown promising results. However, such models are constrained by the limited size of publicly available mammography datasets, in large part due to privacy concerns and the high cost of generating expert annotations. Limited dataset size is further exacerbated by substantial class imbalance since "normal" images dramatically outnumber those with findings. Given the rapid progress of generative models in synthesizing realistic images, and the known effectiveness of simple data augmentation techniques (e.g. horizontal flipping), we ask if it is possible to synthetically augment mammogram datasets using generative adversarial networks (GANs). We train a class-conditional GAN to perform contextual in-filling, which we then use to synthesize lesions onto healthy screening mammograms. First, we show that GANs are capable of generating high-resolution synthetic mammogram patches. Next, we experimentally evaluate using the augmented dataset to improve breast cancer classification performance. We observe that a ResNet-50 classifier trained with GAN-augmented training data produces a higher AUROC compared to the same model trained only on traditionally augmented data, demonstrating the potential of our approach.

1 Introduction

A major enabler of the recent success of deep learning in computer vision has been the availability of massive-scale, labeled training sets (e.g. ImageNet [1]). However, in many medical imaging domains, collecting such datasets is difficult or impossible due to privacy restrictions, the need for expert annotators, and the distribution of data across many sites that cannot share data. The class imbalance naturally present in many medical domains, where "normal" images dramatically outnumber those with findings, further exacerbates these issues (Fig. 1).

A common technique used to combat overfitting is to synthetically increase the size of a dataset through data augmentation, where affine transformations such as flipping or resizing are applied to training images. The success of these

D. Stoyanov et al. (Eds.): RAMBO 2018/BIA 2018/TIA 2018, LNCS 11040, pp. 98–106, 2018.
https://doi.org/10.1007/978-3-030-00946-5_11

Original   GAN Input   Synthetic

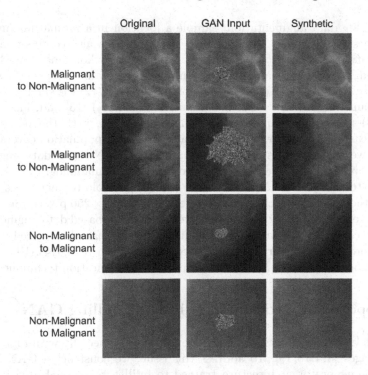

Fig. 1. Generated samples from ciGAN using previously unseen patches as context. Each row contains (from left to right) the original image, the input to ciGAN, and the synthetic example generated for the opposite class. The first two rows contain examples of the GAN synthesizing a non-malignant patch from a malignant lesion. The third and fourth rows are examples of the GAN synthesizing a malignant lesion on a non-malignant patch, using randomly selected segmentations from other malignant patches. We observe that the GAN is able to incorporate contextual information to smooth out borders of the segmentation masks.

simple techniques raises the question of whether one can further augment training sets using more sophisticated methods. One potential avenue could be to synthetically generate new training examples altogether. While generating training samples may seem counterintuitive, rapid progress in designing generative models (particularly generative adversarial networks (GANs) [2–4]) to synthesize highly realistic images merits exploration of this proposal. Indeed, GANs have been used for data augmentation in several recent works [5–9], and investigators have applied GANs to medical images such as magnetic resonance (MR) and computed tomography (CT) [10,11]. Similarly, GANs have been used for data augmentation in liver lesions [12], retinal fundi [13], histopathology [14], and chest x-rays [15].

A particular domain where GANs could be highly effective for data augmentation is cancer detection in mammograms. The localized nature of many tumors in otherwise seemingly normal tissue suggests a straightforward, first-order procedure for data augmentation: sample a location in a normal mammogram and synthesize a lesion in this location. This approach also confers benefits to the generative model, as only a smaller patch of the whole image needs to be augmented. GANs for data augmentation in mammograms is especially promising because of (1) the lack of large-scale public datasets, (2) the small proportion of malignant outcomes in a normal population ($\sim$0.5%) [16] and, most importantly, (3) the clinical impact of screening initiatives, with the potential for machine learning to improve quality of care and global population coverage [17].

Here, we take a first step towards harnessing GAN-based data augmentation for increasing cancer classification performance in mammography. First, we demonstrate that our GAN architecture (ciGAN) is able to generate a diverse set of synthetic image patches at a high resolution (256×256 pixels). Second, we provide an empirical study on the effectiveness of GAN-based data augmentation for breast cancer classification. Our results indicate that GAN-based augmentation improves mammogram patch-based classification by 0.014 AUC over the baseline model and 0.009 AUC over traditional augmentation techniques alone.

2   Proposed Approach: Conditional Infilling GAN

GANs are known to suffer from convergence issues, especially with high dimensional images [3,4,18,19]. To address this issue, we construct a GAN using a multi-scale generator architecture trained to infill a segmented area in a target image. First, our generator is based on a cascading refinement network [20], where features are generated at multiple scales before being concatenated to improve stability at high resolutions. Second, rather than requiring the generator to replicate redundant context in a mammography patch, we constrain the generator to infill only the segmented lesion (either a mass or calcification). Finally, we use a conditional GAN structure to share learned features between non-malignant and malignant cases [21].

2.1   Architecture

Our conditional infilling GAN architecture (here on referred to as ciGAN) is outlined in Fig. 2. The input is a concatenated stack (in blue) of one grayscale channel with the lesion replaced with uniformly random values between 0 and 1 (the corrupted image), one channel with ones representing the location of the lesion and zeros elsewhere (the mask), and two channels with values as $[1, 0]$ representing the non-malignant class or $[0, 1]$ as the malignant class (the class labels). The input stack is downsampled to 4×4 and passed into the first convolutional block (in green), which contains two convolutional layers with 3×3 kernels and ReLU activation functions. The output of this block is upsampled to twice the current resolution (8×8) and then concatenated with an input stack resized to 8×8 before being passed into the second convolutional block. This process is repeated until a final resolution of 256×256 is obtained.

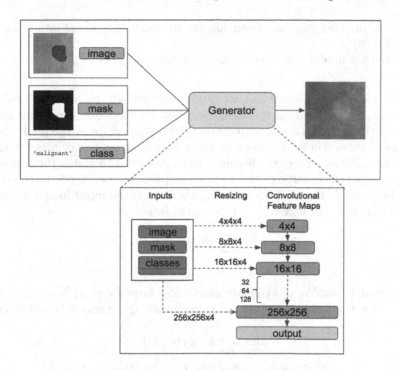

Fig. 2. The ciGAN generator architecture. The inputs consist of four channels (in blue): one context image (where the lesion is replaced with a random noise mask), one lesion mask, and two class channels for indicating a malignant or non-malignant label. Each convolutional block (in green) represents two convolutional layers with an upsampling operation. (Color figure online)

The convolutional layers have 128, 128, 64, 64, 32, 32, and 32 kernels from the first to the last block. We use the nearest neighbors method for upsampling.

The discriminator network has a similar but inverse structure. The input consists of a 256×256 image. This is passed through a convolutional layer with 32 kernels, 3×3 kernel size, and the LeakyReLU [22] activation function, followed by a 2×2 max pooling operation. We apply a total of 5 convolutional layers, doubling the number of kernels each time until the final layer of 512 kernels. This layer is then flattened and passed into a fully connected layer with one unit and a sigmoid activation function.

2.2 Training Details

Patch-Level Training: Given that most lesions are present within a localized area much smaller than the whole breast image (though context & global features may also be important), we focus on generating patches (256×256) containing such lesions. This allows us to more meaningfully measure the effects of GAN-augmented training as opposed to using the whole image. Furthermore, patch-level pre-training has been shown to increase generalization for full images [23–25].

The ciGAN model is trained using a combination of the following three loss functions:

Feature Loss: For a feature loss, we utilize the VGG-19 [26] convolutional neural network, pre-trained on the ImageNet dataset. Real and generated images are passed through the network to extract the feature maps at the $pool_1$, $pool_2$, and $pool_3$ layers, where the mean of the absolute errors is taken between the maps. This loss encourages the features of the generator to match the real image at different spatial resolutions and feature complexities. Letting Φ_i be the collection of layers in Φ, the VGG19 network, where Φ_0 is the input image, we define VGG loss for the real image R and generated image S as:

$$\mathcal{L}_{R,S}(\theta) = \sum_l ||\Phi_l(R) - \Phi_l(S)||_1$$

Adversarial Loss: We use the adversarial loss formulated in [27], which seeks optimize over the following mini-max game involving generator G and discriminator D:

$$\min_G \max_D \mathcal{L}_{GAN}(G, D)$$

$$\mathcal{L}_{GAN}(G, D) = \mathbb{E}_{(c,R)}[\log D(c, R)] + \mathbb{E}_R[\log(1 - D(c, S))]$$

Where c is the class label, R is a real image, and S is the generated image.

Boundary Loss: To encourage smoothing between the infilled component and the context of a generated image, we introduce a boundary loss, which is the L_1 difference between the real and generated image at the boundary:

$$B_{R,S}(\theta) = ||w \odot (R - S)||_1$$

Where R is the real image, S is the generated image, w is the mask boundary with a Gaussian filter of standard deviation 10 applied, and $\odot$ is the element-wise product.

Training Details: In our implementation, we alternate between training the generator and discriminator when the loss for either drops below 0.3. We use the Adam [28] optimizer with $\beta_1 = 0.9$, $\beta_2 = 0.999$, $\epsilon = 10^{-8}$, a learning rate of 1e−4, and batch size of 8. To stabilize training, we first pre-train the generator exclusively on feature loss for 10,000 iterations. Then, we train the generator and discriminator on all losses for an additional 100,000 iterations. We weigh each loss with coefficients 1.0, 10.0, and 10000.0 for GAN loss, feature loss, and boundary loss, respectively.

3   Experiments

3.1   DDSM Dataset

The DDSM (Digital Database for Screening Mammography) dataset contains 10,480 total images, with 1,832 (17.5%) malignant cases and 8,648 (82.5%) non-malignant cases. Image patches are labeled as malignant or non-malignant along with the segmentation masks in the dataset. Both calcifications and masses are used and non-malignant patches contain both benign and non-lesion patches.

We apply a 80% training, 10% validation, and 10% testing split on the dataset. To process full resolution images into patches, we take each image ($\sim$5500 × 3000 pixels) and resize to a target range of 1375 × 750 while ensuring the original aspect ratio is maintained, as described in [23]. For both non-malignant and malignant cases, we generate 100,000 random 256 × 256 pixel patches and only accept patches that consist of more than 75% breast tissue.

3.2   GAN-Based Data Augmentation

We evaluate the effectiveness of GAN-based data augmentation on the task of cancer detection. We choose the ResNet-50 architecture as our classifier network [29]. We use the Adam optimizer with an initial learning rate of 10^{-5} and $\beta_1 = 0.9$, $\beta_2 = 0.999$, $\epsilon = 10^{-8}$. To achieve better performance, we initialize the classifier with ImageNet weights. For each regime, we train for 10,000 iterations on a batch size of 32 with a 0.9 learning rate decay rate every 2,000 iterations. The GAN is only trained on the training data used for the classifier.

For traditional image data augmentation, we use random rotations up to 30 degrees, horizontal flipping, and rescaling by a factor between 0.75 and 1.25. For augmentation with ciGAN, we double our existing dataset via the following procedure: for each non-malignant image, we generate a malignant lesion onto it using a mask from another malignant lesion. For each malignant patch, we remove the malignant lesion and generate a non-malignant image in its place. In total, we produce 8,648 synthetically generated malignant patches and 1,832 synthetically generated non-malignant patches. We train the classifier by initially training on equal proportions of real and synthetic data. Every 1000 iterations, we increase the relative proportion of real data used by 20%, such that the final iteration is trained on 90% real data. We observe that this regime helps prevent early overfitting and greater generalization for later epochs.

3.3   Results

Table 1 contains the results of three classification experiments. ciGAN, combined with traditional augmentation, achieves an AUC of 0.896. This outperforms the baseline (no augmentation) model by 0.014 AUC ($p < 0.01$, DeLong method [30]) and traditional augmentation model by 0.009 AUC ($p < 0.05$). Direct comparison of our results with similar works is difficult given that DDSM does not have standardized training/testing splits, but we find that our models compare on par or favorably to other DDSM patch classification efforts [25,31,32].

Table 1. ROC AUC (Area under ROC curve) for three augmentation schemes.

Data augmentation scheme	AUC
Baseline (no augmentation)	0.882
Traditional augmentation	0.887
ciGAN + Traditional aug	**0.896**

4   Conclusion

Recent efforts for using deep learning for cancer detection in mammograms have yielded promising results. One major limiting factor for continued progress is the scarcity of data, and especially cancer positive exams. Given the success of simple data augmentation techniques and the recent progress in generative adversarial networks (GANs), we ask whether GANs can be used to synthetically increase the size of training data by generating examples of mammogram lesions. We employ a multi-scale class-conditional GAN with mask infilling (ciGAN), and demonstrate that our GAN indeed is able to generate realistic lesions, which improves subsequent classification performance above traditional augmentation techniques. ciGAN addresses critical issues in other GAN architectures, such as training instability and resolution detail. Scarcity of data and class imbalance are common constraints in medical imaging tasks, and we believe our techniques can help address these issues in a variety of settings.

Acknowledgements. This work was supported by the National Science Foundation (NSF IIS 1409097).

References

1. Russakovsky, O., et al.: Imagenet large scale visual recognition challenge. IJCV **115**(3), 211–252 (2015)
2. Goodfellow, I.J., et al.: Generative adversarial nets
3. Gulrajani, I., Ahmed, F., Arjovsky, M., Dumoulin, V., Courville, A.C.: Improved training of Wasserstein GANs. In: NIPS, pp. 5769–5779 (2017)
4. Berthelot, D., Schumm, T., Metz, L.: Began: boundary equilibrium generative adversarial networks. arXiv preprint arXiv:1703.10717 (2017)
5. Peng, X., Tang, Z., Yang, F., Feris, R.S., Metaxas, D.: Jointly optimize data augmentation and network training: adversarial data augmentation in human pose estimation. In: CVPR (2018)
6. Yu, A., Grauman, K.: Semantic jitter: dense supervision for visual comparisons via synthetic images. Technical report (2017)
7. Wang, X., Shrivastava, A., Gupta, A.: A-fast-RCNN: hard positive generation via adversary for object detection. arXiv, vol. 2 (2017)
8. Wang, Y.-X., Girshick, R., Hebert, M., Hariharan, B.: Low-shot learning from imaginary data. arXiv preprint arXiv:1801.05401 (2018)
9. Antoniou, A., Storkey, A., Edwards, H.: Data augmentation generative adversarial networks. arXiv preprint arXiv:1711.04340 (2017)

10. Wolterink, J.M., Dinkla, A.M., Savenije, M.H.F., Seevinck, P.R., van den Berg, C.A.T., Išgum, I.: Deep MR to CT synthesis using unpaired data. In: Tsaftaris, S.A., Gooya, A., Frangi, A.F., Prince, J.L. (eds.) SASHIMI 2017. LNCS, vol. 10557, pp. 14–23. Springer, Cham (2017). https://doi.org/10.1007/978-3-319-68127-6_2
11. Nie, D., et al.: Medical image synthesis with context-aware generative adversarial networks. In: Descoteaux, M., Maier-Hein, L., Franz, A., Jannin, P., Collins, D.L., Duchesne, S. (eds.) MICCAI 2017. LNCS, vol. 10435, pp. 417–425. Springer, Cham (2017). https://doi.org/10.1007/978-3-319-66179-7_48
12. Frid-Adar, M., Klang, E., Amitai, M., Goldberger, J., Greenspan, H.: Synthetic data augmentation using GAN for improved liver lesion classification. arXiv preprint arXiv:1801.02385 (2018)
13. Guibas, J.T., Virdi, T.S., Li, P.S.: Synthetic medical images from dual generative adversarial networks. arXiv preprint arXiv:1709.01872 (2017)
14. Hou, L., Agarwal, A., Samaras, D., Kurc, T.M., Gupta, R.R., Saltz, J.H.: Unsupervised histopathology image synthesis. arXiv (2017)
15. Salehinejad, H., Valaee, S., Dowdell, T., Colak, E., Barfett, J.: Generalization of deep neural networks for chest pathology classification in x-rays using generative adversarial networks. arXiv preprint arXiv:1712.01636 (2017)
16. Cancer.gov: Cancer facts and figures, 2015–2016 (2016)
17. Ribli, D., Horváth, A., Unger, Z., Pollner, P., Csabai, I.: Detecting and classifying lesions in mammograms with deep learning. Sci. Rep. 8(1), 4165 (2018)
18. Salimans, T., Goodfellow, I., Zaremba, W., Cheung, V., Radford, A., Chen, X.: Improved techniques for training GANs. In: NIPS, pp. 2234–2242 (2016)
19. Kodali, N., Abernethy, J., Hays, J., Kira, Z.: How to train your dragan. arXiv preprint arXiv:1705.07215 (2017)
20. Chen, Q., Koltun, V.: Photographic image synthesis with cascaded refinement networks. In: ICCV 2017, pp. 1520–1529. IEEE (2017)
21. Mirza, M., Osindero, S.: Conditional generative adversarial nets. arXiv preprint arXiv:1411.1784 (2014)
22. Xu, B., Wang, N., Chen, T., Li, M.: Empirical evaluation of rectified activations in convolutional network. arXiv (2015)
23. Lotter, W., Sorensen, G., Cox, D.: A multi-scale CNN and curriculum learning strategy for mammogram classification. In: Cardoso, M.J., et al. (eds.) DLMIA/ML-CDS -2017. LNCS, vol. 10553, pp. 169–177. Springer, Cham (2017). https://doi.org/10.1007/978-3-319-67558-9_20
24. Nikulin, Y.: DM challenge yaroslav nikulin (therapixel) (2017). Synapse.org
25. Shen, L.: End-to-end training for whole image breast cancer diagnosis using an all convolutional design. arXiv preprint arXiv:1708.09427 (2017)
26. Simonyan, K., Zisserman, A.: Very deep convolutional networks for large-scale image recognition. arXiv preprint arXiv:1409.1556 (2014)
27. Goodfellow, I., et al.: Generative adversarial nets. In: NIPS
28. Kingma, D.P., Ba, J.: Adam: a method for stochastic optimization. arXiv preprint arXiv:1412.6980 (2014)
29. He, K., Zhang, X., Ren, S., Sun, J.: Deep residual learning for image recognition. In: CVPR, pp. 770–778 (2016)
30. DeLong, E.R., DeLong, D.M., Clarke-Pearson, D.L.: Comparing the areas under two or more correlated receiver operating characteristic curves: a nonparametric approach. Biometrics 44(3), 837–845 (1988)

31. Zhu, W., Lou, Q., Vang, Y.S., Xie, X.: Deep multi-instance networks with sparse label assignment for whole mammogram classification. In: Descoteaux, M., Maier-Hein, L., Franz, A., Jannin, P., Collins, D.L., Duchesne, S. (eds.) MICCAI 2017. LNCS, vol. 10435, pp. 603–611. Springer, Cham (2017). https://doi.org/10.1007/978-3-319-66179-7_69

32. Lévy, D., Jain, A.: Breast mass classification from mammograms using deep convolutional neural networks. arXiv (2016)

A Unified Mammogram Analysis Method
via Hybrid Deep Supervision

Rongzhao Zhang$^{(\boxtimes)}$, Han Zhang, and Albert C. S. Chung

The Hong Kong University of Science and Technology, Kowloon, Hong Kong
rzzhang@ust.hk

Abstract. Automatic mammogram classification and mass segmentation play a critical role in a computer-aided mammogram screening system. In this work, we present a unified mammogram analysis framework for both whole-mammogram classification and segmentation. Our model is designed based on a deep U-Net with residual connections, and equipped with the novel hybrid deep supervision (HDS) scheme for end-to-end multi-task learning. As an extension of deep supervision (DS), HDS not only can force the model to learn more discriminative features like DS, but also seamlessly integrates segmentation and classification tasks into one model, thus the model can benefit from both pixel-wise and image-wise supervisions. We extensively validate the proposed method on the widely-used INbreast dataset. Ablation study corroborates that pixel-wise and image-wise supervisions are mutually beneficial, evidencing the efficacy of HDS. The results of 5-fold cross validation indicate that our unified model matches state-of-the-art performance on both mammogram segmentation and classification tasks, which achieves an average segmentation Dice similarity coefficient (DSC) of 0.85 and a classification accuracy of 0.89. The code is available at https://github.com/angrypudding/hybrid-ds.

Keywords: Whole mammogram classification · Mass segmentation
Deep supervision

1 Introduction

Breast cancer is one of the top causes of cancer death in women. In 2017, it is estimated that there are 252,710 new diagnoses of invasive breast cancer among women in the United States, and approximately 40,610 women are expected to die from the disease [2]. The detection of breast cancer in its early stage by mammography allows patients to get better treatments, and thus can effectively lower the mortality rate. Currently, mammogram screening is still based on experts reading, but this process is laborious and prone to error.

Computer-aided diagnosis (CADx) system is a potential solution to facilitate mammogram screening, and the research on automatic (or semi-automatic) mammogram analysis has been a focus in medical vision field. Given the fact

© Springer Nature Switzerland AG 2018
D. Stoyanov et al. (Eds.): RAMBO 2018/BIA 2018/TIA 2018, LNCS 11040, pp. 107–115, 2018.
https://doi.org/10.1007/978-3-030-00946-5_12

that a mass only occupies a small region (typically 2%) of a whole mammogram (i.e. the needle in a haystack problem [9]), it is very hard to identify a mass from the whole image without introducing a large number of false positives. Therefore, traditionally, both hand-crafted feature based methods [1, 11] and deep learning models [4, 7] require manually extracted regions of interest (ROIs), which, however, affects their usefulness in clinical practice. Recently, Dhungel et al. [3] proposed a sophisticated framework integrating mass detection, segmentation and classification modules to do whole-image classification, which achieved state-of-the-art performance with minimal manual intervention (manually rejecting false positives after detection). Besides, Lotter et al. [9] proposed a 2-stage curriculum learning method to cope with the classification of whole mammograms, and Zhu et al. [14] developed a sparse multi-instance learning (MIL) scheme to facilitate the end-to-end training of convolution neural networks (CNNs) for whole-image classification. Nevertheless, these methods either require manual intervention and multi-stage training, or only focus on the classification problem, while the accurate location and size of masses also play a critical role in a CADx system.

In this paper, we propose a CNN-based model with Hybrid Deep Supervision (Hybrid DS, HDS) to perform whole-mammogram classification and mass segmentation simultaneously. This model is based on a very deep U-Net [12] with residual connections [6] (U-ResNet) which has 45 convolutional layers in the main stream. To facilitate the multi-task training of the deep network and boost its performance, we extend deep supervision (DS) [8] to Hybrid DS by introducing multi-task supervision into each auxiliary classifier in DS, and apply this scheme to the U-ResNet model. To evaluate the proposed method, we performed extensive experiments on a publicly available full-field digital mammographic (FFDM) dataset, i.e. INbreast [10]. The results show that our model achieves state-of-the-art performance in both classification and segmentation metrics, and ablation studies are performed to demonstrate the efficacy of HDS scheme.

2   Method

2.1   Motivation

Due to the very small size of masses, directly training deep CNN models for whole mammogram classification can lead to a severe overfitting problem, where the powerful model may easily memorize the patterns presented in the background area rather than learn the feature of masses, leading to poor generalization performance. To deal with this problem, we propose to employ both image-wise and pixel-wise labels to supervise the training process. The underlying assumption for this multi-task scheme is two-fold. First, since classification (whether there exist any masses in a mammogram) and segmentation (whether each pixel belongs to a mass) are highly correlated tasks, the features learned in one task should also be useful in the other; second, multi-task learning itself can serve as a regularization method as it prevents the training process from biasing towards either task. Therefore, we propose a multi-task CNN model trained with Hybrid DS to attack the whole-mammogram classification and segmentation problems.

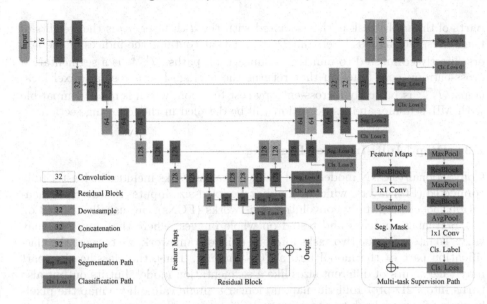

Fig. 1. Architecture of the U-ResNet model with Hybrid DS. Best viewed in color.

2.2 Hybrid Deep Supervision

Similar to DS, Hybrid DS directly supervises intermediate layers via auxiliary classifiers to force the model to learn more discriminative features in early layers. Meanwhile, HDS extends DS by introducing multi-task classifiers into each supervision level. Formally, the optimization objective of HDS is defined as:

$$\mathcal{L}\left(\boldsymbol{X}; \boldsymbol{W}, \widehat{\boldsymbol{w}}\right) = \mathcal{L}^{(\text{seg})}\left(\boldsymbol{X}; \boldsymbol{W}, \widehat{\boldsymbol{w}}^{(\text{seg})}\right) + \alpha \mathcal{L}^{(\text{cls})}\left(\boldsymbol{X}; \boldsymbol{W}, \widehat{\boldsymbol{w}}^{(\text{cls})}\right)$$
$$+ \lambda \left(\|\boldsymbol{W}\|_2 + \|\widehat{\boldsymbol{w}}^{(\text{seg})}\|_2 + \|\widehat{\boldsymbol{w}}^{(\text{cls})}\|_2\right) \tag{1}$$

where $\boldsymbol{X}$ denotes the training dataset, $\boldsymbol{W}$ is the trainable parameters of the main stream, i.e. the U-ResNet model without multi-task supervision pathways, $\widehat{\boldsymbol{w}}^{(\text{seg})}$ and $\widehat{\boldsymbol{w}}^{(\text{cls})}$ respectively denote the parameters of the segmentation and classification parts of the multi-task paths, and α is a constant that controls the relative importance of the classification loss. The third term to the right is a regularization term weighted by a hyper-parameter λ, and $\|\cdot\|_2$ denotes L2-norm. The segmentation loss $\mathcal{L}^{(\text{seg})}$ and classification loss $\mathcal{L}^{(\text{cls})}$ are defined as follow:

$$\mathcal{L}^{(\text{seg})}\left(\boldsymbol{X}; \boldsymbol{W}, \widehat{\boldsymbol{w}}^{(\text{seg})}\right) = \sum_{d \in \mathcal{D}} \eta_d \mathcal{J}_d^{(\text{seg})}\left(\boldsymbol{X}; \boldsymbol{W}_d, \widehat{\boldsymbol{w}}_d^{(\text{seg})}\right) \tag{2}$$

$$\mathcal{L}^{(\text{cls})}\left(\boldsymbol{X}; \boldsymbol{W}, \widehat{\boldsymbol{w}}^{(\text{cls})}\right) = \sum_{d \in \mathcal{D}} \eta_d \mathcal{J}_d^{(\text{cls})}\left(\boldsymbol{X}; \boldsymbol{W}_d, \widehat{\boldsymbol{w}}_d^{(\text{cls})}\right) \tag{3}$$

where $\boldsymbol{W}_d$ denotes the parameter in the first d layers of the main stream, $\widehat{\boldsymbol{w}}_d^{(\text{seg})}$ and $\widehat{\boldsymbol{w}}_d^{(\text{cls})}$ are respectively the weights in the segmentation and the classification parts of the multi-task path associated with the d-th layer, η_d is the weights of the corresponding loss level, and $\mathcal{D}$ is a set that contains the indices of the layers directly connected to multi-task supervision paths. $\mathcal{J}_d^{(seg)}$ is a segmentation cross-entropy cost function that returns the average loss across all pixel locations. $\mathcal{J}_d^{(cls)}$ is basically a cross-entropy cost function, which is made compatible with MIL scheme, and its definition will be detailed in the following section.

2.3   Deep Multi-Instance Learning

Conventionally, CNN models used in classification tasks includes at least 1 fully connected (FC) layers, which can only take fixed-size inputs. However, segmentation models, e.g. fully convolutional networks (FCNs), are usually trained on cropped image patches and tested on whole images, where the input size may vary. To integrate the two tasks into one unified framework, we convert the classification part of the model into a FCN manner. Thus, the classification part may take inputs of different sizes like a segmentation model, but its output also turns into a 2D probabilistic map, no longer a single value. If we map the pixels in such a 2D map back to nonoverlapping patches in the input image, the whole input image can then be regarded as a bag of patches (instances), thus the mammogram classification can be treated as a standard MIL problem. In this case, denoting the pixel values in a 2D probabilistic map as $r_{i,j}$, the mass probability of the input image I is then $p(y = 1|I) = \max_{i,j}\{r_{i,j}\}$. Following the practice of Zhu et al. in [14], we define the classification cost for an input image I as below:

$$\mathcal{J}^{(cls)}(I, y_I; W, w^{(cls)}) = -\log p(y = y_I|I) + \mu \sum_{i,j} r_{i,j} \qquad (4)$$

where y_I is the true label of image I, and $r_{i,j}$ is the pixel value in the 2D probabilistic map. Since masses are sparse in mammograms, the summation of $r_{i,j}$ should be small. Therefore, a sparsity term (the second term to the right) is added to the cost function, which is weighted by μ.

2.4   Network Architecture

The architecture of the proposed neural network model is illustrated in Fig. 1. The model is basically a deep U-ResNet with 45 3×3 convolutional layers (1 convolution and 22 residual blocks), and multi-task supervision pathways are inserted into each scale level for Hybrid DS. We use max pooling in downsampling modules (except for the last downsampling layer in the classification part of each multi-task path, which employs average pooling), and bi-linearly upsample feature maps in upsampling layers. For those transition modules (i.e. downsample, upsample and concatenation), if the input and output channel dimensions are different, 1×1 convolutions are inserted before the operation to change the channel dimension. All max pooling layers have a stride of 2, and the stride of average pooling layers ranges from 2^0 to 2^5 to ensure a total downsampling factor of 2^7 for the output of each classification path (so the size of the output probabilistic map is 4×3 in training and 8×4 in testing). Similarly, All upsampling layers except for the ones in multi-task paths have a stride of 2, and those in multi-task paths range from 2^0 to 2^5 to ensure the output mask have the same size as the input image. Besides, Dropout [13] layers of rate 0.2 (for residual blocks with less than 128 channels) or 0.5 (for others) are inserted into each residual block.

3   Experiments and Results

Dataset. The proposed method was evaluated on a publicly available FFDM dataset, i.e. INbreast [10]. Among the 410 mammograms in INbreast dataset, 107 contain one or more masses, and totally contain 116 benign or malignant masses. In pre-processing, we removed the left or right blank regions by thresholding, resized the mammograms to 1024×512, and then normalized each image to zero-mean and unit-std according to the statistics of training sets. During training, the whole image was randomly flipped vertically or horizontally, and patches of size 512×384 were randomly sampled from it with 50% chance centered on a positive (mass) pixel. The classification label of a cropped patch was set to 1 if the patch contained any pixel from masses, and 0 otherwise. In our experiment, the whole dataset was uniformly divided into 5 folds (82 images per fold), and we used three of them for training, one for validation and one for testing. We first performed ablation study on one data split to demonstrate the efficacy of the proposed method, and then ran a 5-fold cross validation for a fairer comparison with existing methods.

Implementation Details. The proposed method was implemented with PyTorch v0.4.0 on a PC with one NVIDIA Titan Xp GPU. Stochastic gradient descent (SGD) method with a momentum of 0.9 was used to optimize the model, with an initial learning rate of 0.01 and decayed by 0.3 after 1000, 1800, 2400 and 2410 epochs. In all experiments, the model was trained for 2800 epochs, which took about 12.5 h and was long enough for each configuration to converge. The model parameters were initialized by Kaiming method [5]. Other hyper-parameters were set as follows: classification loss weight $\alpha = 0.03$ (such that the segmentation and classification losses of each mini-batch were comparable in magnitude), weight decay $\lambda = 0.0005$, sparsity weight $\mu = 10^{-6}$, and the weights of different supervision levels $(\eta_0, \eta_1, \eta_2, \eta_3, \eta_4, \eta_5) = (1.0, 1.5, 2.0, 2.5, 3.0, 3.5)$, where η_1 to η_5 were gradually decayed to very small values (i.e. $0.005\eta_i$) during training. The losses stemmed from inner layers of the U-Net were initially weighted higher to force the these layers to learn meaningful features, otherwise they tended to be ignored due to the difficulty in learning from low-resolution feature maps.

Metrics. We employed dice similarity coefficient (DSC), sensitivity (SE) and false positives per image (FPI) to evaluate the segmentation results. For classification, accuracy (ACC), area under ROC curve (AUC), F_1 score, precision (Prec) and recall (Recl) were reported.

Table 1. Ablation study

Model	Segmentation			Classification				
	DSC	SE	FPI	ACC	AUC	F_1	Recl	Prec
Multi-task Only	0.787	0.882	0.293	0.829	0.866	0.682	0.714	0.652
Cls + DS	N/A	N/A	N/A	0.878	0.853	0.722	0.619	0.867
Seg + DS*	0.802	**0.910**	0.183	0.842	**0.890**	0.723	**0.810**	0.654
Hybird DS	**0.848**	0.907	0.110	**0.915**	0.887	**0.821**	0.762	**0.889**

*Classification results were retrieved from segmentation masks by assigning the largest activation across the output probabilistic map to the whole image

Ablation Study. To investigate the efficacy of the proposed Hybrid DS scheme, a series of experiments were conducted on one data split. From Table 1, it can be observed that the Hybrid DS model achieves the best performance on several important metrics (e.g. DSC, FPI, ACC, F_1, etc.), and also has high scores on others. HDS outperforms the baseline multi-task model by a large margin (0.848 vs 0.787 in DSC, 0.915 vs 0.829 in ACC), indicating that directly supervising intermediate layers is necessary for training such a deep model. Thanks to the sparse MIL [14] and DS schemes, the Cls+DS model performed well in classification, having an accuracy of 0.878. Meanwhile, HDS achieves even higher classification performance (e.g. ACC: 0.915) than Cls+DS, which evidences the benefit of employing extra pixel-wise supervision. Compared to Seg+DS, HDS achieves better DSC (0.848), accuracy (0.915), F_1 score (0.821) and precision (0.889), which we attribute to the extra image-wise supervision. Since image-wise supervision can force the network to look wider and to learn features based on the whole image (or at least a larger area), the network becomes less sensitive to local patterns that mimic masses and more robust in rejecting false positives, as has been validated by the much higher precision of HDS (0.889) than Seg+DS (0.654). Altogether, these experiments suggest that the proposed Hybrid DS scheme is a promising approach to improve deep model's performance on the mammogram analysis problem.

Comparison with Existing Methods. To compare the proposed model with other mammogram analysis methods, we used 5-fold cross validation to

Table 2. Comparison with state-of-the-art methods

Model	Segmentation			Classification				
	DSC	SE	FPI	ACC	AUC	F_1	Recl	Prec
D. [3]	0.85*	N/A	1.00#	0.91±0.02	0.76±0.23	N/A	N/A	N/A
Z. [14]	N/A	N/A	N/A	0.90±0.02	0.89±0.04	N/A	N/A	N/A
Ours	0.85±0.01	0.88±0.02	0.08±0.02	0.89±0.02	0.85±0.02	0.77±0.04	0.69±0.04	0.87±0.06

*Calculated on correctly detected masses.
#These detection false positives were manually rejected before further processing

evaluate it on the whole INbreast dataset. As shown in Table 2, our model matches the current state-of-the-art performance on both mass segmentation and classification tasks, achieving a high average segmentation DSC of 0.85 and a classification accuracy of 0.89. Besides, our method is fully automatic and easy to deploy, which takes whole mammograms as input and then outputs segmentation masks and image-wise labels simultaneously. In contrast, the method by Dhungel et al. [3] still requires manual intervention to reject false positives after mass detection, and the method by Zhu et al. [14] can only give a very rough location of identified masses. Qualitative segmentation results of our method on several typical testing images have been illustrated in Fig. 2.

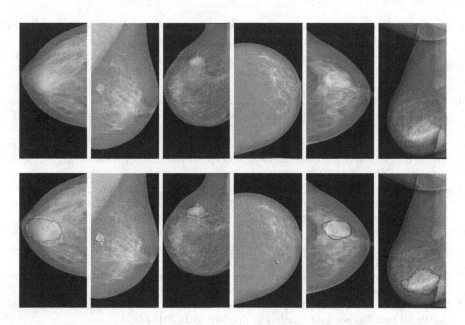

Fig. 2. Qualitative results. The first row is original mammograms. In the second row, red and green boundaries are ground truth delineation and automatic segmentation results, respectively. The fifth column contains a false negative lesion, and the last column has a false positive lesion. Best viewed in color (Color figure online).

4   Conclusion

In this paper, we have developed an end-to-end and unified framework for mammogram classification and segmentation. We seamlessly integrate the two tasks into one model by employing the novel Hybrid DS scheme, which not only inherits the merits of DS but also supports multi-task learning. With such a multi-task learning scheme, pixel-wise labels tell the model where to learn while image-wise labels force the network to make better use of contextual information. We conducted extensive experiments on the publicly available INbreast dataset, and the results show that our method matches the state-of-the-art performance on both segmentation and classification tasks. Ablation study demonstrates that pixel-wise and image-wise supervisions are mutually beneficial, and the proposed Hybrid DS can effectively boost the model's performance on both tasks. Besides, our unified framework is inherently general, which can be easily extended to other medical vision problems.

References

1. Buciu, I., Gacsadi, A.: Directional features for automatic tumor classification of mammogram images. Biomed. Sig. Process. Control **6**(4), 370–378 (2011)
2. DeSantis, C.E., Ma, J., Goding Sauer, A., Newman, L.A., Jemal, A.: Breast cancer statistics, 2017, racial disparity in mortality by state. CA Cancer J. Clin. **67**(6), 439–448 (2017)
3. Dhungel, N., Carneiro, G., Bradley, A.P.: A deep learning approach for the analysis of masses in mammograms with minimal user intervention. Med. Image Anal. **37**, 114–128 (2017)
4. Geras, K.J., Wolfson, S., Shen, Y., Kim, S., Moy, L., Cho, K.: High-resolution breast cancer screening with multi-view deep convolutional neural networks. arXiv preprint arXiv:1703.07047 (2017)
5. He, K., Zhang, X., Ren, S., Sun, J.: Delving deep into rectifiers: surpassing human-level performance on imagenet classification. In: Proceedings of the IEEE International Conference on Computer Vision, pp. 1026–1034 (2015)
6. He, K., Zhang, X., Ren, S., Sun, J.: Deep residual learning for image recognition. In: Proceedings of the IEEE Conference on Computer Vision and Pattern Recognition, pp. 770–778 (2016)
7. Kooi, T., et al.: Large scale deep learning for computer aided detection of mammographic lesions. Med. Image Anal. **35**, 303–312 (2017)
8. Lee, C.Y., Xie, S., Gallagher, P., Zhang, Z., Tu, Z.: Deeply-supervised nets. In: Artificial Intelligence and Statistics, pp. 562–570 (2015)
9. Lotter, W., Sorensen, G., Cox, D.: A multi-scale CNN and curriculum learning strategy for mammogram classification. In: Cardoso, M.J., et al. (eds.) DLMIA/ML-CDS -2017. LNCS, vol. 10553, pp. 169–177. Springer, Cham (2017). https://doi.org/10.1007/978-3-319-67558-9_20
10. Moreira, I.C., Amaral, I., Domingues, I., Cardoso, A., Cardoso, M.J., Cardoso, J.S.: Inbreast: toward a full-field digital mammographic database. Acad. Radiol. **19**(2), 236–248 (2012)
11. Pratiwi, M., Harefa, J., Nanda, S.: Mammograms classification using gray-level co-occurrence matrix and radial basis function neural network. Proc. Comput. Sci. **59**, 83–91 (2015)
12. Ronneberger, O., Fischer, P., Brox, T.: U-Net: convolutional networks for biomedical image segmentation. In: Navab, N., Hornegger, J., Wells, W.M., Frangi, A.F. (eds.) MICCAI 2015. LNCS, vol. 9351, pp. 234–241. Springer, Cham (2015). https://doi.org/10.1007/978-3-319-24574-4_28

13. Srivastava, N., Hinton, G., Krizhevsky, A., Sutskever, I., Salakhutdinov, R.: Dropout: a simple way to prevent neural networks from overfitting. J. Mach. Learn. Res. **15**(1), 1929–1958 (2014)
14. Zhu, W., Lou, Q., Vang, Y.S., Xie, X.: Deep multi-instance networks with sparse label assignment for whole mammogram classification. In: Descoteaux, M., Maier-Hein, L., Franz, A., Jannin, P., Collins, D.L., Duchesne, S. (eds.) MICCAI 2017. LNCS, vol. 10435, pp. 603–611. Springer, Cham (2017). https://doi.org/10.1007/978-3-319-66179-7_69

Structure-Aware Staging for Breast Cancer Metastases

Songtao Zhang[1], Li Sun[1], Ruiqiao Wang[1], Hongping Tang[2], Jin Zhang[1], and Lin Luo[3]([✉])

[1] Southern University of Science and Technology, Shenzhen 518055, China
[2] Department of Pathology, Shenzhen Maternity and Child Healthcare Hospital Affiliated to Southern Medical University, Shenzhen 518028, China
[3] Peking University, Beijing 100871, China
luol@pku.edu.cn

Abstract. Determining the stage of breast cancer metastases is an important component of cancer surveillance and control. It is laborious for pathologist to manually examine large amount of biological tissue and this process is error-prone. Deep learning methods can be used to automatically detect cancer metastases and identify cancer subtypes. However, current deep learning-based methods mainly focus on local patches but ignore the overall structure of lymph tissue, due to the memory limitation and computational cost of processing the gigapixel whole slide histopathological image (WSI) at a time. In this paper, we propose a structure-aware deep learning framework for staging of breast cancer metastases, in which we introduce lymph structure information to guide training patch selection and prediction features design. Our approach achieves 85.1% accuracy on slide-level and 0.80 kappa score on patient level. In addition, we see 6.1% and 5% performance gain on slide level and patient level classification respectively after introducing global structure information.

Keywords: Cancer staging · Structure-aware · Deep learning

1 Introduction

Breast cancer is the most common malignant tumor among the women, whose morbidity has increased fastest compared to other kinds of cancer. Metastatic breast cancer is a kind of breast cancer that has spread beyond the breast to other organs in the body. Metastases staging can contribute to the prediction of the patient prognosis and treatment planning. For example, early-stage cancer may need to be treated with surgery or radiation, while a more advanced cancer may need to be treated with chemotherapy. In addition, early detection for breast cancer has the best prognosis.

S. Zhang, L. Sun—equal contribution.

D. Stoyanov et al. (Eds.): RAMBO 2018/BIA 2018/TIA 2018, LNCS 11040, pp. 116–123, 2018.
https://doi.org/10.1007/978-3-030-00946-5_13

In order to determine the stage for breast cancer metastases, pathologists need to examine histopathological slides manually. But this process is painstaking and error-prone. The last decade has witnessed the advancement of digital pathology, which aims to digitize tissue slides and automatically analyze them using computer algorithms. In recent years, deep convolutional neural network (CNN) has immensely improved performance on a wide range of computer vision tasks such as image recognition, instance detection, and semantic segmentation. Similarly, deep CNNs have been introduced in digital pathology to improve the accuracy of diagnoses.

Several research works [2,7] have applied deep learning to histopathology. But these methods only focus on local characters of lymph node. In this paper, we propose a structure-aware staging framework to determine the metastases stage using gigapixel pathology image of lymph tissue. We observe considerable performance gain after we bring in global structure features of lymph nodes.

2   Related Work

2.1   pN Stage in TNM System

The TNM Classification of Malignant Tumors (TNM) [4] is a notation system that describes the stage of a cancer. In this system, T stands for the original (primary) tumor, N stands for nodes while M stands for metastases. In this paper, we focus on pathology N stands (pN-stage) [1] which describes the extent of cancer spread in nearby lymph nodes. Our diagnosis target is to determine the pN-stage for patients, depending on the categories of lymph node metastases, including macro-metastases, micro-metastases and isolated tumor cells (ITC). Based on the description of diagnosis on WSI level, the pN stage on patient level can be defined as below (Table 1):

Table 1. pN stage on patient level

pN-stage	Description
pN0	No micro-metastases or macro-metastases or ITCs found
pN0(i+)	Only ITCs found
pN1mi	Micro-metastases found, but no macro-metastases found
pN1	Metastases found in 13 lymph nodes, of which at least one is a macro-metastases
pN2	Metastases found in 49 lymph nodes, of which at least one is a macro-metastases

2.2 Previous Methods

In recent years, several research works have applied deep learning to histopathology. Many camelyon17 participants [1] achieve good performance in the challenge of staging lymph node involvement for breast cancer patients. Thagaard et al. [1] from DTU team proposed to detect region-of-interest (ROI) by intensity thresholding. Then they extracted image patches from ROI as training set. The authors trained a InceptionV3 model to classify patches, and trained a random forest classier on 42 hand-engineered local features of morphology for prediction. Liu et al. [7] proposed to extract image patches from multiple magnifications, then input to separate towers and merged for prediction. However, their methods still focus on local patches but ignore the overall structure of lymph tissue.

3 Methodology

3.1 Overview

Our proposed structure-aware staging framework consists of the following steps, as illustrated in the figure below. The surrounding box shows a typical learning process of pathological image classification, which includes patch selection, patch-level classification, heatmap composition and processing, feature engineering, slide-level classification and patient diagnosis. The center area in the figure shows how lymph structure is extracted and then applied to guide the steps in the whole learning process. We extract the overall lymph structure from WSIs. The segmented lymph region is used to guide patch selection while the contour information is used for feature engineering.

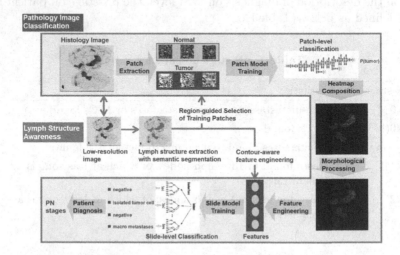

Fig. 1. Overview of our proposed structure-aware staging framework

3.2 Lymph Structure Extraction with Semantic Segmentation

We use semantic segmentation to extract the overall structure of lymph tissue, which is used to guide the selection of relevant patches for training and feature engineering. Traditionally patch selection is done by thresholding method, which is transferring the original image to the HSV color space, then use the Otsu algorithm to select the optimal threshold values in each channel. But this method produces rather coarse result. We use semantic segmentation to understand the slide by assigning a class for each pixel. It can delineate the boundaries of lymph tissue and obtain the overall structure. In natural image processing, convolutional neural networks (CNN) have achieved great success on segmentation problems. We leverage the current state of the art method for semantic segmentation, DeepLab-v3+ model [3], to extract the overall structure of lymph tissue. DeepLab-v3+ model employs the encoder-decoder structure. For the encoder module, rich contextual information is extracted using atrous convolution, which is capable of encoding features at an arbitrary resolution. The decoder module is used to recover the boundaries of lymph tissue.

3.3 Lymph Region-Guided Selection of Training Patches

We use overall structure of lymph tissue to guide the patch selection for training. With aim of training a dedicated model, all patches are selected from the lymph tissue region. In addition, we extract similar number of positive and negative patches to deal with class imbalance. The size of training patches is 256 * 256.

3.4 Patch-Level Classification

This step mainly consists of three parts which are data argumentation, evaluation of convolution neural network and hard example mining. Because these slides are from different medical centers, the H&E stained color on the slide may also be slightly different. We preprocessed images by adjusting the brightness, saturation, hue and contrast randomly in a limited range. In addition, we applied random rotation and random flip to the patches.

Then we evaluated the predicting performance of different deep CNN architectures for the patch-based classification task, including VGG16 [5], GoogLeNet [9], InceptionV3 [10], ResNet101 [6] and Inception-ResNet [8]. The validation performance is shown in the experiment section. We found that ResNet101 and InceptionV3 architectures achieve the best performance. Based on the trade off between performance and speed, InceptionV3 is chosen as our final model.

Since our training set only consists of a small portion of all patches, it may not be sufficient to represent the entire diversity of different tissue. We enriched the training set by adding additional normal patches that are wrongly predicted in cross-validation stage. The patch-level classifier is trained again using the enriched training set. Based on the patch-level classifier, we transformed each whole slide image into a tumor possibility heatmap in which each pixel represents the tumor possibility of patch from original whole slide.

3.5 Contour-Aware Feature Engineering for Slide-Level Classification

We extracted both structure level features and local features from tumor probability heatmap to grade breast cancer metastasis on slide level and patient level. We in total designed 50 features based on medical criteria, which can be divided into three categories: size, shape and depth of tumor invasion. The shape features include relative size of tumor, absolute size of tumor, number of tumor regions. The shape features include eccentricity, major axis length, minor axis length, perimeter, extent and other features. Depth of tumor invasion is an important indicator of metastases state. So we incorporate the overall structure of lymph tissue to characterize the extent of tumor invasion, which is defined as the distance of tumor region to the contour of lymph node. We introduced the features of maximum invasion depth, mean invasion depth and minimum invasion depth.

In order to select the important features for prediction and reduce overfitting, recursive feature selection method is used. Then we use random forest classifier to determine the metastasis state on slide level. Finally, based on classification result of five lymph node slides belonging to each patient, we can determine the patient-level pN-stage according to the criteria mentioned before.

4 Experiment

4.1 Dataset

We use the whole-slide images of histological lymph node sections from Camelyon challenge provided by the Diagnostic Image Analysis Group (DIAG) and Radboud University medical center. Both Camelyon16 and Camelyon17 datasets are used. The Camelyon16 dataset [2] consists of 400 WSIs from 2 different centers, including 170 tumor WSIs and 230 normal WSIs. The Camelyon17 dataset [1] consists of a total of 1000 whole slides images (WSIs) from 200 patients (each patient has five whole-slide images of histological lymph node sections). All slides were annotated by professional pathologists where annotations are considered as lesion-level ground truth.

4.2 Segmentation of Lymph Structure

We manually annotate 400 slides as training set for the DeepLab-v3+ model. Horizontal and vertical flipping is used to augment the data. We also use the contrast limited adaptive histogram equalization method to enhance the local contrast of the image. Due to the memory limitation, we resize the slides to 1408*1408. We train the model using momentum optimizer with initial learning rate of 10^{-6}. For the testing phase, we also resize the slides and enhance the local contrast. Then we use trained DeepLab-v3+ model to segment the tissue region. Finally, we resize the segmentation result back to the original slide size. Our experiment shows that semantic segmentation can precisely extracted the overall structure of lymph tissue.

Original image   Lymph structure extraction by segmentation

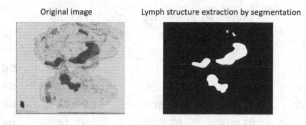

Fig. 2. Illustration of lymph tissue extraction result

The DeepLab-v3+ model converges after 20 epochs training. It achieves Dice coefficient of 0.95 for lymph tissue segmentation, which demonstrated it can be used to extract the lymph tissue precisely.

4.3 Patch-Level Classification

In the patch-level classifier, the validation dataset is split from camelyon16 dataset. Particularly, all patches are extracted in lymph region detected by semantic segmentation. And the sample of positive and negative is balanced when sampling.

The table below show the evaluation result of the patch-level classifier (Table 2).

Table 2. Evaluation result of different architectures

CNN-architecture	Validation accuracy	Test accuracy
VGG-19	96.12%	93.11%
GoogLeNet	97.12%	96.17%
InceptionV3	97.80%	97.23%
Inception-ResNet	97.90%	97.21%
ResNet101	98.01%	97.33%

4.4 Performance Gain by Semantic Segmentation

This table show the evaluation result of the patch-level classifier comparing threshold processing method and lymph region guided method for patch extraction.

We found that most of the false positive patches appear out of lymph tissue region in WSI when using thresholding method for patch extraction. This explains the reason that our proposed lymph region guided method is superior.

Methods	Threshold processing method		Lymph region guided	
Category	Validation accuracy	Test accuracy	Validation accuracy	Test accuracy
VGG-19	96.12%	93.11%	**97.31%**	**96.81%**
GoogLeNet	97.12%	96.17%	**98.51%**	**98.21%**
InceptionV3	97.80%	97.23%	**98.73%**	**98.35%**
Inception-ResNet	97.90%	97.21%	**99.14%**	**98.71%**
ResNet101	98.01%	97.33%	**98.94%**	**98.40%**

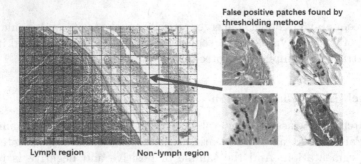

Fig. 3. Examples of false positive patches found by thresholding method

4.5 Evaluation Metric

We use multi-class quadratic weighted kappa for evaluation where the classes are the pN-stages.

$$\kappa = \frac{\sum_{i=1}^{k} \sum_{j=1}^{k} w_{ij}\, x_{ij}}{\sum_{i=1}^{k} \sum_{j=1}^{k} w_{ij}\, m_{ij}} \tag{1}$$

where k stands for number of classes and w_{ij}, x_{ij}, and m_{ij} are elements in the weight, observed, and expected matrices, respectively.

4.6 Slide-Level and Patient-Level Evaluation

For training of slide-level classifier, we use 500 slides with five-fold cross validation. For patient-level prediction, 500 WSIs are used as test set. We compare the performance of our structure-aware method with the traditional thresholding method, and the result demonstrates that incorporating overall structure information brings considerable performance gain (Table 3).

4.7 Implementation Details

To implement the algorithm framework, we use Tensorflow framework and We train a fine tuning model without any pre-trained weight running on a NVIDIA Tesla M40 GPU. We use SGD with momentum 0.9 and set initial learning rate

Table 3. Slide and patient-level evaluation result

Category	Result without structure guidance	Result with structure guidance
Slide-level accuracy	0.793	**0.851**
Patient-level Kappa score	0.75	**0.80**

to 0.01. We also set the number of epoch to decay at 70, decay to 0.001 and batch size to 32 for training.

5 Conclusion

In this paper, we presented a structure-aware staging framework for breast cancer metastases which can take the global structure information into account compared to existing method. Results shows impressive improvement by introducing lymph structure information to guide patch selection and to design prediction features. The proposed framework can also be applied to tasks related to staging other cancer metastases based on the whole slide histopathological images. In the future, we will explore more possibilities of introducing hierarchical information to the computer-aided diagnosis of the slide histopathological images.

References

1. CAMELYON17 Workshop (2017). https://camelyon17.grand-challenge.org/. Accessed 4 June 2018
2. Bejnordi, B.E., et al.: Diagnostic assessment of deep learning algorithms for detection of lymph node metastases in women with breast cancer. Jama **318**(22), 2199–2210 (2017)
3. Chen, L.-C., et al.: Encoder-decoder with atrous separable convolution for semantic image segmentation. arXiv preprint arXiv:1802.02611 (2018)
4. Goldstraw, P., et al.: The IASLC lung cancer staging project: proposals for the revision of the TNM stage groupings in the forthcoming (seventh) edition of the TNM classification of malignant tumours. J. Thorac. Oncol. **2**(8), 706–714 (2007)
5. Han, S., Mao, H., Dally, W.J.: Deep compression: compressing deep neural networks with pruning, trained quantization and Huffman coding. arXiv preprint arXiv:1510.00149 (2015)
6. He, K., Zhang, X., Ren, S., Sun, J.: Deep residual learning for image recognition. In: Proceedings of the IEEE Conference on Computer Vision and Pattern Recognition, pp. 770–778 (2016)
7. Liu, Y., et al.: Detecting cancer metastases on gigapixel pathology images. arXiv preprint arXiv:1703.02442 (2017)
8. Szegedy, C., Ioffe, S., Vanhoucke, V., Alemi, A.A.: Inception-v4, inception-ResNet and the impact of residual connections on learning. In: AAAI, vol. 4, p. 12 (2017)
9. Szegedy, C., et al.: Going deeper with convolutions. In: CVPR (2015)
10. Szegedy, C., Vanhoucke, V., Ioffe, S., Shlens, J., Wojna, Z.: Rethinking the inception architecture for computer vision. In: Proceedings of the IEEE Conference on Computer Vision and Pattern Recognition, pp. 2818–2826 (2016)

Reproducible Evaluation of Registration Algorithms for Movement Correction in Dynamic Contrast Enhancing Magnetic Resonance Imaging for Breast Cancer Diagnosis

I. A. Illan[1,2(✉)], J. Ramirez[2], J. M. Gorriz[2], K. Pinker[3,4],
and A. Meyer-Baese[1]

[1] Scientific Computing Department, Florida State University, Tallahassee, USA
[2] Department of Signal Theory, Networking and Communications,
DaSCI (Data Science and Computational Intelligence Research Institute),
Universidad de Granada, Granada, Spain
illan@ugr.es
[3] Department of Radiology, Memorial Sloan-Kettering Cancer Center,
New York, USA
[4] Department of Biomedical Imaging and Image-guided Therapy,
Division of Molecular and Gender Imaging,
Medical University of Vienna/AKH Wien, Vienna, Austria

Abstract. Accurate methods for computer aided diagnosis of breast cancer increase accuracy of detection and provide support to physicians in detecting challenging cases. In dynamic contrast enhancing magnetic resonance imaging (DCE-MRI), motion artifacts can appear as a result of patient displacements. Non-linear deformation algorithms for breast image registration provide with a solution to the correspondence problem in contrast with affine models. In this study we evaluate 3 popular non-linear registration algorithms: MIRTK, Demons, SyN Ants, and compare to the affine baseline. We propose automatic measures for reproducible evaluation on the DCE-MRI breast-diagnosis TCIA-database, based on edge detection and clustering algorithms, and provide a rank of the methods according to these measures.

Keywords: Medical image processing · Reproducibility · DCE-MRI
Registration · Diffeomorphism · Optical flow · Non-affine registration

1 Introduction

Early and accurate detection is a key factor in maximizing probability of survival of breast cancer, the second most common cause of cancer death, after lung cancer [17]. Computer aided diagnosis (CAD) systems support the physicians

© Springer Nature Switzerland AG 2018
D. Stoyanov et al. (Eds.): RAMBO 2018/BIA 2018/TIA 2018, LNCS 11040, pp. 124–131, 2018.
https://doi.org/10.1007/978-3-030-00946-5_14

in decision making by means of imaging processing techniques. Dynamic contrast enhancing magnetic resonance imaging (DCE-MRI) allows to obtain non-invasive information about tissue dynamics that allows for cancer identification, and CAD systems have been developed to assist clinicians in the analysis. Accuracy of such CADs depend on the preprocessing steps such as registration. Registration is a challenging task due to the highly deformable nature of the breast, and linear methods are unsuitable.

Nowadays, with the impetuous advance of data-sharing and code-sharing in science, reproducibility has become a key factor in new developments and analysis. Medical image processing traditionally has been focused in giving a solution to the registration problem, together with the segmentation problem. In the field of DCE-MRI of the breast, there has been considerable interest in non-linear deformation modeling to solve the correspondence problem due to the deformable nature of the breast. Although successful methods for enhancement subtraction have been developed [11], the non-rigid registration step in DCE-MRI is often performed using state-of-the art approaches, such as diffeomorphic based ones, or partial-differential-equations-based ones [6,7,13,18]. However, there is no clear argument for a preferable choice nor a systematic comparison of the proposed solutions. Led by the neuroimaging community, a large variety of high quality software tools, projects and analysis are publicly available to the medical imaging community that solve the registration problem. Concretely, consistent effort has been dedicated in the last decade to evaluate registration algorithms, such as with the projects the mindboggle (http://www.mindboggle.info) and NIREPS (http://www.nirep.org/links).

Given the importance and challenges in nonlinear deformation algorithms for breast image registration, a systematic analysis with reproducible results can provide an evaluation of the available registration tools and its efficacy in the aforementioned task, setting a baseline for ulterior developments. Existing evaluations of registration methods are often based on landmarks. Landmarks require some expert intervention, and are prone to subjectivity and non-reproducibility. We propose an automatic method for registration evaluation based on an algorithmic-driven extraction of morphological features: contours and volume. For the extraction of contours we propose the use of the Canny edges detection algorithm and k-means algorithm to extract tissue-specific volumes. We evaluate 3 popular non-linear registration algorithms: MIRTK, Demons, SyN Ants, and compare to the affine baseline. We use a publicly available DCE-MRI breast database and rank the tested registration algorithms according to the measures proposed.

2   Methods

2.1   TCIA Database

The data used in this work is the Breast-Diagnosis collection [3] from the cancer imaging archive (TCIA)[4]. The Breast-Diagnosis collection contains cases that are high-risk normals, DCIS, fibroids and lobular carcinomas. Each case has 3 or more distinct MR pulse sequences from a Phillips 1.5 T, such as T2, STIR and BLISS. For the DCE-MRI, the volume of Magnevist (Bayer) gadolinium contrast injected into the brachial vein is based on a rule of thumb which in ml's is 10% of the patient weight. The injection itself is 6 or 7 s, at a rate of 3cc per second. The first dynamic sequence is started 1 min after the injection is started.

2.2   The Registration Problem

One of the main medical image processing problems is the registration problem. The goal of the registration is to find the transformation T that maps each point x of a fixed image F to a point y = T(x) in image moving image M, so that some measure of similarity $E(F, M)$ between F and M is minimized. In the affine case, this transformation can be parametrized by a small set of parameters (12 in 3D). When non-rigid transformations are allowed, a non-parametric characterization of the transformation must be given, usually in terms of a displacement field.

This study will consider well established deformable techniques for deformable registration: Diffeomorfic Demons, MIRTK, SyN [8]:

- **Diffeomorphic Demons** is a non-parametric algorithm based in optical flow theory that generalizes Thirion's Demons algorithm with a diffeomorphic spatial transformation [20]. This method alternates between the computation of warping forces and smoothing. The Demons algorithm may be related to a Taylor expansion of the squared difference between the fixed and moving image, with some regularization in the form of fluid-like equations.
- **MIRTK** [15, 16] uses a combined transformation T which consists of a global affine transformation and a local transformation. The local transformation describes any local deformation required to match the anatomies of the subjects using a free-form deformation (FFD) model based on B-splines. The basic idea of FFDs is to deform an object by manipulating an underlying mesh of control points. The resulting deformation controls the shape of the 3-D object and can be written as the 3-D tensor product of the familiar 1-D cubic B-splines. The lattice of control points is defined as a grid with uniform spacing which is placed on the underlying reference image. The optimal transformation is found using a gradient descent minimization of a cost function associated with the global transformation parameters as well as the local transformation parameters. The cost function comprises two competing goals: The first term represents the cost associated with the voxel-based similarity measure, in this case normalised mutual information, while the second term corresponds to a regularization term which constrains the transformation to be smooth.
- **The symmetric normalization (SyN)** methodology uses a symmetric parameterization of the shortest path of diffeomorphisms connecting two anatomical configurations [2]. The SyN formulation uses a bidirectional gradient descent optimization which gives results that are unbiased with respect to the input images. SyN also provides forward and inverse continuum mappings that are consistent within the discrete domain and enables both large

and subtle deformations to be captured. Specific performance characteristics depend upon the range of similarity metrics chosen for the study and the velocity field regularization.

2.3 Automatic Contour and Volume Estimation

For evaluation purposes, two features are extracted from the 3D MRI images: contours and volumes. Contours are extracted by a Canny edge detector algorithm, that provides the external surface as well as interior structures. The Canny filter is a multi-stage edge detector that uses a derivative-of-a-Gaussian in order to compute the intensity of the gradients. We used the simpleITK [10, 21] implementation and set the variance of the Gaussian $[\sigma_x, \sigma_y, \sigma_z]$ to [25, 25, 25]. The Canny edge detector has been reported to have superior capabilities as other edge detectors as Sobel [14].

In brain imaging, registration evaluation is usually performed by evaluating the overlap between different brain structures, as the thalamus or the hippocampus, defined in some standard atlas. The differences on breast density, shape and randomness of breast lesion locations makes the definition of a breast atlas inviable. Therefore, the volume overlap evaluation of the registration algorithm lacks of a natural volume subdivision of the breast to compare to. Consequently, subvolumes and structures must be either manually defined case by case, a task prone to inaccuracies and subjectivity, or extracted automatically from a clustering algorithm. Here, different breast structures are extracted by the k-means algorithm. Since the number of different tissues is expected to be low, following Thirion et al. [19], the k-means algorithm performs better than other competitive alternatives, as the Ward agglomerative clustering with spatial constraints. We use the k-means implementation from nilearn [1] with standardization and smoothing (FWHM = 10) and 3 clusters.

3 Results

For file preparation, the first step is convert the DICOM files to NIFTI format. All the tested algorithms require NIFTI files as input, since it is the standard format in neuroimaging. This task is performed with the use of dcm2niix [9]. Next, the images are masked to remove the strong signals from internal organs. It is important for a registration algorithm to remove the signals from interior cavities of the chest. In the case of non-affine transformations, the variability of these regions produces the highest metric values on those localized regions, thus dominating in the optimization algorithm. The mask is defined as the middle plane in the axial direction, and all the voxels inside the plane are set to background.

The masked images are registered to the pre-contrast images using the different tested algorithms. Contours and volumes are extracted from each sequence and two metrics are employed to evaluate the overlap between solutions:

- **Dice similarity score (DCS)** Also known as F1-score, the DSC evaluates the overlap between the true labels in the fixed image (F) and the test labels in the moving image (M) by:

$$DSC(F, M) = \frac{2|F \cap M|}{|F| + |M|} \tag{1}$$

- **Jaccard similarity score (JCS)** Evaluates the overlap between the fixed image and the moving image with respect to the whole volume of both.

$$JSC(F, M) = \frac{|F \cap M|}{|F \cup M|} = \frac{|F \cap M|}{|F| + |M| - |F \cap M|} \tag{2}$$

A Welch t-test is performed between the values obtained by each algorithm and the best performance, in order to detect significant differences. Figure 1 shows a boxplot of the evaluation parameters on different algorithms, while Fig. 2 shows the adequacy of the DSC parameter to evaluate the registration performance: in time point 5 a movement is registered and not corrected by the affine transformation, while the deformation transformation minimizes the differences in subsequent times in the sequence (Table 1).

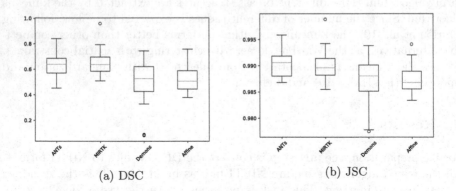

(a) DSC   (b) JSC

Fig. 1. DSC and Jaccard scores for contour overlap evaluation

Table 1. Average performance parameters on validating data for contour and volume

	Contour		Volume
	DSC	JSC	DSC
Affine	0.517 ± 0.007	0.9873 ± 0.0001	0.975 ± 0.001
ANTs	0.631 ± 0.009	0.9904 ± 0.0001	0.979 ± 0.001
MIRTK	0.646 ± 0.007	0.9898 ± 0.0001	0.982 ± 0.006
Diffeomorphic Demons	0.497 ± 0.029	0.987 ± 0.001	0.965 ± 0.001

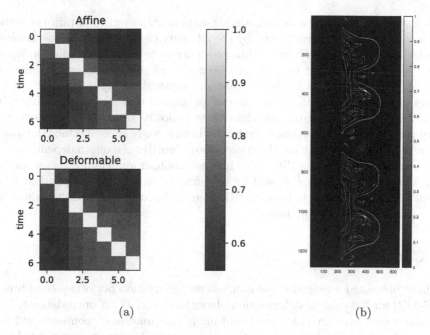

Fig. 2. (a) DSC comparison of an example affine and deformable registration for 6 timepoints in the DCE-MRI sequence. Pre and post contrast differences can be noted, as well as post-contrast motion correction with the deformable model. (b) Center axial slice of mean contour overlap after deformable registration (up) and affine registration (down). Increase in sharpness in chest-wall lines can be noted in deformable-registration mean contours.

4   Discussion

The results presented here combine two independent measures of 3 registration algorithms. Taking altogether, diffeomorphic Demons appear to be the registration algorithm with less consistent performance. In the contour evaluation, ANTs and MIRTK provide similar performance. Although MIRTK reaches the maximum DSC, ANTs has the maximum JSC. This fact can be explained from the effect on chest-wall contours, where ANTs algorithm produces larger deformations to remove dissimilarities, not related to motion artifacts. When performing a Welch t-test, the null hypothesis of having equal values for ANTs and MIRTK can not be rejected (p-value 0.32), while is rejected when comparing with the other methods. Regarding the volumetric measures, it is remarkable that independent measures show a consistent behavior, suggesting that this results may generalize to other databases. These results are in coherence with other performance studies involving some of the studied algorithms [5,8].

For registration evaluation its implicitly assumed in this work that within subject differences due to enhancing tissues do not modify substantially the contour and volume of organic structures. However, one of the limitations of the present study relies on the automatic algorithms employed to obtain the structure measures, as they are affected by the intensity changes due to enhancement. To alleviate this effect, results within pre-contrast images are studied independently from post-contrast ones. It has been argued that the intensity enhancement of MRI signals has itself an effect on registration algorithms [12]. From the results presented in this work, it can be argued that the effect of intensity enhancement on the registration algorithms is not as dramatic as the effect of interior chest organs, as preliminary results in this study showed. Once the masking preprocessing step is done, the registration algorithms seem to depend weakly on the enhancement, as the difference between contour and volume measures display. A future line of research will be to define an enhancing-independent measure of structure features in breast MRI to quantitatively evaluate the enhancing effect on registration algorithms.

5   Conclusion

We have presented a reproducible analysis on registration performance in breast DCE-MRI for 3 non-rigid deformation algorithms on a TCIA open dataset. Two automatic measures are calculated containing information on contours and volume overlap, and manual intervention is avoided. Results suggest that ANTs and MIRTK should be between the preferable choices for registration, and this result may generalize to other datasets.

Acknowledgments. This work has received funding from the European Unions Horizon 2020 research and innovation programme under the Marie Skodowska-Curie grant agreement No. 656886.

References

1. Abraham, A.: Machine learning for neuroimaging with scikit-learn. Front. Neuroinform. **8**, 1–14 (2014)
2. Avants, B.B., Epstein, C.L., Grossman, M., Gee, J.C.: Symmetric diffeomorphic image registration with cross-correlation: evaluating automated labeling of elderly and neurodegenerative brain. Med. Image Anal. **12**(1), 26–41 (2008)
3. Bloch, Nicolas, B., Jain, Ashali, Jaffe, C.C.: Data from breast-diagnosis. The Cancer Imaging Archive (2015)
4. Clark, K., et al.: The Cancer Imaging Archive (TCIA): maintaining and operating a public information repository. J. Digit. Imaging **26**(6), 1045–1057 (2013)
5. Diez, Y., et al.: Comparison of methods for current-to-prior registration of breast DCE-MRI. In: Fujita, H., Hara, T., Muramatsu, C. (eds.) IWDM 2014. LNCS, vol. 8539, pp. 689–695. Springer, Cham (2014). https://doi.org/10.1007/978-3-319-07887-8_95
6. Ebrahimi, M., Martel, A.L.: A general PDE-framework for registration of contrast enhanced images. In: Yang, G.-Z., Hawkes, D., Rueckert, D., Noble, A., Taylor, C. (eds.) MICCAI 2009. LNCS, vol. 5761, pp. 811–819. Springer, Heidelberg (2009). https://doi.org/10.1007/978-3-642-04268-3_100

7. Kim, M., Wu, G., Shen, D.: Hierarchical alignment of breast DCE-MR images by groupwise registration and robust feature matching. Med. Phys. **39**(1), 353–366 (2012)
8. Klein, A., et al.: Evaluation of 14 nonlinear deformation algorithms applied to human brain MRI registration. NeuroImage **46**(3), 786–802 (2009)
9. Li, X., Morgan, P.S., Ashburner, J., Smith, J., Rorden, C.: The first step for neuroimaging data analysis: DICOM to NIfTI conversion. J. Neurosci. Methods **264**, 47–56 (2016)
10. Lowekamp, B.C., Chen, D.T., Ibanez, L., Blezek, D.: The design of SimpleITK. Front. Neuroinform. **7**, 1–45 (2013)
11. Martel, A.L., Froh, M.S., Brock, K.K., Plewes, D.B., Barber, D.C.: Evaluating an optical-flow-based registration algorithm for contrast-enhanced magnetic resonance imaging of the breast. Phys. Med. Biol. **52**(13), 3803 (2007)
12. Melbourne, A., Atkinson, D., White, M.J., Collins, D., Leach, M., Hawkes, D.: Registration of dynamic contrast-enhanced MRI using a progressive principal component registration (PPCR). Phys. Med. Biol. **52**(17), 5147 (2007)
13. Ong, R.E., Ou, J.J., Miga, M.I.: Non-rigid registration of breast surfaces using the laplace and diffusion equations. BioMed. Eng. OnLine **9**, 8 (2010)
14. Othman, Z., Haron, H., Kadir, M.R.A., Rafiq, M.: Comparison of Canny and Sobel edge detection in MRI images. Comput. Sci. Biomech. Tissue Eng. Group Inf. Syst. 133–136 (2009)
15. Rueckert, D., Sonoda, L.I., Hayes, C., Hill, D.L.G., Leach, M.O., Hawkes, D.J.: Nonrigid registration using free-form deformations: application to breast MR images. IEEE Trans. Med. Imaging **18**(8), 712–721 (1999)
16. Schnabel, J.A., et al.: Validation of nonrigid image registration using finite-element methods: application to breast MR images. IEEE Trans. Med. Imaging **22**(2), 238–247 (2003)
17. Siegel, R.L., Miller, K.D.: Cancer statistics. CA Cancer J. Clin. **68**(1), 7–30 (2018)
18. Sotiras, A., Davatzikos, C., Paragios, N.: Deformable medical image registration: a survey. IEEE Trans. Med. Imaging **32**(7), 1153–1190 (2013)
19. Thirion, B., Varoquaux, G., Dohmatob, E., Poline, J.B.: Which fMRI clustering gives good brain parcellations? Front. Neurosci. **8**, 1–13 (2014)
20. Vercauteren, T., Pennec, X., Perchant, A., Ayache, N.: Diffeomorphic demons: efficient non-parametric image registration. NeuroImage **45**(1, Suppl. 1), S61–S72 (2009)
21. Yaniv, Z., Lowekamp, B.C., Johnson, H.J., Beare, R.: SimpleITK image-analysis notebooks: a collaborative environment for education and reproducible research. J. Dig. Imaging **31**(3), 290–303 (2018)

First International Workshop on Thoracic Image Analysis, TIA 2018

Robust Windowed Harmonic Phase Analysis with a Single Acquisition

Santiago Sanz-Estébanez[1(✉)], Lucilio Cordero-Grande[2],
Marcos Martín-Fernández[1], and Carlos Alberola-López[1]

[1] Laboratorio de Procesado de Imagen, Universidad de Valladolid, Valladolid, Spain
ssanest@lpi.tel.uva.es, {marcma,caralb}@tel.uva.es
[2] Biomedical Engineering Department, King's College, London, UK
lucilio.cordero_grande@kcl.ac.uk

Abstract. The HARP methodology is a widely extended procedure for cardiac tagged magnetic resonance imaging since it is able to analyse local mechanical behaviour of the heart; extensions and improvements of this method have also been reported since HARP was released. Acquisition of an over-determined set of orientations is one of such alternatives, which has notably increased HARP robustness at the price of increasing examination time. In this paper, we explore an alternative to this method based on the use of multiple peaks, as opposed to multiple orientations, intended for a single acquisition. Performance loss is explored with respect to multiple orientations in a real setting. In addition, we have assessed, by means of a computational phantom, optimal tag orientations and spacings of the stripe pattern by minimizing the Frobenius norm of the difference between the ground truth and the estimated material deformation gradient tensor. Results indicate that, for a single acquisition, multiple peaks as opposed to multiple orientations, are indeed preferable.

Keywords: Cardiac tagged magnetic resonance imaging
Harmonic phase · Multi-harmonic analysis
Robust strain reconstruction

1 Introduction

Measures of local myocardial deformation are essential for a deeper comprehension of heart functionalities for both normal and pathologic subjects [1]. Tagged magnetic resonance (MR-T) is a noninvasive method for assessing the displacement of heart tissue over time [2]. This modality is based on the generation of a set of saturated magnetization planes on the imaged volume, so that material points may be tracked throughout the cardiac cycle [3] and local functional indicators, such as the strain tensor [4], can be estimated.

Regarding the analysis of MR-T images [5], we can differentiate two main families of methods, image-based and k-space-based techniques. The image-based

© Springer Nature Switzerland AG 2018
D. Stoyanov et al. (Eds.): RAMBO 2018/BIA 2018/TIA 2018, LNCS 11040, pp. 135–146, 2018.
https://doi.org/10.1007/978-3-030-00946-5_15

techniques are devised to directly process and analyse the tagged images by identifying the tag lines and tracking their deformation between frames. Examples of such techniques are optical flow [6] or deformable models [7] methodologies. Alternatively, the k-space-based techniques focus on the Fourier Transform (FT) of the tagged images. Compared to the image-based, k-space-based techniques have proven to be much faster and less prone to artifacts [8]. Most notable methodologies in this category are sinewave modeling (SinMod) [9] and HARmonic Phase (HARP) [10] analysis. Recent studies have reported that, although both techniques are consistent in motion estimates, an exaggeration in measurements is often observed for SinMod [8], leading to larger biases. Therefore, we have focused on HARP-based methods. These methods are grounded on the extraction of the complex image phase obtained by band-pass (BP) filtering the spectral peaks introduced by the applied modulation; they rely on the fact that the extracted harmonic phase is linearly related to a directional component of the true motion [10]. Hence, dense displacement fields can be recovered on the basis on a constant local phase assumption, which turns out to be more reliable than a constant pixel brightness assumption.

An in-depth study of the HARP method is provided in [11]; the author uses a communications-based approach to analyze the method in detail, including resolution, dynamic range and noise. Signal processing solutions based on the Windowed Fourier Transform (WFT) [12] have been proposed to balance the spatial and spectral localization of the image, thus obtaining smooth local phase estimations. Adaptive approaches have been subsequently proposed in [13, 14] in order to accommodate tag local properties both in window and filter designs, respectively. However, slight improvements have been reported with respect to non-adaptive methods, taking into account the considerable computational cost increasing.

Techniques to synthesize more desirable tag patterns have also been proposed using multiple harmonic peaks, both with different tag spacings [15] and new profiles [16]. Methodologies that make use of multiple orientations [17–19] have also been devised to improve the quality of the estimated motion at the prize of increasing acquisition time. Besides, these methodologies require of non-trivial image registration techniques to align the multiple acquisitions, which itself may also have an important impact on processing conclusions.

In this paper we depart from the reported idea that using an overdetermined set of orientations (MO) significantly increases the quality of the estimated deformation gradient tensor [19]; however, our purpose is to convey information within a single acquisition at the expense of a worse performance with respect to multiple acquisitions. Therefore, we have explored performance of using two peaks with two orthogonal orientations within a single acquisition, as opposed to multiple single-peaked orientations in multiple acquisitions, and we quantify performance loss. Then, we find out through optimization both tag orientation and spacing of two stripes patterns that are set free when another two are set beforehand. Interestingly, our results indicate that the latter approach converges to the former, i.e., two orthogonal orientations with two peaks is the preferable solution when a unique acquisition is pursued.

2 Materials

MR-T is usually performed by SPAtial Modulation of Magnetization (SPAMM) [20], which is grounded on the ability of altering the magnetization of the tissue in presence of motion. This process will generate a modulation with different sinusoidal functions. Each of these sinusoids will be given by its wave vector $\mathbf{k}_i$ with $\mathbf{k}_i = k_i \mathbf{u}_i$, where k_i is the wave number (related to its frequency) and $\mathbf{u}_i$ its orientation vector (corresponding to the orientation of the applied gradient).

We have acquired a medial slice on an adult volunteer using a MR SPAMM SENSitivity Encoding (SENSE) Turbo Field Echo sequence on a Philips Achieva 3T scanner. The image has a spatial resolution of $1.333 \times 1.333\,\mathrm{mm}^2$ and a slice thickness of $8\,\mathrm{mm}$. The acquisition parameters are $T_E = 3.634\,\mathrm{ms}$, $T_R = 6.018\,\mathrm{ms}$ and $\alpha = 10°$. Regarding the tagging parameters, the tag spacing has been set to $\lambda = 7\,\mathrm{mm}$, with its different harmonic peaks at $\mathbf{k} = \{1,2\}/\lambda$ and different orientations $u_i = (\cos(\theta_i), \sin(\theta_i))$. The specific orientations are $\theta_i = -85° + i \cdot 5°$ with $0 \leq i \leq 35$, therefore with $-85° \leq \theta_i \leq 90°$. Two grid patterns have also been acquired with $\{45°\text{--}135°\}$ and $\{0°\text{--}90°\}$ orientations.

Simulated SPAMM sequences [21] have also been launched both with one (1D) and two orientations (2D), with different λ values and multiple spectral peaks, some examples of which are shown in Fig. 1. Harmonic coefficients have been set according to [16].

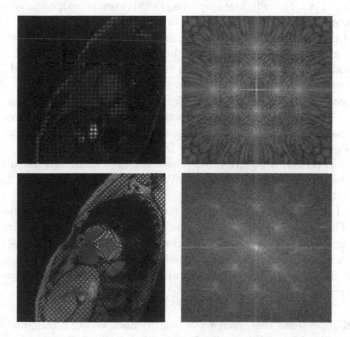

Fig. 1. The two upper images show synthetic data (2D) while real dataset is sketched below for 2D in a $\{45°\text{--}135°\}$ grid. All intermodulations for the 2D case are present.

Optimization experiments have been performed on the synthetic data; the computational phantom consists in an annulus centered at the myocardium with $R_i = 28$ and $R_o = 40$ as its inner and its outer radii, respectively. An incompressible radially varying deformation has also been applied according to $r = \sqrt{R^2 - \gamma R_i^2}$, where γ controls the degree of deformation and r and R represent the spatial and material radial coordinates, respectively. Notice that for the simulated SPAMM synthetic data, we have not included noise, tag fading or other undesired effects. We have preferred not to simulate these confounding factors, which are present in real data, in order to remove its influence in the final tag pattern design.

3   Method

3.1   Reconstruction Pipeline

As stated in [10], HARP motion reconstruction using SPAMM requires a minimum of 2 linearly independent wave vectors. The proposed approach allows us to accommodate multiple wave vectors stemming from the different orientations and harmonic peaks. Reconstruction pipeline can be summarized in the following steps (see Fig. 2):

- **Calculation of the local phase of the image.** For a given cardiac phase, we compute the 2D discrete WFT [19] to obtain the local spectrum $S[\mathbf{m}]$ for each image $I[\mathbf{x}]$. The window employed at this step is real, even, of unit norm, and monotonically decreasing for positive values of its argument. Hence, the obtained discrete WFT can be seen as a set of discrete FTs applied to the result of windowing an image throughout its support.

  Once local spectrum is calculated, a complex BP filter is applied to extract the corresponding phase to each wave vector i. Therefore, for each pixel of the image, we have built a circumferential spectral filter, whose radius is linearly related to a previously defined bandwidth, which has been centered at the maximum of the spectra inside a predefined region located in the surroundings of the reference spatial frequency of the tags.

  The final WHARP image, for each wave vector, can be reconstructed in the spatial domain by using an inverse WFT (IWFT) from which its phase is readily extracted, i.e., $\phi_i[\mathbf{x}] = \angle \hat{I}_i[\mathbf{x}]$.

- **Material deformation gradient tensor estimation at end-systolic phase.** The material deformation gradient tensor $\mathbf{F}(\mathbf{x})$ can be estimated from the gradient of the phase image $\mathbf{Y}(\mathbf{x})$ as stated in [10]. Robust estimation of $\mathbf{F}(\mathbf{x})$ is achieved through Least Absolute Deviation (LAD) procedure [22]. Reconstruction is performed via Iteratively Reweighted Least Squares:

$$\mathbf{F}_{l+1}(\mathbf{x}) = (\mathbf{Y}^T(\mathbf{x})\mathbf{W}_l(\mathbf{x})\mathbf{Y}(\mathbf{x}))^{-1}\mathbf{Y}^T(\mathbf{x})\mathbf{W}_l(\mathbf{x})\mathbf{K}, \tag{1}$$

where $\mathbf{K}$ represents the given wave vectors and $\mathbf{W}_l(\mathbf{x})$ a diagonal weighting matrix updated at each iteration by considering the fitting residuals [19]. For illustration purposes, the Green-Lagrange strain tensor is also computed in the polar coordinate system.

3.2   Optimal Tag Pattern Search

In order to find the optimal tag pattern, we have carried out an optimization procedure on the synthetic data; the procedure is schematically shown in Fig. 2. The upper part shows how the ground truth data is obtained. First, the stripe patterns, consisting in two sets of two orthogonal directions are generated. Each pattern is then applied to a previously acquired cine sequence. Each pattern is applied in isolation so that no interference arises. Then, the methodology described in Sect. 3.1 is applied to calculate $\mathbf{F}^{GT}$.

The stripes are oriented as $\{0°, 45°, 90°, 135°\}$ with $\lambda = 7.15$ mm and only the DC component and the two symmetric peaks are included in the simulation. The analysis window w of the WFT is defined as stated in Sect. 3.1 and its size has been set to $\mathbf{Q} = [32, 32]$.

The BP filter parameters, for each pixel $\mathbf{x}$ and wave vector i, are represented as $\beta_i[\mathbf{x}] = (\hat{\mathbf{k}}_i[\mathbf{x}], \rho)$, where ρ is the radius of the filter, which is centered at $\hat{\mathbf{k}}[\mathbf{x}]$. The filter bandwidth is normalized with respect to the wave number ($\mu = \rho/k$, $k = 2\pi/\lambda$) so that area of all filters remains the same along the pipeline.

As for the lower part of the figure, the tags are multiplied to each other as well as to the cine sequence; intermodulations are therefore present in the problem. Then, the aforementioned reconstruction procedure is performed but for the fact that the WFT is applied to the image degraded by interference. When the BP filter bank is applied, channels are processed in parallel. In this case, two stripes ($\{0°, 90°\}$) remain fixed with its tag spacing at $\lambda_{1,2} = 7.15$ mm. The other two stripes are considered as variables in the optimization problem, both in tag orientation and spacing ($\theta_3, \theta_4, \lambda_3, \lambda_4$). The objective function to be minimized is defined upon the Frobenius Norm Difference (FND) between a ground-truth tensor F^{GT} and the estimated tensor with a specific value of the variable Θ (see below); this function is integrated over a predefined region of interest χ that encloses the myocardium. Formally:

$$\Theta^* = \arg\min_{\Theta} \int_{\chi} FND(\mathbf{x}, \Theta)^2 d\chi$$

$$= \arg\min_{\Theta} \int_{\chi} \sum_{m=1}^{2} \sum_{n=1}^{2} (F_{mn}^{GT}(\mathbf{x}) - F_{mn}(\mathbf{x}, \Theta))^2 d\chi \qquad (2)$$

with $\Theta = [\theta_3, \theta_4, \lambda_3, \lambda_4]$.

The solution has been obtained by means of the Nelder-Mead algorithm [23]. This algorithm does not require derivatives of the objective function. Simulation has been limited to four stripes to avoid an overwhelming peak interference.

4   Evaluation and Discussion

The importance of the number of orientations is measured in Fig. 3 in terms of reproducibility for the real dataset. Estimated tensors should be equal irrespective of the stripe pattern used; therefore, a useful measure of reproducibility is

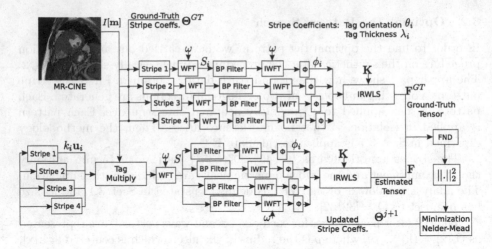

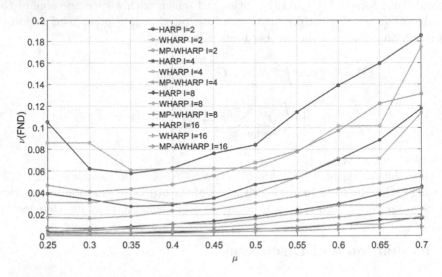

Fig. 2. Flowchart of the optimization procedure for optimal stripes parameter search. Notice that connections from the Nelder-Mead algorithm to stripes 1 and 2 do not undergo any variation.

the FND defined above but applied in this case to two instances of the reconstructed tensor with two different, albeit comparable, stripe sets. Specifically, given two stripe sets with the same number of orientations and their respective reconstructed tensors, we have calculated the median of the $FND(\mathbf{x})$ with both for $\mathbf{x} \in \chi$.

Figure 3 shows the impact on reproducibility of using either additional orientations or additional harmonic peaks.

Fig. 3. Median of the FND $\forall \mathbf{x} \in \chi$ obtained with different number of images as a function of the filter bandwidth μ.

As previously described [19], an overdetermined set of stripes increases reproducibility at the price of a higher number of acquisitions. For a given number of orientations the multi-peak (MP) windowed approach (WHARP) shows additional improvement for moderate bandwidths. HARP analysis has also been added showing lower figures. When bandwidth is excessive, interference from nearby peaks reduces the stability of results. MP-WHARP obtained with $I = 2$ is located halfway between the other results with $I = 2$ and those with $I = 4$. This solution would require a single acquisition while $I = 4$ requires at least two, for a grid pattern.

For the synthetic dataset, Fig. 4 shows the mean squared error (MSE) of the strain tensor principal components $(\hat{E}^{rr})$ and $(\hat{E}^{cc})$ for different options (windowed, MP, MO) as a function of the degree of deformation γ. In these figures solid lines are obtained with multiple images $(I = 18)$ and dashed lines with only two orthogonal directions $(I = 1)$; in both, grid patterns have been used. As can be observed, MO and MP play a satisfactory role for moderate values of γ. It is worthy to say that MP approach presents a notable performance, even with a unique grid-like acquisition. On the other side, when severe deformation is applied to the $I = 1$ cases, non-MP approaches depart dramatically from the ground truth while LAD algorithm maintains quality fairly unaltered for the MP version (dashed-red line).

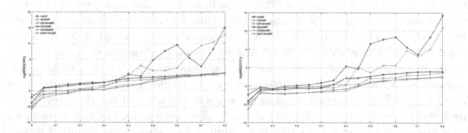

Fig. 4. Log-mean squared error of $(\hat{E}^{rr})$ (left) and $(\hat{E}^{cc})$ (right) for $\mu = 0.35$. Solid line denotes reconstruction error with 18 images while dashed lines are obtained with only two. (Color figure online)

In Fig. 5, we show the output of the optimization procedure described in Sect. 3.2. According to the figure, the two free orientations turn out to align with the two that remained fixed, although spectral separation is lower than the separation of the steady peaks with respect to the DC component; specifically, the steady peaks are located at $k = (7.15\,\mathrm{mm})^{-1} = 0.14\,\mathrm{mm}^{-1}$, while the other two turn out to be located (on average) $k \sim \frac{1.6}{7.15}\,\mathrm{mm}^{-1}$. This output, however, is not directly available in equipments routinely used in clinical settings.

Therefore, we have carried out an additional two-fold experiment in order to test relevance of peak separation or, equivalently, tag spacing. For this purpose, we have calculated the MSE in E^{rr} estimation for both 1D and 2D cases; for the former, we have simulated a pattern with two peaks in the same direction, where

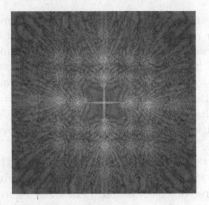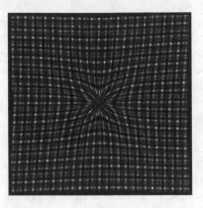

Fig. 5. Final configuration of the tag pattern obtained with Nelder-Mead algorithm both on k-space (left figure) and spatial domain (centered at right figure) with $\gamma = 0.45$.

the first peak is located at $\lambda_1 = 7.15$ mm and the second peak is translated, in k-space, along that direction. For the latter, the pattern consists of a multiplication of two such 1D patterns in orthogonal directions. Results, as shown in Fig. 6, indicate that optimal separation depends on the degree of deformation γ, with higher sensitivity in the 1D case, whereas, for 2D, sensitivity is much lower for $\gamma \geq 0.3$. In this interval, performance is fairly constant so a $\frac{1}{\lambda_1} = 0.14\,\text{mm}^{-1}$ separation, i.e., location of harmonically related peaks, seems an appropriate design choice. This is the case of a grid pattern with second order SPAMM acquisition, which is a commonly available sequence. Presence of noise and tag fading in simulation will presumably increase smearing in k-space, making this space more crowded, so this conclusions tend to reinforce. With this in mind, it may be appealing to include even more peaks in the acquisition. However, growing between-peak-interference may severely affect estimates. For that reason, we have limited our experiments to a maximum of four stripes per acquired image. Further research should be developed in this direction to assess the influence of heavily-peaked acquisitions in the robustness of reconstructions.

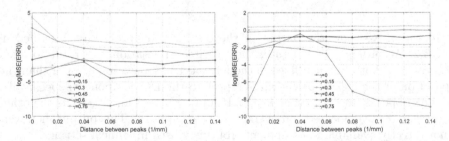

Fig. 6. Log-mean squared error in E^{rr} estimation as a function of the distance between peaks in presence of different degrees of deformation with a fixed $\mu = 0.35$. 1D and 2D cases have been plotted in left and right figures, respectively

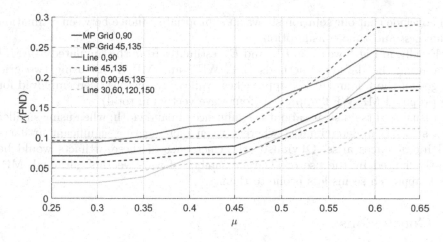

Fig. 7. Median of the FND obtained with different stripe sets as a function of μ.

Additionally, in Fig. 7 we show the FND obtained on real data with different stripe sets for different bandwidths; we have used as a silver estimate of $\mathbf{F}$ the one obtained with the eight 1D orientations indicated in Sect. 2. Specifically, we have tried the following subsets: $\{45°\text{--}135°\}$ and $\{0°\text{--}90°\}$ in a grid (2D) pattern with two peaks per orientation, and $\{45°\text{--}135°\}$, $\{0°\text{--}90°\}$, $\{45°\text{--}135°\text{--}0°\text{--}90°\}$ and $\{30°\text{--}60°\text{--}120°\text{--}150°\}$ for line (1D) acquisitions with a unique peak. The figure reveals that harmonic MP solution with a single acquisition overcomes the solution obtained with two orthogonal line acquisitions and it provides a reasonable performance loss with respect to four-orientation reconstructions, i.e., those needing two acquisitions, at least, in commercial equipments. Therefore, we

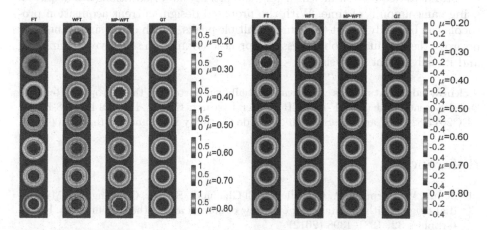

Fig. 8. E^{rr} (left) and E^{cc} (right) strain components for synthetic data obtained for different bandwidths and methodologies. Ground-truth (GT) is also shown for the sake of comparison.

can conclude that our solution shows an appropriate balance between estimation robustness and time consumption.

Finally, in Fig. 8 we show E^{rr} and E^{cc} estimates from the simulated SPAMM data using the different methods (FT, WFT and MP-WFT) using two grid images for the FT and WFT approaches, while only one has been employed for the proposed MP-WFT approach (four wave vectors in total).

Visual results illustrate about the influence of bandwidth; when using smaller ones strain is underestimated whereas when incrementing significant artifacts and interferences arise. Obviously, the emergence of these artifacts would be greatly limited by the use of a larger number of wave vectors, although MP-WFT approach seems less prone to them.

5   Conclusions

In this paper we have described a robust alternative to the original HARP method, intended for a single acquisition. To this end, we have observed that information comprised by various peaks of the stripe pattern is useful for achieving robust results despite using a unique acquisition. We have quantified performance of this solution with respect to multi-oriented solutions.

Simulation results indicate that four orientations converge into an orthogonal grid with harmonically related peaks (in a mid to high deformation degree interval) for an optimal performance, so multiple peaks as opposed to multiple stripes is a preferable solution. The proposed pattern has also shown comparable results, for the case of a single acquisition, to those obtained with two different grid acquisitions, while the latter doubles the scan time.

Furthermore, the proposed multi-peaked method has significantly improved both the accuracy and the reproducibility of strain measurements with respect to the standard acquisition in which just two orthogonal orientations are acquired, using same amount of time. With the proposed design, current acquisition protocols can be easily recast to include multiple peaks, which could simultaneously improve the resolution, robustness and precision of motion sensitive MR imaging and its subsequent analysis.

Acknowledgments. This work was partially supported by the European Regional Development Fund (ERDF-FEDER) under Research Grants TEC2014-57428-R and TEC2017-82408-R and the Spanish Junta de Castilla y León under Grant VA069U16.

References

1. Jeung, M., Germain, P., Croisille, P., El Ghannudi, S., Roy, C., Gangi, A.: Myocardial tagging with MR imaging: overview of normal and pathologic findings. Radio-Graphics **32**, 1381–1398 (2012)
2. Shehata, M., Cheng, S., Osman, N., Bluemke, D., Lima, J.: Myocardial tissue tagging with cardiovascular magnetic resonance. J. Cardiovasc. Magn. Reson. **11**(1), 55 (2009)

3. Ibrahim, E.: Myocardial tagging by cardiovascular magnetic resonance: evolution of techniques pulse sequences, analysis, algorithms and applications. J. Cardiovasc. Magn. Reson. **13**, 36 (2011)

4. Simpson, R., Keegan, J., Firmin, D.: MR assessment of regional myocardial mechanics. J. Cardiovasc. Magn. Reson. **37**, 576–599 (2013)

5. Axel, L., Montillo, A., Kim, D.: Tagged magnetic resonance imaging of the heart: a survey. Med. Image Anal. **9**, 376–393 (2005)

6. Horn, B., Schunck, B.: Determining optical flow. Artif. Intell. **17**, 185–203 (1981)

7. Young, A., Axel, L.: Three-dimensional motion and deformation of the heart wall: estimation with spatial modulation of magnetization-a model-based approach. Radiology **185**(1), 241–247 (1992)

8. Ibrahim, E., Swanson, S., Stojanovska, J., Duvernoy, C., Pop-Busui, R.: Harmonic phase versus sine-wave modulation for measuring regional heart function from tagged MRI images. In: 13th IEEE ISBI, Prague, Czech Republic (2016)

9. Arts, T., Prinzen, F., Delhaas, T., Milles, J., Rossi, A., Clarysse, P.: Mapping displacement and deformation of the heart with local sine-wave modeling. Trans. Med. Imag. **29**, 1114–1123 (2010)

10. Osman, N., McVeigh, E., Prince, J.: Imaging heart motion using harmonic phase MRI. IEEE Trans. Med. Imaging **19**(3), 186–202 (2000)

11. Parthasarathy, V.: Characterization of harmonic phase MRI: theory, simulations and applications. Ph.D. thesis, Doctoral dissertation, Johns Hopkins University (2006)

12. Cordero-Grande, L., Vegas-Sánchez-Ferrero, G., Casaseca-de-la-Higuera, P., Alberola-López, C.: Improving harmonic phase imaging by the windowed Fourier transform. In: 8th IEEE International Symposium on Biomedical Imaging: From Nano to Macro, Chicago, USA, pp. 520–523, March-April 2011

13. Fu, Y., Chui, C., Teo, C.: Accurate two-dimensional cardiac strain calculation using adaptive windowed Fourier transform and Gabor wavelet transform. Int. J. Comput. Assist. Radiol. Surg. **8**(1), 135–144 (2013)

14. Sanz-Estébanez, S., Cordero-Grande, L., Martín-Fernández, M., Aja-Fernández, S., Alberola-López, C.: Spatial and spectral anisotropy in HARP images: an automated approach. In: IEEE International Symposium on Biomedical Imaging: From Nano to Macro, Prague, Czech Republic, pp. 1105–1108 (2016)

15. Atalar, E., McVeigh, E.: Optimization of tag thickness for measuring position with magnetic resonance imaging. IEEE Trans. Med. Imag. **13**(1), 152–160 (1994)

16. Osman, N., Prince, J.: Regenerating MR tagged images using harmonic phase (HARP) methods. IEEE Trans. Biomed. Eng. **51**(8), 1428–1433 (2004)

17. Mosher, T., Smith, M.: A DANTE tagging sequence for the evaluation of translational sample motion. Magn. Reson. Med. **15**, 334–339 (1990)

18. Agarwal, H., Prince, J., Abd-Elmoniem, K.: Total removal of unwanted harmonic peaks (TruHARP) MRI for single breath-hold high-resolution myocardial motion and strain quantification. Magn. Reson. Med. **64**(2), 574–585 (2010)

19. Cordero-Grande, L., Royuela-del-Val, J., Sanz-Estébanez, S., Martín-Fernández, M., Alberola-López, C.: Multi-oriented windowed harmonic phase reconstruction for robust cardiac strain imaging. Med. Image Anal. **29**, 1–11 (2016)

20. Axel, L., Dougherty, L.: MR imaging of motion with spatial modulation of magnetization. Radiology **171**(3), 841–845 (1989)

21. Rutz, A., Ryf, S., Plein, S., Boesiger, P., Kozerke, S.: Accelerated whole-heart 3D CSPAMM for myocardial motion quantification. Magn. Reson. Med. **59**, 755–763 (2008)

22. Cordero-Grande, L., Royuela-del-Val, J., Martín-Fernández, M., Alberola-López, C.: MOWHARP: multi-oriented windowed harp reconstruction for robust strain imaging. In: 22nd Proceedings of the International Society on Magnetic Resonance in Medicine, Milan, Italy, p. 7540, May 2014
23. Nelder, J., Mead, R.: A simplex method for function minimization. Comput. J. **7**, 308–313 (1965)

Lung Structures Enhancement in Chest Radiographs via CT Based FCNN Training

Ophir Gozes[✉] and Hayit Greenspan

Faculty of Engineering, Department of Biomedical Engineering,
Medical Image Processing Laboratory, Tel Aviv University, 69978 Tel Aviv, Israel
ophirgozes@mail.tau.ac.il

Abstract. The abundance of overlapping anatomical structures appearing in chest radiographs can reduce the performance of lung pathology detection by automated algorithms (CAD) as well as the human reader. In this paper, we present a deep learning based image processing technique for enhancing the contrast of soft lung structures in chest radiographs using Fully Convolutional Neural Networks (FCNN). Two 2D FCNN architectures were trained to accomplish the task: The first performs 2D lung segmentation which is used for normalization of the lung area. The second FCNN is trained to extract lung structures. To create the training images, we employed Simulated X-Ray or Digitally Reconstructed Radiographs (DRR) derived from 516 scans belonging to the LIDC-IDRI dataset. By first segmenting the lungs in the CT domain, we are able to create a dataset of 2D lung masks to be used for training the segmentation FCNN. For training the extraction FCNN, we create DRR images of only voxels belonging to the 3D lung segmentation which we call "Lung X-ray" and use them as target images. Once the lung structures are extracted, the original image can be enhanced by fusing the original input x-ray and the synthesized "Lung X-ray". We show that our enhancement technique is applicable to real x-ray data, and display our results on the recently released NIH Chest X-Ray-14 dataset. We see promising results when training a DenseNet-121 based architecture to work directly on the lung enhanced X-ray images.

Keywords: Deep learning · Image synthesis · CT · X-ray
Lung nodules · CAD

1 Introduction

Chest X-ray is the most frequently performed diagnostic x-ray examination. It produces images of the heart, lungs, airways, blood vessels and the bones of the spine and chest. It aides in the diagnosis and evaluation of chest diseases such as lung cancer, pneumonia, emphysema, fibrosis, pleural effusion, pneumothorax and tuberculosis. Lung cancer is the leading cause of cancer death among men

D. Stoyanov et al. (Eds.): RAMBO 2018/BIA 2018/TIA 2018, LNCS 11040, pp. 147–158, 2018.
https://doi.org/10.1007/978-3-030-00946-5_16

and women in the United States and around the world. In the U.S, according to the American Cancer Society [1], in 2018 alone, lung cancer is expected to account for 25% of cancer related deaths, exceeding breast, prostate, colorectal, skin melanoma and bladder cancers combined.

It was found that approx. 90% of presumed mistakes in pulmonary tumor diagnosis occur in chest radiography, with only 5% in CT examinations [2]. For this reason, missed lung cancer in chest radiographs is a great source of concern in the radiological community.

In 2006 Suzuki et al. [7] introduced a method for suppression of ribs in chest radiographs by means of Massive Training Artificial Neural Networks (MTANN). Their work relied on Dual energy X-ray in the creation of training images. Other recently published works have used Digitally Reconstructed Radiographs (DRR) for training CNN models. Albarqouni et al. [10] used DRR image training for decomposing CXR into several anatomical planes, while Campo et al. [9] used the DRR image training to quantify emphysema severity. In recent years, with the rapid evolution of the field of deep learning, hand in hand with the release of large datasets [3,4], an opportunity to create a data driven approach for X-ray lung structures enhancement as well as lung pathology CAD has been enabled [5].

The current work focuses on enhancement of lung structures in chest X-ray. Our training approach is based on CT data and is focused on extraction of lung tissues and their enhancement in combination with the original radiograph. The enhanced result maintains a close appearance to a regular x-ray, which may be attractive to radiologists. The proposed methodology is based on neural networks trained on synthetic data: To produce training images, we use DRRs that we generated from a subset of LIDC-IDRI dataset. The LIDC-IDRI dataset (Lung Image Database Consortium image collection) [3] consists of diagnostic and lung cancer screening thoracic computed tomography (CT) scans with marked-up annotated lesions.

Given a chest X-ray as input, we introduce a method that allows extraction of lung structures as well as synthesis of an enhanced radiograph.

The contribution of this work includes the following:

- We present a novel CT based approach to automatically generate lung masks which can be used for training 2D lung segmentation algorithms.
- We present a novel CT based approach to automatically extract lung structures in CXR which we term "lung X-ray" synthesis. The training process for this method makes use of nodule segmentations contained in LIDC-IDRI dataset to introduce a novel nodule weighted reconstruction loss. This assures lungs nodules are not suppressed by the extraction FCNN.
- Combining the above mentioned methods, we present a scheme for lung structures enhancement in real CXR.

The proposed method is presented in Sect. 2. Experimental results are shown in Sect. 3. In Sect. 4, a discussion of the results is presented followed by a conclusion of the work.

2   Methods

The principal methods presented in the work are the following:

- **Synthetic chest X-ray generation for training**
- **2D segmentation of the lungs:** We present an algorithm for 2D segmentation of the lungs in synthetic X-ray. The algorithm is trained using masks retrieved from CT 3D lung segmentation.
- **Generation of "lung X-ray" for training:** Given a CT case as input, we describe a process for the creation of a synthetic X-ray of exclusively the lungs. We term the resulting reconstruction "lung X-ray" and use it for training.
- **Lung structures extraction:** Given a synthetic X-ray as input, a FCNN based algorithm for the synthesis of "lung X-ray" is presented.
- **Lung structures enhancement:** Combining the above mentioned methods, we present a scheme for lung structures enhancement on real CXR.

Given real chest X-ray as input, the resulting trained lung enhancement method is presented in Fig. 1. The solution is comprised of a lung segmentation FCNN, a lung structures extraction FCNN, and a fusion block to create the final enhanced radiograph.

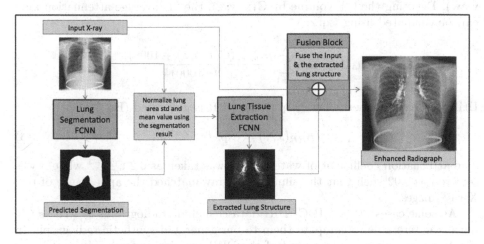

Fig. 1. A description of the enhancement algorithm structure.

2.1   Synthetic X-Ray: Digitally Reconstructed Radiographs

We begin by introducing the method for generating digitally reconstructed radiographs (DRRs).

Our neural networks are trained by using 2D DRRs which serve as input images during the training process. These synthetic X-ray images are generated by reconstructing a three dimensional CT case such that the physical process of 2D X-ray generation is simulated. In the following subsection we review the physical process which governs chest X-ray generation and review our method for simulating it.

DRR Generation: Our DRR generation method is based on the recently published work by Campo et al. [9]. As X-rays propagate through matter, their energy decreases. This attenuation in the energy of the incident X-ray depends on the distance traveled and on the attenuation coefficient. This relationship is expressed by Beer Lambert's law, where I_0 is the incident beam, I is the Intensity after traveling a distance x and A is the attenuation coefficient:

$$I = I_0 \exp^{Ax} \tag{1}$$

In order to simulate the X-ray generation process, calculation of the attenuation coefficient is required for each voxel in the CT volume. In a CT volume, each voxel is represented by its Hounsfield unit (HU) value, which is a linear transformation of the original linear attenuation coefficient. Therefore the information regarding the linear attenuation is maintained. We assume for simplicity a parallel projection model and compute the average attenuation coefficient along the y axis ranging from [1, N] (where N is the pixel length of the posterior anterior view). Denoting the CT volume by G(x, y, z), the 2D average attenuation map can be computed using Eq. 2:

$$\mu_{av}(x, z) = \sum_{y=1}^{N} \frac{\mu_{water}(G(x, y, z) + 1000)}{(N \cdot 1000)} \tag{2}$$

Utilizing Beer Lambert's law (Eq. 1) the DRR is generated (Eq. 3):

$$I_{DRR}(x, z) = \exp^{\beta \cdot \mu_{av}(x,z)} \tag{3}$$

The attenuation coefficient of water μ_{water} was taken as $0.2 \ CM^{-1}$ while β was selected as 0.02 such that the simulated X-ray matched the appearance of real X-ray images.

As some cases in the LIDC-IDRI dataset include radiographs as well as CT data, we were able to compare them to our generated synthetic radiograph. In Fig. 2, we present a sample result of the DRR creation process. The real X-ray and the DRR appear similar in structure. Since our CT dataset contains cases with slice thickness as high as 2.5 mm, the DRR is less detailed then the CXR.

2.2   Lung Segmentation in Synthetic X-Ray

In the next step of the process, our goal is to segment the lung region in a given synthetic X-ray (DRR). For this we employ a FCNN and train it as detailed next.

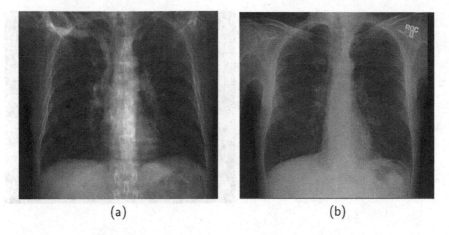

(a)   (b)

Fig. 2. (a) DRR(simulated X-ray) for LIDC-007 (b) CXR for LIDC-007

Creation of 2D Lungs Masks for Training: For each synthetic X-ray, a 2D training mask can be generated by a 2D projection of the 3D lung mask matching the CT case used for DRR generation. In order to create a 3D lung mask of the lung volume in CT, we first perform binarization of the CT scan $G(x, y, z)$ with a threshold of $-500[\text{HU}]$. For each axial slice we extract the filled structure of the largest connected component. The 2D axial segmentations are then stacked to create a 3D binary mask $M_{lung}3D$ of the entire volume. In order to create 2D masks to accompany the 2D DRR's we project the binary $M_{lung}3D$ along the y axis, yielding a 2D mask which we denote $M_{lung}2D$.

In contrast to 2D masks usually employed in the process of training 2D lung field segmentation algorithms [8], the masks generated by our method reflect the exact position the of lungs in the image even when occluded by other structures. As a result, the subdiaphagramatic and retrocardiac areas which are known as hidden spots for nodule detection [2] are included in the mask. An example of a 3D mask and a 2D mask is given in Fig. 3.

Segmentation FCNN: The networks we use in this work are based on the U-net FCNN architecture [6]. We specify here the modifications which we made to the original architecture: The inputs size to the segmentation network is 512×512 with 32 filters in the first convolution layer. In order to improve generalization of the network, we add a Gaussian noise layer(std $= 0.2$) which operates on the input. We use dilated convolutions (dilation rate $= 2$) in order to enlarge the receptive field of the network. Batch normalization layers were not used. For nonlinearity, RELU activation is used throughout the net, while at the network output we use a sigmoid activation. The output size is 512×512. The loss function we used is weighted binary cross entropy.

Training was performed on batches of size 8. ADAM optimizer was used. The optimal initial learning rate was found to be 1E–4. Validation loss converged after

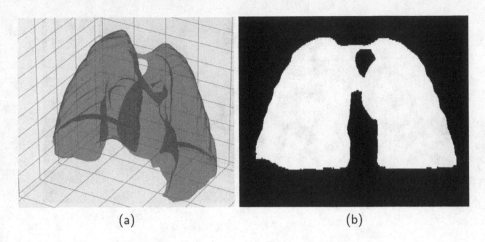

(a)   (b)

Fig. 3. (a) 3D lung segmentation mask (b) 2D projection of the lung mask

80 epochs. To augment the dataset during the training we utilized random data augmentation for both the source and the lung mask. We used random rotations by 2°, width shift with range 0.1, height shift with range 0.2, random zooming with factor 0.3.

2.3   Lung Structures Extraction Method

The input to the lung structures extraction algorithm is a synthetic X-ray. The output is an image which includes only the lung structures appearing in the original image. In order to teach a FCNN to perform this decomposition task, we make use of the 3D CT data. A DRR of the lungs which we term "Lung X-ray" is created and used as the training target image. Training pairs of source and target images are generated as detailed next:

Source "Synthetic X-Ray" DRR Image Generation: For each CT case we produce a DRR (Eq. 3) which serves as a "Synthetic X-ray" source image.

Target "Lung X-Ray" Image Generation: Utilizing the 3D segmentation map M_{lung}, we mask out all non Lung voxels yielding G_{Lung}.

$$G_{Lung} = M_{lung} \cdot G(x, y, z) \qquad (4)$$

A DRR can now be generated as before for G_{Lung} using Eq. 3. As a consequence, the DRR generation process is now limited to the lung area. An example result of the "Lung X-ray" generation process is given in Fig. 4. It is noticeable that only inner lung structures appear, excluding overlapping anatomical structures.

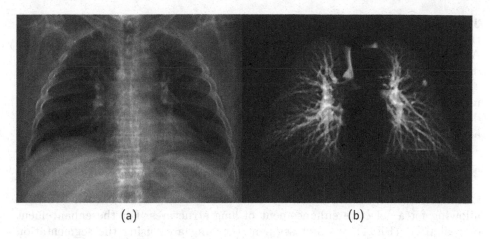

(a)   (b)

Fig. 4. (a) DRR source image: (b) "Lung X-ray" target image for training

Lung Structures Extraction FCNN: By training a FCNN to synthesize a "Lung X-ray" matching a DRR input, we are able to extract the lung structures from the input image.

In the following we describe the FCNN used in the lung structures extraction algorithm. We used the U-Net Architecture [6] with the following modifications: The inputs size is 512×512 with 32 filters in the first convolution layer. We use RELU activation functions throughout the net while at the network output we use the Tanh activation. The output size is 512×512.

In order to ensure small structures such as nodules appear in the synthesized "Lung X-ray", we assigned higher loss weight to image areas which contained nodules. For each DRR, a matching 2D binary mask of nodules was generated by projecting the 3D CT nodule annotations which are available in the LIDC dataset.

The resulting loss function (Eq. 5) is a weighted L1 loss computed between the FCNN output y_{pred} and the GT target "Lung X-ray" image.

$$L1_{weighted} = \|(y_{pred} - target) \cdot (1 + w_{noduleLoss} \cdot noduleMask)\|_1 \qquad (5)$$

Nodules with the following features were selected: median texture greater then 3, median subtlety greater then 4, level of agreement of at least 2 radiologists. This was performed in order to ensure that the nodules used are actually visible in the DRR. A suitable $w_{noduleLoss}$ was found to be 30.

Preprocessing. Images have been normalized to be in the range of [0,1] and have been equalized using by first HE, then CLAHE with window of [40,40] and contrast clip limit 0.01. When working with real X-ray, before feeding the images to the extraction network, we use the segmentation FCNN to segment the lungs and then normalize the lung area to mean 0, and std 0.5.

Training of the Lung Extraction FCNN. The network was trained to synthesize the required target image using training with batches of size 8 and with ADAM optimizer. The optimal initial learning rate was found to be 1E–4. Validation loss converged after 200 epochs.

To augment the dataset during the training we utilized random data augmentation for both the source and the target. We used random rotations by 4 degrees, width and height shift with range 0.1, random zooming with factor 0.2, and horizontal flipping.

2.4   A Scheme for Lung Structures Enhancement in Real CXR

Once extracted, the lung structures can be added to the original DRR image, allowing for a selective enhancement of lung structures. For the enhancement of real CXR (Fig. 1), we first segment the lung area using the segmentation FCNN. We proceed by normalizing the lung area to mean 0, std 0.5. Following the normalization procedure, we use the lung structures extraction FCNN to extract lung structures from the input image (i.e. prediction of a "Lung X-ray"). The input CXR image and the synthesized "Lung X-ray" are scaled to the range of [0,1]. We fuse the two images by performing a weighted summation (Eq. 6).

$$I_{Enhanced} = I_{CXR} + w \cdot I_{LungXray} \tag{6}$$

In Fig. 5 we display example results on a real chest X-ray image. An enhancement weight factor w is used to factor the extracted lung image. By controlling w, multiple enhancement levels can be achieved.

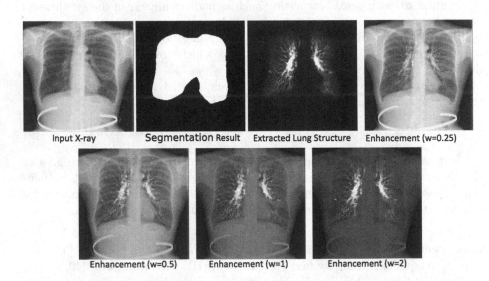

Input X-ray   Segmentation Result   Extracted Lung Structure   Enhancement (w=0.25)

Enhancement (w=0.5)   Enhancement (w=1)   Enhancement (w=2)

Fig. 5. NIH chest X-Ray-14 case #1555 enhancement results

3   Experiments and Results

3.1   Lung Segmentation

A total of 990 CT cases were used to create pairs of DRR and Lung mask for training the segmentation FCNN. Data was split in 80-20 training validation ratio. We threshold the continuous output of the segmentation network to get a binary segmentation prediction (threshold=0.95). An example result of the segmentation algorithm is given in Fig. 6. The Dice coefficient was chosen as the segmentation metric. On the training set the Dice score was **0.971** while on the validation set the Dice score was **0.953**. Since our lung segmentation algorithm is used for normalization of the input to the extraction FCNN we were satisfied with the result. To the best of our knowledge, this is the first work that performs lung segmentation using CT ground truth. As a result, we were not able to perform a comparison to other works.

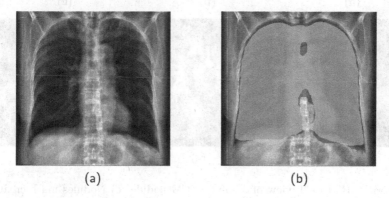

(a)   (b)

Fig. 6. (a) Original DRR (b) Segmentation result (Red: GT mask derived from CT, Yellow: segmentation result, Orange: overlap) (Color figure online)

3.2   Lung Structures Extraction

A subset of 516 CT scans belonging to LIDC dataset was used for training. For each CT case we generate a DRR and a "Lung X-ray" pair which we denote by I_{Source} and I_{Target}. In addition, we generate a 2D binary mask of the nodules that belong to the case and use it for the computation of the loss function(Eq. 5). We split the dataset to 465 training pairs and 51 validation pairs. We evaluate our results on 51 validation cases and report MAE (Mean Absolute Error), MSE, PSNR, and SSIM. Results are given in Table 1. An example result of the extraction algorithm is given in Fig. 7. In this case, the CT (7b) contained one nodule which was projected to create the nodules mask (7c). Notice that the introduction of our weighted nodule loss function greatly improves the visibility of the nodule in the extracted result(7e vs 7f).

Table 1. Extraction network performance results

	MAE	MSE	PSNR [dB]	SSIM
Average	0.082	0.03	24.98	0.80
Std	0.017	0.007	1.41	0.04

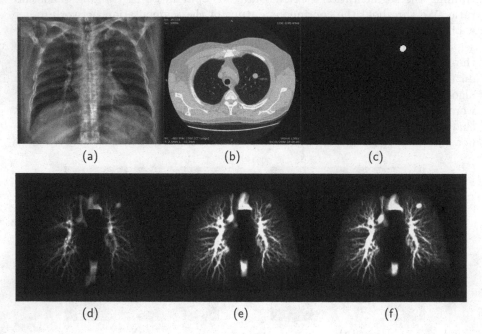

(a)   (b)   (c)

(d)   (e)   (f)

Fig. 7. (a) DRR (b) CT view of a solid 1.6CM nodule (c) Nodules mask created by projecting LIDC annotations to 2D (d) Target GT- "Lung X-ray" (e) Synthesized result without nodule weighted L1 loss (f) Synthesized result ($w_{noduleLoss} = 30$)

3.3 Applicability to Real X-Ray

In order to explore the applicability of our algorithm to real X-ray and to examine whether the enhancement scheme introduces artifacts detrimental to CAD detection performance, we chose to perform the lung enhancement algorithm as a preprocessing step on nodule and mass CAD input images.

To accomplish this, we trained and tested a CheXNet [5] based network on 67,313 images released in ChestX-ray14 dataset(subset of PA images). In Fig. 8 we show the results of the enhancement on an image from NIH ChestX-ray14 dataset [4]. The architecture we chose was a DenseNet-121 based network, with 512×512 input size. Network weights were initialized with pretrained ImageNet weights and training was performed independently for enhanced images and non-enhanced images.

The dataset was split to 44,971 training, 11,245 validation and 11,097 test images. Results are given on the official test set in terms of average precision

(AP) for the labels mass and nodule. We see a moderate increase in AP scores for the mass detection task (Table 2).

Table 2. Effect of lung structure enhancement preprocessing on CAD AP%. Evaluated using 5000 bootstrap replicates, given as mean(std).

	Mass	Nodule
Non enhanced	36.83 (1.58)	29.25 (1.53)
Enhanced	**39.65 (1.74)**	**29.73 (1.56)**

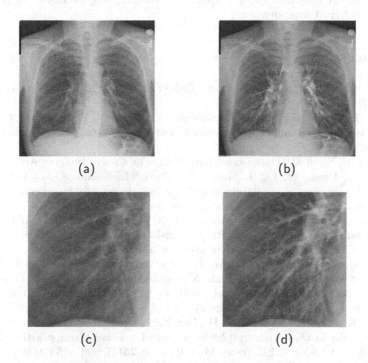

(a)   (b)

(c)   (d)

Fig. 8. Enhancement result on NIH ChestX-Ray14 image. One network was trained on the original X-ray and a second network was trained on the enhanced X-ray (a) Original X-ray (b) Enhanced X-ray (c) Zoom (d) Zoom-Enhanced

4   Discussion and Conclusion

In this work we presented a novel method for enhancement of lung structures in chest X-ray. We demonstrated that 3D CT data, along with 3D nodule annotations, can be used to train a 2D lung structures enhancement algorithm. By generating our own synthetic data, we enable neural networks to train on ground truth images which are not achievable by current X-ray techniques. Initial results suggest a moderate improvement of lung mass CAD can be achieved by performing the proposed lung enhancement scheme as a preprocessing step. The results also indicate that the effect of artifacts that may have been introduced by the enhancement scheme is minimal. We plan to study next the impact that the enhancement algorithm can have on a human reader performance. In future work, we plan to improve the robustness of our method by performing unsupervised domain adaptation between the CXR domain and the synthetic DRR domain.

Acknowledgments. We thank Prof. Edith Marom from Sheba Medical Center for providing clinical consultation. We appreciate valuable suggestions from Avi Ben-Cohen in Tel-Aviv University.

References

1. Siegel, R.L., Miller, K.D., Jemal, A.: Cancer statistics, 2018. CA Cancer J. Clin. **68**, 7–30 (2018)
2. del Ciello, A., Franchi, P., Contegiacomo, A., Cicchetti, G., Bonomo, L., Larici, A.R.: Missed lung cancer: when, where, and why? Diagn. Interv. Radiol. **23**(2), 118 (2017)
3. Armato III, S., et al.: Data from LIDC-IDRI. The Cancer Imaging Archive (2015)
4. Wang, X., Peng, Y., Lu, L., Lu, Z., Bagheri, M., Summers, M.: Chestx-ray8: hospital-scale chest x-ray database and benchmarks on weakly-supervised classification and localization of common thorax diseases. In: 2017 IEEE Conference on Computer Vision and Pattern Recognition (CVPR), pp. 3462–3471. IEEE (2017)
5. Rajpurkar, P., et al.: CheXNet: Radiologist-Level Pneumonia Detection on Chest X-Rays with Deep Learning. arXiv preprint arXiv:1711.05225 (2017)
6. Ronneberger, O., Fischer, P., Brox, T.: U-Net: convolutional networks for biomedical image segmentation. In: Navab, N., Hornegger, J., Wells, W.M., Frangi, A.F. (eds.) MICCAI 2015. LNCS, vol. 9351, pp. 234–241. Springer, Cham (2015). https://doi.org/10.1007/978-3-319-24574-4_28
7. Suzuki, K., Abe, H., MacMahon, H., Doi, K.: Image-processing technique for suppressing ribs in chest radiographs by means of massive training artificial neural network (MTANN). IEEE Trans. Med. Imaging **25**(4), 406–416 (2006)
8. Van Ginneken, B., Stegmann, M.B., Loog, M.: Segmentation of anatomical structures in chest radiographs using supervised methods: a comparative study on a public database. Med. Image Anal. **10**(1), 19–40 (2006)
9. Campo, M.I., Pascau, J., Estpar, R.S.J.: Emphysema quantification on simulated X-rays through deep learning techniques. In: IEEE 15th International Symposium on Biomedical Imaging (ISBI 2018), pp. 273–276. IEEE (2018)
10. Albarqouni, S., Fotouhi, J., Navab, N.: X-Ray in-depth decomposition: revealing the latent structures. In: Descoteaux, M., Maier-Hein, L., Franz, A., Jannin, P., Collins, D.L., Duchesne, S. (eds.) MICCAI 2017. LNCS, vol. 10435, pp. 444–452. Springer, Cham (2017). https://doi.org/10.1007/978-3-319-66179-7_51

Improving the Segmentation of Anatomical Structures in Chest Radiographs Using U-Net with an ImageNet Pre-trained Encoder

Maayan Frid-Adar[1](✉), Avi Ben-Cohen[2], Rula Amer[2], and Hayit Greenspan[1,2]

[1] RADLogics Ltd., Tel Aviv, Israel
[2] Faculty of Engineering, Department of Biomedical Engineering, Medical Image Processing Laboratory, Tel Aviv University, 69978 Tel Aviv, Israel
maayan@radlogics.com

Abstract. Accurate segmentation of anatomical structures in chest radiographs is essential for many computer-aided diagnosis tasks. In this paper we investigate the latest fully-convolutional architectures for the task of multi-class segmentation of the lungs field, heart and clavicles in a chest radiograph. In addition, we explore the influence of using different loss functions in the training process of a neural network for semantic segmentation. We evaluate all models on a common benchmark of 247 X-ray images from the JSRT database and ground-truth segmentation masks from the SCR dataset. Our best performing architecture, is a modified U-Net that benefits from pre-trained encoder weights. This model outperformed the current state-of-the-art methods tested on the same benchmark, with Jaccard overlap scores of 96.1% for lung fields, 90.6% for heart and 85.5% for clavicles.

Keywords: Chest radiographs · Lung segmentation
Clavicle segmentation · Heart segmentation
Fully convolutional networks

1 Introduction

Approximately 3.6 billion diagnostic radiological examinations, such as radiographs (x-rays), are performed globally every year [1]. Chest radiographs are performed to evaluate the lungs, heart and thoracic viscera. They are crucial for diagnosing various lung disorders in all levels of health care. Computer-aided diagnostic (CAD) tools serve an important role to assist the radiologists with the growing number of chest radiographs. Accurate segmentation of anatomical structures in chest radiographs is essential for many analysis tasks in CAD. For example: segmentation of the lungs field can help detecting lung diseases and shape irregulars; segmentation of the heart outline can help to predict

© Springer Nature Switzerland AG 2018
D. Stoyanov et al. (Eds.): RAMBO 2018/BIA 2018/TIA 2018, LNCS 11040, pp. 159–168, 2018.
https://doi.org/10.1007/978-3-030-00946-5_17

cardiomegaly; and the segmentation of clavicles can improve the diagnosis of pathologies near the apex of the lung.

Evaluating a chest radiograph is a challenging task due to the high variability between patients, unclear and overlapping organs borders, and image artifacts. A clear and high quality radiograph is not easy to acquire. This challenge drew many researchers over the years to improve the segmentation of anatomical structures in chest radiographs [2–5]. An open benchmark dataset that was provided by Ginneken et al. [6] facilitated over the years an objective comparison between the different segmentation methods. Classic approaches include active shape and appearance models, pixel classification methods, hybrid models and landmark based models. More recently deep learning approaches were suggested [2,3] based on the successful employment of convolutional neural networks (CNNs) on various detection and segmentation tasks in the medical imaging domain [7].

CNN architectures for semantic segmentation usually incorporate encoder and decoder networks [8,9] that reduce the resolution of the image to capture the most important details and then restore the resolution of the image. Another semantic segmentation approach is to keep the resolution of the network by incorporating dilated convolutions [10] that enlarge the global receptive field of the CNN to larger context information. In both approaches, the CNN can output single-class or multiple-class segmentation masks. The resolution of the output mask is the same as the input radiograph image. The training process of each CNN is affected by several training features: One is the selection of the loss function that guides the optimization process during the training process (with different loss functions effecting differently the final output segmentation performance results); The other is the initialization of the network weights - random initialization or weights transferred from another trained network (transfer learning from a totally different task).

In this paper, we explore the segmentation of anatomical structures in chest radiographs, namely the lungs field, the heart and the clavicles, using a set of the most advanced CNN architectures for multi-class semantic segmentation. We propose an improved encoder-decoder style CNN with pre-trained weights of the encoder network and show its superiority over other state of the art CNN architectures. We further examine the use of multiple loss functions for training the best selected network and the effect of multi-class vs. single-class training. We present qualitative and quantitative comparisons on a common benchmark data, based on the JSRT database [11]. Our best performing model, the U-net with an ImageNet pre-trained encoder, outperformed the currently state-of-the-art segmentation methods for all anatomical structures.

2   Methods

2.1   Fully Convolutional Neural Network Architectures

Fully convolutional networks (FCN) are extensively used for semantic segmentation tasks. In this study, four different state of the art architectures have been tested as follows:

FCN - The first FCN architecture that we used in this work is based on the FCN-8s net that uses the VGG-16 layer net [9,12]. The VGG-16 net is converted into an FCN by decapitating the final classification layer and converting fully connected layers into convolution. Deconvolution layers are then used to upsample the coarse outputs to pixel-dense outputs. Skip connections are used to merge output from previous pooling layers in the network which was shown to improve the segmentation quality [9].

Fully Convolutional DenseNet - The second network architecture that was tested is based on the fully convolutional DenseNet shown in [13]. DenseNet architecture [14] proposes intensive layer fusion. Each dense block consists of a set of convolution layers using a similar scale where each convolution layer processes the concatenation of all its previous layers thus enabling the fusion of numerous representation levels. For the fully convolutional DenseNet architecture a decoding path is added to generate the segmentation output. The fusion between different layers consists of intra dense block layers fusion as well as the concatenation of the preceding high level feature maps and the ones coming from the encoding block at the same scale.

Dilated Residual Networks - The dilated residual network (DRN) [10] uses dilated convolution [15] to increase the resolution of output feature maps without reducing the receptive field of individual neurons. It was shown to improve the performance compared to the standard residual networks presented in [16]. We have implemented the DRN-C-26 as stated in [10].

U-Net with VGG-16 Encoder - The U-Net architecture [8] has been extensively used for different image-to-image tasks in computer vision with a major contribution to the image segmentation task. The U-Net includes a contracting path (the encoder) with several layers of convolution and pooling for downsampling. The second half of the network includes an expansion path (the decoder) that uses up-sampling and convolution layers sequentially to generate an output with a similar size as the input image. Additionally, the U-Net architecture combines the encoder features with the decoder features in different levels of the network using skip connections. Iglovikov et al. [17] proposed to use a VGG11 [12] as an encoder which was pre-trained on ImageNet [18] dataset and showed that it can improve the standard U-Net performance in binary segmentation of buildings in aerial images. A similar concept was used in the current study with the more advanced VGG16 [12] as an encoder. Figure 1 shows a diagram of our proposed network. The chest X-ray image is duplicated to obtain an input image with 3 channels similar to the RGB images that are used as input to the VGG-16 net (which is the encoder in the proposed architecture).

2.2 Objective Loss Functions

The loss function is used to guide the training process of a convolutional network by measuring the compatibility between the network prediction and the ground truth label. Let us denote S as the estimated segmentation mask and G as the ground truth mask. In a multi-class semantic segmentation task including

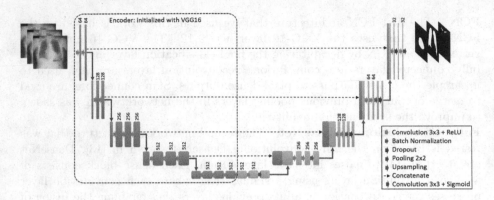

Fig. 1. The proposed U-Net architecture with a VGG-16 based encoder.

$C = \{c_1, ..., c_m\}$ classes, the total loss (TS) between S and G is defined as the sum of losses in every class:

$$TL(S, G) = \sum_{c=1}^{m} L_c(S, G) \tag{1}$$

In this study we explore the influence of using different loss functions in the FCNs training process. The Dice similarity coefficient (DSC) and Jaccard similarity coefficient (JSC) are two well known measures in segmentation and can be used as objective loss functions in training. These segmentation measures between S and G are defined as:

$$DSC(S, G) = 2\frac{|SG|}{|S| + |G|} \tag{2}$$

$$JSC(S, G) = \frac{|SG|}{|S| + |G| - |SG|} \tag{3}$$

when used as loss in training, both measures weights FP and FN detections equally. The Tversky loss [19] introduces weighting into the loss function for highly imbalanced data, where we want to segment small objects. The Tversky index is defined as:

$$Tversky(S, G; \alpha, \beta) = \frac{|SG|}{|SG| + \alpha|S/G| + \beta|G/S|} \tag{4}$$

where α and β control the magnitude of penalties for FPs and FNs, respectively. In our study we used $\alpha = 0.3$ and $\beta = 0.7$.

An additional loss function tested is the Binary Cross-Entropy (BCE). BCE was calculated separately for each class segmentation map. For each pixel $s_i \in S$ and pixel $g_i \in G$ that share the same pixel position i, the loss is averaged over all pixels N as follows:

$$BCE(S, G) = \frac{1}{N} \sum_{i=1}^{N} g_i \log(s_i) + (1 - g_i) \log(1 - s_i) \tag{5}$$

3 Segmentation of Anatomical Structures

3.1 Dataset

Evaluation of the chest anatomical structures segmentation was done on chest radiographs from the JSRT database [11]. This public database includes 247 posterior-anterior (PA) chest radiograph images of size 2048×2048 pixels, 0.175 mm pixel spacing and 12-bit gray levels. Ginneken et al. [6] publicized the Segmentation in Chest Radiographs (SCR) database, a benchmark set of segmentation masks for the lungs field, heart and clavicles (see Fig. 2). The annotations were made by two human observers and a radiologist consultant. The segmentations of the first observer generate the ground-truth segmentation masks and the other - human observer results. The benchmark data is split into two folds of 124 and 123 cases, each containing equal amount of normal cases and cases with lung nodules. Following the suggested instructions for comparison between the segmentation results, images in one fold were used for training and images from the other fold were used for testing, and vise versa. The final evaluation is defined as the average performance over the two folds.

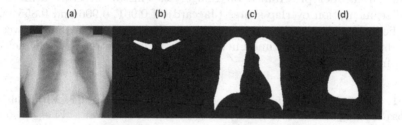

Fig. 2. Data sample from [6]: (a) chest radiograph image; (b) clavicles segmentation mask; (c) lung segmentation mask; (d) heart segmentation mask.

For training, we resize the images to 224×224 pixels and normalize each image by its mean and standard deviation. The networks are trained using Adam optimizer with initial learning rate of 10^{-5} and default parameters for 100 epochs. We use augmentations of scaling, translation and small rotations. In testing, We threshold the output score maps with $threshold = 0.25$ to generate binary segmentation masks of each anatomical structure.

3.2 Performance Measures

To measure the performance of the proposed architectures and compare to state-of-the-art results, we use well accepted metrics for segmentation: Dice similarity coefficient, jaccard index (also known as intersection over union) and mean absolute contour distance (MACD). MACD is a measure of distance between two contours. For each point on contour A, the closest point on contour B is computed by the euclidean distance $d(a_i, B) = min_{b_j \in B}\|b_j - a_i\|$. The distance values are then averaged over all points. Since distances from A to B are not the same as B to A, we derive a common average between the two averages as follows:

$$MACD(A, B) = \frac{1}{2}\left(\frac{\sum_{i=1}^{n} d(a_i, B)}{n} + \frac{\sum_{i=1}^{m} d(b_i, A)}{m}\right) \tag{6}$$

Because MACD measure is given in millimeters, we multiply the original pixel spacing by a factor of 2048/224 to match the target image resolution.

3.3   Experimental Results

Table 1 compares the segmentation performance of the four state of the art fully convolutional networks for semantic segmentation as listed in Sect. 2.1. All models are trained for multi-class segmentation into three classes: *lungs field, heart, clavicles*. We use the *sigmoid* activation function after the last layer of each network with *Dice* as the loss function. An additional column in Table 1 shows if the network is fine-tunned (FT) from a pre-trained network.

The results show that the best performing architecture for the segmentation of all anatomical structures in chest radiograph, is the U-Net including the VGG16 encoder pre-trained on ImageNet. This architecture achieved the highest segmentation overlap scores (Jaccard) of 0.961, 0.906 and 0.855 for the Lungs field, Heart and Clavicles respectively. It is noticeable that between all four architectures, the fine-tuned networks performed better than the networks trained from scratch.

Table 1. Segmentation results of four compared architectures trained with multi-class Dice loss showing the Dice (D), Jaccard (J) and MACD metrics. Fine tuned (FT) architectures include a pre-trained VGG16 as an initial encoder.

Architecture	FT	Lungs			Heart			Clavicles		
		D	J	MACD	D	J	MACD	D	J	MACD
FCN	v	0.976	0.953	1.341	0.944	0.895	3.099	0.884	0.795	1.277
U-Net (VGG16)	v	**0.980**	**0.961**	**1.121**	**0.950**	**0.906**	**2.569**	**0.921**	**0.855**	**0.871**
FC DenseNet		0.973	0.947	1.511	0.934	0.879	3.396	0.884	0.796	1.349
DRN		0.966	0.935	1.842	0.936	0.881	3.365	0.840	0.727	1.860

For the top performing architecture, the U-Net based network, we further analyzed several training features. Table 2 summarizes the multi-class segmentation performance using different objective loss functions. It is evident that structures with smaller pixel area, like the clavicles, benefits from loss metrics with pixel weighing such as Tversky loss function. We also tested the performance of training a single-class network for each of the three classes vs. the multi-class training. For the lungs, the single class training did not resolve in significant improvement. However, for the heart and clavicles, the Dice and Jaccard scores in a single-class training were improved each by 1% in comparison to

Table 2. Multi-class segmentation results using different loss functions including DSC, JSC, Tversky and BCE (rows). The Dice (D), Jaccard (J) and MACD are used as metrics (columns) for each anatomical structure

Loss Function	Lungs			Heart			Clavicles		
	D	J	MACD	D	J	MACD	D	J	MACD
DSC	**0.980**	**0.961**	1.121	**0.950**	**0.906**	**2.569**	0.921	0.855	**0.871**
JSC	0.979	0.960	**1.082**	0.949	0.905	2.602	0.921	0.855	0.920
Tversky	0.979	0.960	1.139	**0.950**	0.905	2.581	**0.923**	**0.858**	0.987
BCE	**0.980**	**0.961**	1.119	**0.950**	**0.906**	2.592	0.911	0.838	1.145

the multi-class training. The last improvement in performance of the multi-class segmentation was achieved using post-processing including small objects removal and hole fill. While the Dice and Jaccard metrics were not improved, the MACD metric showed an improvement from 1.121, 2.569 and 0.871 [mm] for the lungs, heart and clavicles to 1.019, 2.549 and 0.856 [mm] respectively. Figure 3 shows a few segmentation examples of our best performing model. A comparison of our U-Net based model trained with multi-class dice loss to existing state-of-the-art methods, validated on the same benchmark of chest radiographs and a human observer, is presented in Table 3.

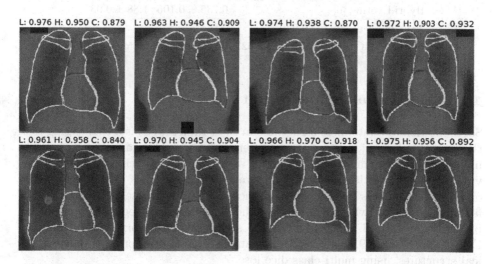

L: 0.976 H: 0.950 C: 0.879   L: 0.963 H: 0.946 C: 0.909   L: 0.974 H: 0.938 C: 0.870   L: 0.972 H: 0.903 C: 0.932

L: 0.961 H: 0.958 C: 0.840   L: 0.970 H: 0.945 C: 0.904   L: 0.966 H: 0.970 C: 0.918   L: 0.975 H: 0.956 C: 0.892

Fig. 3. Segmentation results of our best performing architecture with Jaccard score above each image for the Lungs(L), Heart(H) and Clavicles(C); Ground-truth segmentation is shown in blue, CNN segmentation in red and the overlap (true detections) in green. (Color figure online)

Table 3. Our best performing architecture compared to state-of-the-art models; "-" means that the score was not reported; (*) used different data split than suggested in SCR benchmark

	Dice	Jaccard	MACD (mm)
Lungs			
Human observer [6]	-	0.946 ± 0.018	1.64 ± 0.69
Hybrid voting [6]	-	0.949 ± 0.020	1.62 ± 0.66
Ibragimov et al. [4]	-	0.953 ± 0.020	1.43 ± 0.85
Hwang and Park [3]	0.980 ± 0.008	0.961 ± 0.015	1.237 ± 0.702
Novikov et al. [2](*)	0.974	0.950	-
Yang et al. [5]	0.975 ± 0.001	0.952 ± 0.018	1.37 ± 0.67
U-Net (VGG16)	0.980 ± 0.008	0.961 ± 0.014	1.019 ± 0.564
Heart			
Human observer [6]	-	0.878 ± 0.054	3.78 ± 1.82
Hybrid voting [6]	-	0.860 ± 0.056	4.24 ± 1.87
Novikov et al. [2](*)	0.937	0.882	-
U-Net (VGG16)	0.950 ± 0.021	0.906 ± 0.038	2.549 ± 1.126
Clavicles			
Human observer [6]	-	0.896 ± 0.037	0.68 ± 0.26
Hybrid voting [6]	-	0.736 ± 0.106	1.88 ± 0.93
Novikov et al. [2](*)	0.929	0.868	-
U-Net (VGG16)	0.921 ± 0.027	0.855 ± 0.045	0.855 ± 0.322

4 Discussion and Conclusion

Segmentation of anatomical structures in chest radiographs is a challenging task that attracted considerable interest over the years. The advantages of newly introduced CNN architectures, together with the public benchmark dataset provided in [6] on the JSRT images, motivated further studies in this field. Some of the recent studies focused only on the problem of lung segmentation, and a few have also dealt with the problem of heart and clavicles segmentation. In this paper, we employed and evaluated the segmentation performance of four top FCN architectures [9,10,13,17] for semantic segmentation for all three anatomical structures, using multi-class dice loss.

The network architectures presented in this study are well known and showed promising results in many computer vision semantic segmentation tasks. The FCN [9] and the U-Net [8] are considered classical approaches while the FC DenseNet and the DRN are more advanced and relatively new approaches for semantic segmentation. Hence, it was interesting to see in Table 1 that the classic U-Net and FCN showed superior segmentation performance over the more advanced approaches. The advantage of using pre-trained networks for medical imaging tasks has already been shown in several studies [7], and even though only the encoder part of the FCN and U-Net (VGG16 encoder) networks was pre-trained using the ImageNet database in our case, it seemed to be advantageous. The best segmentation performance was obtained using the proposed U-Net based architecture including the pre-trained VGG16 encoder (Table 1).

Next, we explored the effect of training multi-class segmentation model using different loss functions (Table 2). We demonstrated that small structures such as the clavicles can benefit from weighted loss functions such the Tversky loss function while the larger structures (lung and heart) achieved the best segmentation results using Dice or Binary Cross-Entropy loss functions. Applying additional minor post-processing resulted in further decrease of the MACD measure with cleaner and more precise segmentations for all three structures as displayed in Fig. 3.

Table 3 presents the final comparison between our top selected model, the multi-class U-Net VGG16 with dice loss, to state-of-the-art methods [2–6] and human observer segmentations [6]. Our model outperformed all state-of-the-art methods tested in this study and the human observer for the lungs and heart segmentation. For the clavicles segmentation, fewer studies were conducted. Novikov et al. [2] reported results on different data split than the benchmark recommendation so its not an objective comparison. However, our proposed network outperformed an additional top reported method [6].

In conclusion, we presented an experimental study in which four top segmentation architectures and several losses were compared for the task of segmenting anatomical structures on chest X-Ray images. Results were evaluated quantitatively with qualitative examples of our best performing model. Improving the segmentation of the lung field, heart and clavicles is the foundation for better CAD tools and the development of new applications for medical thoracic images analysis.

References

1. United Nations. Scientific Committee on the Effects of Atomic Radiation. Report of the United Nations Scientific Committee on the Effects of Atomic Radiation: Fifty-sixth Session (10–18 July 2008) (No. 46). United Nations Publications (2008)
2. Novikov, A.A., Lenis, D., Major, D., Hladuvka, J., Wimmer, M., Bühler, K.: Fully convolutional architectures for multiclass segmentation in chest radiographs. IEEE Trans. Med. Imaging **37**(8), 1865–1876 (2018)
3. Hwang, S., Park, S.: Accurate lung segmentation via network-wise training of convolutional networks. In: Cardoso, M.J., et al. (eds.) DLMIA/ML-CDS -2017. LNCS, vol. 10553, pp. 92–99. Springer, Cham (2017). https://doi.org/10.1007/978-3-319-67558-9_11
4. Ibragimov, B., Likar, B., Pernu, F., Vrtovec, T.: Accurate landmark-based segmentation by incorporating landmark misdetections. In: 2016 IEEE 13th International Symposium on Biomedical Imaging (ISBI), pp. 1072–1075. IEEE (2016)
5. Yang, W., et al.: Lung field segmentation in chest radiographs from boundary maps by a structured edge detector. IEEE J. Biomed. Health Inf. **22**(3), 842–851 (2018)

6. Van Ginneken, B., Stegmann, M.B., Loog, M.: Segmentation of anatomical structures in chest radiographs using supervised methods: a comparative study on a public database. Med. Image Anal. **10**(1), 19–40 (2016)
7. Greenspan, H., van Ginneken, B., Summers, R.M.: Guest editorial deep learning in medical imaging: overview and future promise of an exciting new technique. IEEE Trans. Med. Imaging **35**(5), 1153–1159 (2016)
8. Ronneberger, O., Fischer, P., Brox, T.: U-Net: convolutional networks for biomedical image segmentation. In: Navab, N., Hornegger, J., Wells, W.M., Frangi, A.F. (eds.) MICCAI 2015. LNCS, vol. 9351, pp. 234–241. Springer, Cham (2015). https://doi.org/10.1007/978-3-319-24574-4_28
9. Long, J., Shelhamer, E., Darrell, T.: Fully convolutional networks for semantic segmentation. In: Proceedings of the IEEE Conference on Computer Vision and Pattern Recognition, pp. 3431–3440 (2015)
10. Yu, F., Koltun, V., Funkhouser, T.: Dilated residual networks. In: Computer Vision and Pattern Recognition, vol. 1 (2017)
11. Shiraishi, J., et al.: Development of a digital image database for chest radiographs with and without a lung nodule: receiver operating characteristic analysis of radiologists' detection of pulmonary nodules. Am. J. Roentgenol. **174**(1), 71–74 (2000)
12. Simonyan, K., Zisserman, A.: Very deep convolutional networks for large-scale image recognition. arXiv preprint arXiv:1409.1556 (2014)
13. Jgou, S., Drozdzal, M., Vazquez, D., Romero, A., Bengio, Y.: The one hundred layers tiramisu: Fully convolutional densenets for semantic segmentation. In: IEEE Conference on Computer Vision and Pattern Recognition Workshops (CVPRW), pp. 1175–1183. IEEE (2017)
14. Huang, G., Liu, Z., Weinberger, K.Q., van der Maaten, L.: Densely connected convolutional networks. In: Proceedings of the IEEE conference on computer vision and pattern recognition, vol. 1, no. 2, p. 3 (2017)
15. Chen, L.C., Papandreou, G., Kokkinos, I., Murphy, K., Yuille, A.L.: DeepLab: semantic image segmentation with deep convolutional nets, atrous convolution, and fully connected CRFs. IEEE Trans. Pattern Anal. Mach. Intell. **40**(4), 834–848 (2018)
16. He, K., Zhang, X., Ren, S., Sun, J.: Deep residual learning for image recognition. In: Proceedings of the IEEE Conference on Computer Vision and Pattern Recognition, pp. 770–778 (2016)
17. Iglovikov, V., Shvets, A.: TernausNet: U-Net with VGG11 encoder pre-trained on ImageNet for image segmentation. arXiv preprint arXiv:1801.05746 (2018)
18. Deng, J., Dong, W., Socher, R., Li, L.J., Li, K., Fei-Fei, L.: ImageNet: a large-scale hierarchical image database. In: IEEE Conference on Computer Vision and Pattern Recognition, CVPR 2009, pp. 248–255. IEEE (2009)
19. Salehi, S.S.M., Erdogmus, D., Gholipour, A.: Tversky loss function for image segmentation using 3D fully convolutional deep networks. In: Wang, Q., Shi, Y., Suk, H.-I., Suzuki, K. (eds.) MLMI 2017. LNCS, vol. 10541, pp. 379–387. Springer, Cham (2017). https://doi.org/10.1007/978-3-319-67389-9_44

Tuberculosis Histopathology on X Ray CT

Ana Ortega-Gil[1,2(✉)], Arrate Muñoz-Barrutia[1,2],
Laura Fernandez-Terron[1], and Juan José Vaquero[1,2]

[1] Departamento de Bioingeniería e Ingeniería Aeroespacial,
Universidad Carlos III de Madrid, Leganés, Spain
anaorteg@ing.uc3m.es
[2] Instituto de Investigación Sanitaria Gregorio Marañón, Madrid, Spain

Abstract. Cutting-edge translational research on preclinical models of lung infectious diseases, such as Tuberculosis disease uses computed tomography (CT) images for assessing infection burden and drug efficacy over treatment. Biomarkers which characterize the distribution and extent of the disease-associated tissue are commonly based on the analysis of the intensity histogram as the involved tissues present abnormal densities in the organ being diagnosed. Often the cellular composition of the tissue represented by those grey-levels is ignored. Our hypothesis is that an accurate CT segmentation of the disease-associate tissue components could be based on the histopathological analysis of the sample. Drug development studies would then benefit of the efficacy assessment by lesion compartment response. We present here a protocol that allows to segment the healthy parenchyma, foamy macrophages and neutrophil foci in excised lung samples of healthy and tuberculous animal models.

Keywords: Tuberculosis · Micro-CT · X-ray histology · HU segmentation

1 Introduction

The increase of drug-resistant strains of Mycobacterium Tuberculosis (Tb) claims for new effective antibiotic combinations. The selection of compound candidates is speeded up by the use of animal models that accurately reflect the pathological progression of pulmonary tuberculosis [1–3].

The hallmark of tuberculosis is the formation of organized aggregates of immune cells, known as granulomas. In the presence of stimuli, tuberculous granulomas are the host-protective structures formed to contain infection. These containments act as barriers preventing the penetration of chemotherapeutic eradication agents, and also as an incubator for bacillus proliferation.

In granulomas, bacteria are predominantly found evading immune defences: intracellularly, inside macrophages and neutrophils and extracellularly, in interstitial tissue. Necrotizing granulomas present a caseous centre which constitutes the reservoir from which large bacterial numbers emerge. Furthermore, Tb can also provoke an inflammatory response in lung tissue which is subjected to repair, a niche that is often ignored [4, 5].

© Springer Nature Switzerland AG 2018
D. Stoyanov et al. (Eds.): RAMBO 2018/BIA 2018/TIA 2018, LNCS 11040, pp. 169–179, 2018.
https://doi.org/10.1007/978-3-030-00946-5_18

Thus, drug efficacy depends on its ability to reach both their extracellular and intracellular targets, penetrating and permeating complex lung lesion compartments.

The classical bacteriological examination used for human subjects such as the tuberculin skin test or the sputum culture are not available for mouse models. Classically, histopathological tests are performed at significant points during the experiment to estimate the number of viable bacteria or fungal cells in the samples [1, 6–12].

In drug development studies, in vivo low-dose high-resolution micro-CT imaging allows to follow up the advance/recession of the infection in terms of disease tissue extent [13, 14], independently on the type of lesion. Well established biomarkers are based on the intensity thresholding between the healthy and diseased lung parenchyma in thoracic micro-CT scans [6–9, 11, 12, 15]. Among the variety of texture features, the ones based on the grey level co-occurrence matrix (GLCM) [16] are proved to be especially useful in our context [17–20]. The information provided by these biomarkers allows to follow up the host response over time per subject of the experimental protocol, reducing the need of the histopathological evaluation. The strength of longitudinal studies is the deep understanding of the disease mechanisms and the structural changes it causes in the damaged parenchymal tissue.

The nomenclature stablished by CT biomarkers defines the mid-high intensity lung regions as soft diseased tissue and the high intensity lung regions as hard diseased tissue, remarking that the higher the diseased volume, the higher the disease burden (soft and hard). More specifically, the larger the hard volume, the lower responsiveness to treatment [10]. However, the relationship between grey levels and cellular composition of the lesion is not yet defined. We believe that the prognosis information given by those known biomarkers reflects underlying histopathology of the disease. For this reason, in this work, we propose a thresholding protocol which translates the histopathological segmentation to the CT images for the classification of granuloma intensities by their cellular composition. This approach enables the detection and stratification of tuberculosis involvement in micro-CT volumes of excised mouse lungs and opens the door to the assessment of treatment efficacy per granuloma composition.

2 Materials

For this work, we used lungs excised from two females C57BL/6J mice using procedures approved by the Animal Experimentation Ethics Committee of Hospital General Universitario Gregorio Marañón, Madrid, Spain and performed according to EU directive 2010/63/EU and national regulations (RD 53/2013). One was inoculated with the virulent strain of Tb H37Rv at the age of ten weeks. Both subjects were sacrificed eight weeks after the intratracheal insult. At that time, the infected mouse reached the chronic phase of the disease.

The preparation for histology consists on the immersion of the whole organ in paraffin blocks. The tissue was processed for fixation, dehydration, and wax immersion treatment. An iodinated-based staining step was added to the cycle before the wax immersion to enhance the CT contrast of the embedded organs.

When embedded in paraffine and before histology slicing, the two lungs were screened by micro CT scan. A standard micro-CT subsystem of a SuperArgus scanner

(Sedecal Molecular Imaging, Madrid) was used (settings: 68 kV, 420 uA and soft-tissue filtering). We selected a 0.5° step-and-shoot protocol covering 360° and a multi-frame rate of eight frames per gantry position at 20 frames per second. These acquisition parameters lead to a total volume data of 4.27 GB (2.84 MB per frame, 80 frames in total) and a total acquisition time of sixteen minutes. Data-sets were reconstructed using the filtered back-projection (FBP) algorithm and an isotropic voxel resolution of 44 um. The axial CT slices were acquired parallel to the microtome slicing plane.

Once the acquisitions were finished, we processed four infected histological glass slides (from the disease model lung) and one healthy histological glass slide (from the healthy organ) with haematoxylin and eosin (He) stain which adds the contrast for nuclei, cytoplasm and extracellular matrix. The five slides were digitalized using the Aperio CS2 image capture device (Leica Biosystems, Nussloch, Germany) in tiled multi-resolution format. This format is the standard for virtual slides. By default, it is composed by three images of different resolution and each one stored as a separate layer within the image file. For the files on this work, the first layer corresponds to the full resolution image (at 40x magnification and 0.251 microns-per-pixel), the second level to a 25% of the original slide, meaning a 4:1 ratio, and the last level corresponds to a preview image called thumbnail.

3   Methods

The main steps of the proposed algorithm are presented in Fig. 1. The 3D micro-CT volumes and the 2D mid resolution histology images are the input datasets for the registration, annotation and Hounsfield Unit (HU) thresholding steps which result in the cellular segmentation of the micro-CT volume. The dissected Tb-infected mouse lung served as training sample for the protocol in Fig. 1 and the dissected healthy mouse lung served as thresholding testing sample.

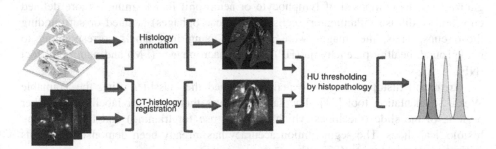

Fig. 1. Thresholding algorithm: The paraffine block with the embedded organ is scanned by CT and then the block is sliced and digitalized. The CT slices are registered with the annotated histology slides. HU-based segmentation is done using the histopathological labelling information.

3.1 Histological Annotation

An He slide (Fig. 2) corresponding to the right upper lobe of the infected animal was used to create and train the classifier of the information concerning lung tissue: healthy alveolar tissue appears as light pink and diseased tissue as dark violet. Other structures such as the airways and tracheal walls appear as the diseased tissue stained with a dark violet colour.

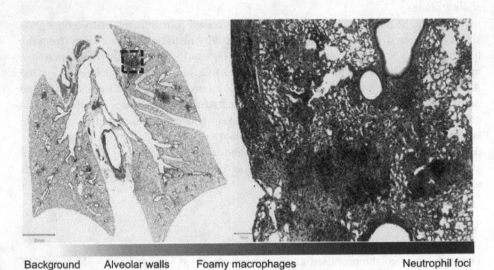

Background   Alveolar walls   Foamy macrophages   Neutrophil foci

Fig. 2. Lung tissue appearance in histological images. Detail of lesions and cells represented by the colour scale in haematoxylin and eosin stain. Scale bars represent 2 mm and 100 um. (Color figure online)

The granulomas from the murine model under study are characterized by unorganized lesions composed of lymphocyte or neutrophil foci forming a more defined cup, and of diffuse inflammatory cells (foamy macrophages) isolated or surrounding those cups. Thus, the images were annotated using four labels corresponding to background, healthy parenchyma (HP), foamy macrophages (FM) and neutrophil foci (NF).

An expert histopathologist created and trained the classifier using the Trainable Weka Segmentation tool [21]. The same tool was then used for labelling the other regions of the slide (the lobes which were not use for training) and the remaining histological slides. The segmentation accuracy has already been demonstrated by its utilization in microscopy [22–28].

3.2 CT-Histology Registration

Owing that the same excised sample has been acquired by CT and by microscopy imaging of the histology preparations, datasets are affine sets even after manipulating the paraffin block. The possible deformations may involve rotations, translations, scaling, and/or shears, which leads us to use the affine registration. By preserving collinearity and ratios of distances, the histological slide is deformed using a gradient descent optimization until the mutual information between it and the reference image is maximized. The mutual information is the similarity measure commonly used for registration of multimodality images and it is the parameter considered for the assessment of the optimum registration.

By finding the micro-CT slice correspondence and the transformation matrix, we can compare the structures and lesion compartments in the 2D histology slide and in the 3D micro-CT slice.

3.3   HU Thresholding by Histopathology

A preliminary slice segmentation based on the CT volume histogram served as basis for the fine threshold determination using the histopathological annotations. This step consisted on the identification of three tuberculosis-related tissue classes by iso-data thresholding: healthy tissue, soft tissue and hard tissue. An extra class is added for the background identification. The segmentation was done according to the classes defined in literature [9, 11, 29] and its main purpose is to delimit the regions of interest to avoid the misclassification induced by noise and image artefacts.

The four CT classes applied to each slice were then registered with their corresponding four histology classes using the previously derived affine transformation (Sect. 3.2). By separating the CT slices into four masks each corresponding to a normal distribution per tissue.

The intersection points of their probability density functions determine the HU thresholds. Radiodensity ranges can then be applied to the 3D CT volumes of the paraffin blocks to stratify the pulmonary tissues.

All methods presented in this section were developed in Matlab (Matlab Inc., Natick, MA, USA).

4   Results

The four histological slides from tuberculosis-infected subjects were classified using WEKA and registered with their corresponding 3D micro-CT slices (Fig. 3). From the four micro-CT slices, the HU tissue masks were extracted and the resulting normal distributions per tissue are shown in Fig. 4. The points of intersections of their probability density function are the micro-CT thresholds. These thresholds were used for the segmentation of the 3D micro-CT volumes, comprising the remaining 75 slices of the Tb-infected mouse lung and the 80 slices of dissected healthy mouse lung.

To evaluate and validate the proposed histopathological thresholding protocol, two metrics were defined: the visual assessment of the resulting segmented volumes for both the infected and the healthy samples, and their quantitative assessment by the Jaccard index, a well-known similarity index.

The diagnostic ground truth used for evaluation is the manual segmentation of the 3D CT volumes by an expert radiologist, who used the intensity segmentation approach described in Gordaliza et al. [29] for evaluating disease burden. Table 1 gives a

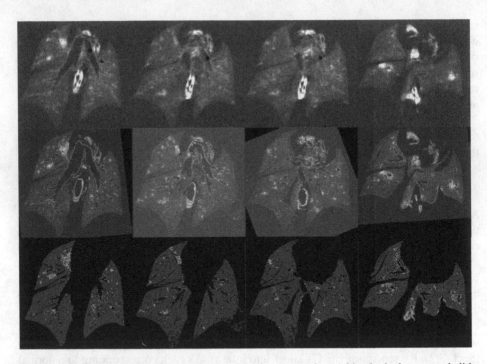

Fig. 3. Registered images: (first row) micro-CT slice, (second row) histological annotated slide registered with the micro-CT and (third row) the composite result with colour code: **Black,** background; **blue,** healthy parenchyma; **green,** foamy macrophages and **red** neutrophil foci. This leads to HU tissue masks guided by histological annotations. Image size 256 × 256 px. (Color figure online)

Table 1. Thresholds for segmentation of 3D micro-CT volumes (HU).

Tissue	Ground truth	Histological thresholding
Healthy parenchyma	$-384 \leq HP < -198$	$-345 \leq HP < -185$
Foamy macrophages	$-198 \leq FM < 157$	$-185 \leq FM < 103$
Neutrophil foci	$157 \leq NF < max$	$103 \leq NF < max$

Table 2. Jaccard indexes between histology-based segmentation and radiologist decision.

Tissue	Healthy organ	TB infected organ
Healthy parenchyma	0,95	0,91
Foamy macrophages	0,75	0,71
Neutrophil foci	0,79	0,73
Total	0,90	0,85

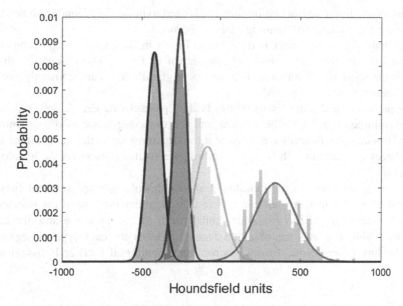

Fig. 4. Histogram per tissue of the CT-histology registered slices (bars) and their derived probability distribution function (curves) of the normal distribution. Labels from the histology annotation have been preserved: **black,** background; **blue,** healthy parenchyma; **green,** foamy macrophages and **red** neutrophil foci. (Color figure online)

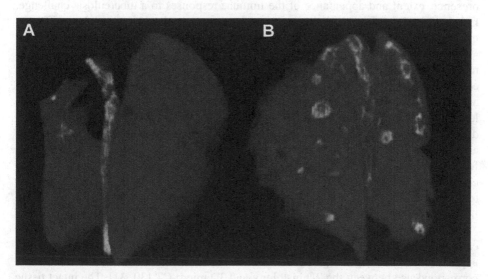

Fig. 5. Composite of the classified 3D micro CT based on the HU distribution of the three tuberculosis-associated tissue volumes in **a,** healthy organ and in **b,** an infected organ. **Black,** background; **blue,** healthy parenchyma; **green,** foamy macrophages and **red** neutrophil foci. (Color figure online)

summary of the tissue segmentation thresholds used to build the ground truth and those computed by the presented histology-based approach.

The qualitative assessment is depicted in Fig. 5 in which the composition of the segmented masks uses the colour scheme shown in Fig. 4. The absence of disease tissue (in the form of inflammatory response or of granulomas) can be visually assessed on the healthy volume (Fig. 5A).

The presence of disease tissue within healthy parenchyma can be assessed on the infected volume (Fig. 5B). The trachea and the oesophagus are also segmented as diseased tissue, since the radiodensities of those structures lay in the same ranges as the macrophages or the neutrophils. This circumstance is also present on the histological annotations.

The similarity between the radiologist and the histology-based segmentation was measured using the Jaccard index, a metric that quantifies the size of the intersection divided by the union of the sets under comparison: the closer to the unit, the higher similarity. Table 2 shows the obtained Jaccard indexes for each type of segmented tissue (healthy parenchyma, foamy macrophages, neutrophil foci) and all segmented tissue.

5 Discussion

Our results confirm that the proposed histopathology on x ray CT provides a satisfactory estimation of the granuloma cellular structure by statistically modelling the HU distribution and by registering the CT with histological slides. The proposed methodology automatically assigns thresholds to 3D micro-CT for revealing the presence, extent and appearance of the immune responses to a tuberculosis challenge. Lobes and tuberculous granulomas were segmented by healthy parenchyma, foamy macrophages (predominant in inflammatory response) and neutrophil foci.

Histological annotations based in intensity have misidentifications owing that multiple tissues are coded with the same colour range. In our case, the characteristic cells composing the walls of collapsed alveoli, trachea and airways are automatically annotated as diseased tissue, both in the 3D micro CT volume and in the 2D histological slide. Spots in the digitalized histology slide due to dust in the lens were also detected by the classifier as diseased tissue. Furthermore, the staining concentration also interferes the classification, preventing the extraction of a global set of thresholds for CT slices or He slides. Approaches worth to explore are those using texture to classify the different cell components on the histological slides and those using histogram equalization strategies to further generalize the HU thresholds for Tb-related tissues.

The correspondence between standard histology and molecular imaging techniques can be estimated using registration techniques tailored for multimodal images. Most approaches rely on rigid registrations (i.e., affine transformation), for the initial slice correspondence between the 2D histology and 3D micro-CT [30, 31]. The intact tissue preservation and the digitalization quality are critical aspects for an optimum registration.

There are multiple image-based procedures which benefit from the 3D/2D registration of the whole organ image volume with histological slides. For example, the correspondence between MRI and histopathology in prostate cancer detection [32, 33]. In this type of cancer, it is generally difficult to differentiate the cancerous and non-cancerous regions directly on the preoperative in vivo MR images and the information that histopathological images offer ease the planning tasks.

It has also been demonstrated that is a good method to compare bone structure measurements performed on micro-CT images and to check that the diagnosis is correct [30, 31]. As far as we know, few results have been presented for soft tissue imaging tasks such as the pulmonary tissue [34–36].

It must also be considered that there is not exact correspondence between the histology image and a slice in the micro-CT. The voxel size of our 2D micro-CT slice is 40 um, meaning that the image is a flat cross-section which integrates all the structures within 40 um depth, whereas the width of the histology samples is 3 um. This may lead to misclassification of lesions or patterns that appear in the histology slide but not in the CT slice. One common event is the edge effect. Edges in histology have high intensity values and sometimes misclassified as neutrophil focus. However, those patterns are not expressed at the micro-CT scale. The limitations mentioned will be addressed in future studies by considering multiple disease models, strains and disease mechanisms, which will extend the robustness and accuracy of the granuloma stratification. We will focus on increasing the sample size of the training dataset with the goal of translating the approach to in-vivo longitudinal studies for a robust prediction of treatment outcome. With such studies, the efficacy of a compound to penetrate any type of lesion can be tested and therefore, the time to find plausible candidates for clinical trials can be reduced.

To conclude, we have proposed a fully automatic method for a virtual histopathological analysis based on the radiodensities of tuberculosis involvement on whole mouse lungs. The statistical model profits from the expert's semiquantitative histopathological annotations. The method has the potential to define the correspondence between the grey-level intensity-based biomarkers and the pathological manifestations of infectious diseases involving any organ.

Acknowledgement. The research leading to these results received funding from the Innovative Medicines Initiative (www.imi.europa.eu) Joint Undertaking under grant agreement no. 115337, whose resources comprise funding from the European Union Seventh Framework Programme (FP7/2007-2013) and EFPIA companies in kind contribution. This work was partially funded by projects RTC-2015-3772-1, TEC2015-73064-EXP and TEC2016-78052-R from the Spanish Ministry of Economy, TOPUS S2013/MIT-3024 project from the regional government of Madrid and by the Department of Health, UK. This study (was supported by the Instituto de Salud Carlos III (Plan Estatal de I+D+i 2013–2016) and cofinanced by the European Social Fund (ESF) "ESF investing in your future". The authors would like to acknowledge Dr. Guembe from CIMA-Universidad de Navarra for preparing and staining the tissue sections and to Dr. Guerrero-Aspizua and Prof. Conti of the Department of Bioengineering, Universidad Carlos III de Madrid for the pathology evaluation.

References

1. Rayner, E.L., et al.: Early lesions following aerosol infection of rhesus macaques (macaca mulata) with mycobacterium tuberculosis strain H37RV. J. Comput. Pathol. **149**(4), 475–485 (2013)
2. Irwin, M.S., et al.: Presence of multiple lesion types with vastly different microenvironments in C3HeB/FeJ mice following aerosol infection with Mycobacterium tuberculosis. Dis. Model Mech. **8**(6), 591–602 (2015)
3. Sharpe, S., et al.: Ultra low dose aerosol challenge with Mycobacterium tuberculosis leads to divergent outcomes in rhesus and cynomolgus macaques. Tuberculosis **96**(Suppl. C), 1–12 (2016)
4. Dartois, V.: The path of anti-tuberculosis drugs: from blood to lesions to mycobacterial cells. Nat. Rev. Microbiol. **12**(3), 159–167 (2014)
5. Pai, M., et al.: Tuberculosis. Nat. Rev. Dis. Prim. **2**, 16076 (2016)
6. Via, L.E., et al.: Infection dynamics and response to chemotherapy in a rabbit model of tuberculosis using [(1)(8)F]2-fluoro-deoxy-D-glucose positron emission tomography and computed tomography. Antimicrob. Agents Chemother. **56**(8), 4391–4402 (2012)
7. Galbán, C.J., et al.: Computed tomography–based biomarker provides unique signature for diagnosis of COPD phenotypes and disease progression. Nat. Med. **18**(11), 1711–1715 (2012)
8. Chen, R.Y., et al.: PET/CT imaging correlates with treatment outcome in patients with multidrug-resistant tuberculosis. Sci. Transl. Med. **6**(265), 166 (2014)
9. Via, L.E., et al.: A sterilizing tuberculosis treatment regimen is associated with faster clearance of bacteria in cavitary lesions in marmosets. Antimicrob. Agents Chemother. **59**(7), 4181–4189 (2015)
10. Volkman, H.E., Pozos, T.C., Zheng, J., Davis, J.M., Rawls, J.F., Ramakrishnan, L.: Tuberculous granuloma induction via interaction of a bacterial secreted protein with host epithelium. Science (80-) **327**(5964), 466–469 (2010)
11. Via, L.E., et al.: Differential virulence and disease progression following mycobacterium tuberculosis complex infection of the common marmoset (callithrix jacchus). Infect. Immun. **81**(8), 2909–2919 (2013)
12. Wallis, R.S., et al.: Tuberculosis biomarkers discovery: developments, needs, and challenges. Lancet Infect. Dis. **13**(4), 362–372 (2013)
13. Nachiappan, A.C., et al.: Pulmonary tuberculosis: role of radiology in diagnosis and management. RadioGraphics **37**(1), 52–72 (2017)
14. Lin, P.L., et al.: Radiologic responses in cynomolgous macaques for assessing tuberculosis chemotherapy regimens. Antimicrob. Agents Chemother. **57**(9), 4237–4244 (2013)
15. Mansoor, A., et al.: Segmentation and image analysis of abnormal lungs at CT: current approaches, challenges, and future trends. RadioGraphics **35**(4), 1056–1076 (2015)
16. Haralick, R.M.: Statistical and structural approaches to texture. Proc. IEEE **67**(5), 786–804 (1979)
17. Mansoor, A., et al.: A generic approach to pathological lung segmentation. IEEE Trans. Med. Imaging **33**(12), 2293–2310 (2014)
18. Artaechevarria, X., et al.: Longitudinal study of a mouse model of chronic pulmonary inflammation using breath hold gated micro-CT. Eur. Radiol. **20**(11), 2600–2608 (2010)
19. Nock, R., Nielsen, F.: Statistical region merging. IEEE Trans. Pattern Anal. Mach. Intell. **26**(11), 1452–1458 (2004)

20. Depeursinge, A., Foncubierta-Rodriguez, A., Van De Ville, D., Müller, H.: Three-dimensional solid texture analysis in biomedical imaging: Review and opportunities. Med. Image Anal. **18**(1), 176–196 (2014)
21. Arganda-Carreras, I., et al.: Trainable Weka Segmentation: a machine learning tool for microscopy pixel classification. Bioinformatics **33**(15), 2424–2426 (2017)
22. Laptev, D., Vezhnevets, A., Dwivedi, S., Buhmann, J.M.: Anisotropic ssTEM image segmentation using dense correspondence across sections, pp. 323–330 (2012)
23. Villa, M.M., Wang, L., Huang, J., Rowe, D.W., Wei, M.: Visualizing osteogenesis in vivo within a cell-scaffold construct for bone tissue engineering using two-photon microscopy. Tissue Eng. Part C. Methods **19**(11), 839–849 (2013)
24. Frank, M., et al.: Mitophagy is triggered by mild oxidative stress in a mitochondrial fission dependent manner. Biochim. Biophys. Acta - Mol. Cell Res. **1823**(12), 2297–2310 (2012)
25. Anuranjeeta, A., Shukla, K.K., Tiwari, A., Sharma, S.: Classification of histopathological images of breast cancerous and non cancerous cells based on morphological features. Biomed. Pharmacol. J. **10**(1), 353–366 (2017)
26. Wollatz, L., Johnston, S.J., Lackie, P.M., Cox, S.J.: 3D Histopathology—a lung tissue segmentation workflow for microfocus x-ray-computed tomography scans. J. Digit. Imaging **30**(6), 772–781 (2017)
27. Zhan, L., Tang, J., Sun, M., Qin, C.: Animal models for tuberculosis in translational and precision medicine. Front. Microbiol. **8**, 717 (2017)
28. Meng, T., Lin, L., Shyu, M.-L., Chen, S.-C.: Histology image classification using supervised classification and multimodal fusion. In: 2010 IEEE International Symposium on Multimedia, pp. 145–152 (2010)
29. Gordaliza, P.M., Muñoz-Barrutia, A., Via, L.E., Sharpe, S., Desco, M., Vaquero, J.J.: Computed tomography-based biomarker for longitudinal assessment of disease burden in pulmonary tuberculosis. Mol. Imaging Biol. 1–6 (2018)
30. Thomsen, J.S., Laib, A., Koller, B., Prohaska, S., Mosekilde, L., Gowin, W.: Stereological measures of trabecular bone structure: comparison of 3D micro computed tomography with 2D histological sections in human proximal tibial bone biopsies. J. Microsc. **218**(2), 171–179 (2005)
31. Particelli, F., Mecozzi, L., Beraudi, A., Montesi, M., Baruffaldi, F., Viceconti, F.: A comparison between micro-CT and histology for the evaluation of cortical bone: effect of polymethylmethacrylate embedding on structural parameters. J. Microsc. **245**(3), 302–310 (2012)
32. Xiao, G., et al.: Determining histology-MRI slice correspondences for defining MRI-based disease signatures of prostate cancer. Comput. Med. Imaging Graph. **35**, 568–578 (2010)
33. Bart, S., et al.: MRI-histology registration in prostate cancer. In: Proceedings of Surgetica, pp. 361–367 (2005)
34. Dullin, C., et al.: μCT of ex-vivo stained mouse hearts and embryos enables a precise match between 3D virtual histology, classical histology and immunochemistry. PLoS ONE **12**(2), 1–15 (2017)
35. Kak Slaney, M.A.C., et al.: Optimized murine lung preparation for detailed structural evaluation via micro-computed tomography. J. Appl. Phys. **12**(3), 466–469 (2015)
36. Johnson, C., et al.: 3D human lung histology reconstruction and registration to in vivo imaging. In: Medical Imaging 2018: Digital Pathology, vol. 10581, p. 30 (2018)

A CT Scan Harmonization Technique
to Detect Emphysema and Small
Airway Diseases

Gonzalo Vegas-Sánchez-Ferrero[⊠] and Raúl San José Estépar

Applied Chest Imaging Laboratory (ACIL), Brigham and Women's Hospital,
Harvard Medical School, Boston, MA, USA
{gvegas,rsanjose}@bwh.harvard.edu

Abstract. Recent studies have suggested the central role of small airway
destruction in the pathogenesis of COPD leading to further parenchymal
destruction. This evidence has sparked the interest in in-vivo assessment
of small airway disease overall at the early onset of the disease. The
parametric response mapping (PRM) technique has been proposed to
distinguish gas trapping due to small airway disease from low attenuation
areas due to emphysema. Despite its success, the PRM technique shows
some limitations that are precluding the interpretation of its results.
The density value used to assess gas trapping highly depends on acquisition parameters, such as dose and reconstruction kernel, and changes in
body size, that introduce inhomogeneous photon absorption patterns. In
particular, many studies using PRM employ inspiratory and expiratory
images that are obtained at different dose levels. Emphysema impact in
early disease may be confounded with the gas trapping due to the noise
introduced by differences in the acquisition during the PRM. In this
work, we propose a CT harmonization technique to remove the nuisance
factors to distinguish between small airway disease and emphysema. Our
results show that the measurements based on CT harmonization provide
an increase in the detection of both emphysema and airway disease,
resulting in a statistically significant impact of both components and a
better association with lung function measures.

Keywords: CT scans · Emphysema · Lung disease
Statistical characterization

1 Introduction

Chronic Obstructive Pulmonary Disease (COPD) is a complex syndrome with
widely varying clinical and imaging characteristics. The chronic airflow limitation of COPD is caused by a mixture of small airway disease and parenchymal

This study was supported by the National Institutes of Health NHLBI awards
R01HL116931, R01HL116473 and R21HL140422.

D. Stoyanov et al. (Eds.): RAMBO 2018/BIA 2018/TIA 2018, LNCS 11040, pp. 180–190, 2018.
https://doi.org/10.1007/978-3-030-00946-5_19

destruction (emphysema). COPD is a major cause of morbidity and mortality. Despite declines in smoking, mortality from COPD continues to increase and is now the third leading cause of death in the US. Recent studies have suggested that the central role of small airway disease in the pathogenesis of COPD leads to additional parenchymal destruction [1]. This evidence has sparked the interest in in-vivo assessment of small airway disease overall at the early onset of the disease.

Computed Tomography (CT) is the main imaging modality for thoracic conditions due to its high tissue-air contrast. CT has been proven to be effective in the quantification of emphysema [2]. However, direct measurements of the dimensions of small airways using CT scanning is beyond current imaging resolution [3]. One option to indirectly assess the effects of smaller airways is to quantify gas trapping by measuring the percent of voxels in the lung lower than -856 Hounsfield Units (HU) on an expiratory CT scan [4]. A technique named Parametric Response Mapping (PRM) has been proposed to distinguish gas trapping due to small airway disease from low attenuation areas due to emphysema [5]. The technique employs both inspiratory and expiratory CT scans. After the co-registration of both images and the application of established CT density thresholds, one can distinguish between functional small airway disease (FSAD) and emphysema.

The COPD imaging community has extensively used PRM since its introduction. However, despite its success, the PRM technique shows some limitations that are precluding the interpretation of its results. The density value used to assess gas trapping highly depends on acquisition parameters, such as dose and reconstruction kernel, and changes in body size, that introduce inhomogeneous photon absorption patterns. In particular, many studies using PRM employ inspiratory and expiratory images that are obtained at different dose levels and introduce a spatially variant noise and bias across the image [6]. These effects are nuisance factors that affect the inter-scanner and inter-subject variability in CT density and confounds CT-derived metrics by PRM. As an example, Fig. 1 shows the expiratory and inspiratory scans of the same subject and the local

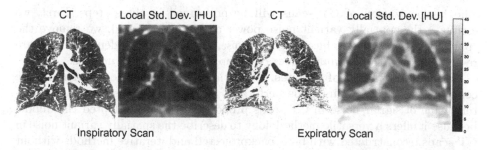

Fig. 1. Inspiratory and expiratory scans used for PRM analysis. Note that the noise variance remarkably increases in the expiratory scan due to the lower dose applied. Additionally, the noise changes across the image affecting the PRM analysis.

standard deviation in each image. Note that the noise changes across the image and that the expiratory scan shows a higher variance of noise due to the lower dose applied.

Researchers are aware of the importance of these nuisance factors and much effort has been done in reducing the spatially variant noise for both iterative and back projection reconstruction techniques [7,8]. Spatial discrepancies in the attenuation levels have been largely observed in clinical studies, especially for air [9]. Some approaches using anatomical references like trachea and aorta densities have been proposed with promising results [9–11]. The inter-scanner deviations due to calibration are also an important factor that has been studied in [12].

A recent PRM study has successfully associated functional respiratory decline with FSAD in the mild-moderate stage of COPD [13]. Surprisingly, the emphysema in this early stage has no effect. The detection of FSAD has been useful in the early detection of rapid lung function decline. However, if the mentioned nuisance factors that affect the interpretation of PRM are precluding the distinction between FSAD and emphysema, we could be losing valuable information about the emphysema and FSAD interplay that can help identify trajectories of rapid decline.

In this work, we propose a harmonization methodology that simultaneously minimizes the spatially variant noise and biases. We employ the harmonization in both inspiratory and expiratory scans for the PRM analysis. Results show that our technique is able to detect the impact of both emphysema and airway disease in contrast to other reference methods used to palliate the effect of noise. Correlation analyses with lung function show a better fit with the harmonized data that cannot be achieved with other conventional noise reduction methodologies. This result evidences the importance of scan harmonization for clinical data and shows that the role of emphysema is still significant in early disease and can be distinguished from FSAD.

2   Harmonization of CT Scans

The harmonization of CT scans will be performed in three steps. First, we estimate the spatially variant noise power and signal. Second, we remove the spatially variant bias induced by the noise, and finally the density levels are re-calibrated to the nominal values of apparent anatomical structures.

Characterization of Tissues. The estimation of both the signal and noise components of the CT image is performed by adopting the statistical characterization of signal/noise in CT scans proposed in [8]. We adopted this model because it offers a versatile methodology to describe the spatially variant noise in CT scans reconstructed with both backprojected and iterative methods without the need of sinograms or any interaction with the reconstruction method.

This model consists in a non-central Gamma distribution (nc-Γ) for each voxel $X(r)$ of the image:

$$f_X(x|\alpha, \beta, \delta) = \frac{(x-\delta)^{\alpha-1}}{\beta^\alpha \Gamma(\alpha)} e^{-\frac{x-\delta}{\beta}}, \qquad x \geq \delta \text{ and } \alpha, \beta > 0 \qquad (1)$$

where α, β are the spatially variant shape, scale parameters; and δ is location parameter usually set to the minimum value of the CT scan (usually -1024 HU).

The heterogeneous nature of lung parenchyma is effectively described by means of a mixture model of nc-Γ distributions:

$$p(x(r)) = \sum_{j=1}^{J} \pi_j(r) f_X(x(r)|\alpha_j(r), \beta_j(r), \delta) \qquad (2)$$

for J components, where π_j are the weights of the mixture and α_j, β_j the parameters of each component. To ensure that the heterogeneous composition of the lung is properly described in the mixture model, we set $J = 9$ components from -1000 to 400 HU. This is a reasonable range of attenuations considering that the normal lung attenuation is between -600 and -700 HU, and also allows us to model other tissues within the CT image such as vasculature, muscle, fat or bone.

The estimation of the parameters for each component is achieved through the Expectation-Maximization method for known mean values for each component, $\{\mu_j\}_{j=1}^{J}$, which reduces the problem to solve a non-linear equation in each iteration at each location. The estimation of the shape parameters for each component, α_j, are obtained for each location r by solving the following non-linear equation derived from the maximum likelihood estimation in the local neighborhood $\eta(r)$ (see [8] for more details):

$$\log(\alpha_j(r)) - \psi(\alpha_j(r)) = \frac{\sum\limits_{s \in \eta(r)} \gamma_j(s) \frac{x_i(s) - \delta}{\mu_j}}{\sum\limits_{s \in \eta(r)} \gamma_j(s)} - \frac{\sum\limits_{s \in \eta(r)}^{N} \gamma_j(s) \log\left(\frac{x_i(s) - \delta}{\mu_j}\right)}{\sum\limits_{s \in \eta(r)} \gamma_j(s)} - 1 \quad (3)$$

with $\psi(\cdot) = \Gamma'(x)/\Gamma(x)$ being the digamma function, and $\gamma_j(r) = P(j|x(r))$ are the posterior probabilities for the j-th tissue class at location r:

$$\gamma_j(r) = \frac{\pi_j(r) f_X(x(r)|\alpha_j(r), \beta_j(r), \delta)}{\sum_{k=1}^{J} \pi_k(r) f_X(x(r)|\alpha_k(r), \beta_k(r), \delta)}. \qquad (4)$$

Then, the scale factor is calculated as $\beta_j = \mu_j/\alpha_j$ and the priors π_j are updated as $\pi_j = \frac{1}{N} \sum_{i=1}^{N} \gamma_{i,j}$.

Equations (3 and 4) are iteratively applied until convergence is reached. This convergence is usually achieved in very few iterations due to the constraint imposed by the mean $\{\mu_j\}_{j=1}^{J}$ for each tissue. A suitable initialization of parameters for the iterative optimization is $\pi_j = 1/J$, $\alpha_j = 2$ and $\beta_j = \mu_j/\alpha_j$ for each component.

Estimation of the Signal and Local Variance of Noise. The characterization of tissues allows us to calculate the sample conditioned moments to each tissue class as follows:

$$\langle X^k(\mathbf{r})|j\rangle = \frac{\sum_{\mathbf{s}\in\eta(\mathbf{r})} x(\mathbf{s})^k \gamma_j(\mathbf{s})}{\sum_{\mathbf{s}\in\eta(\mathbf{r})} \gamma_j(\mathbf{s})}. \tag{5}$$

This formulation provides a more robust estimate of conditioned local moments since it just considers the samples belonging to the j-th tissue class.

Finally, the moments for each location can be calculated as the weighted average of the conditioned moments as:

$$E\{X(\mathbf{r})^k\} = \sum_{j=1}^{J} \pi_j(\mathbf{r})E\{X(\mathbf{r})^k|j\} \approx \sum_{j=1}^{J} \pi_j(\mathbf{r})\langle X(\mathbf{r})^k|j\rangle. \tag{6}$$

Correction of Spatially Variant Bias. The estimation of the local mean $E\{X(\mathbf{r})\}$ and local variance of noise $\hat{\sigma}^2(\mathbf{r}) = E\{X^2(\mathbf{r})\} - E\{X(\mathbf{r})\}^2$ allow us to remove any bias derived from the noise. This bias has been previously reported in the literature [9–11]. As an example of this effect, in Fig. 2a we show the linear dependence between local mean and local variance.

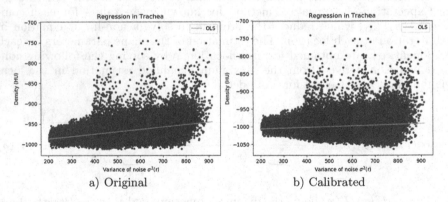

a) Original   b) Calibrated

Fig. 2. Linear regression between local mean and local variance in the trachea before and after calibration.

This dependence is corrected by estimating the linear coefficient of the ordinary least squares (OLS) linear regression, β, in the trachea. This coefficient decreases as the tissue becomes denser as a consequence of the more symmetric distribution of tissues with higher attenuation value than the lung (blood, fat, bone).

One of the advantages of adopting the noise model of Eq. 2 is that there is a functional relationship between the linear coefficient and the CT number: $\beta(\mu) = K/(\mu - \delta)$, where μ is the attenuation coefficient and K is a constant to be determined [11]. In this work, we take advantage of the linear regression in the trachea to determine K. This way, the linear coefficient becomes:

$$\beta(\mu) = \begin{cases} \beta_{\text{trachea}} \dfrac{\mu_{\text{trachea}} - \delta}{\mu - \delta} & \text{if } \mu > \mu_{\text{trachea}} \\ \beta_{\text{trachea}} & \text{if } \mu \le \mu_{\text{trachea}} \end{cases} \tag{7}$$

where μ_{trachea} is the mean value of samples in the trachea. Now, the spatially variant bias can be removed as follows:

$$\widetilde{X}(r) = E\{X(r)\} - \beta\left(E\{X(r)\}\right)\widehat{\sigma}^2(r) \tag{8}$$

It is important to note that a systematic bias still can be present in the image since Eq. (8) removes the linear relationship with the local variance, but not the intercept. We remove the intercept by adjusting the mean values to the nominal densities of tissues in anatomical references. The most evident structures are the descending aorta, (Ω_{aorta}), where the blood attenuation level $(\mu_{\text{blood}} = 50$ HU) is usually adopted [10]; and the trachea, $(\Omega_{\text{trachea}})$, where the air is set to $\mu_{\text{air}} = -1000$ HU by definition. Then, the harmonized image is obtained by linear interpolation for those attenuation levels:

$$\widehat{X}(r) = (1 - \lambda(r))\mu_{\text{air}} + \lambda(r)\mu_{\text{blood}}; \text{ with } \lambda(r) = \frac{\widetilde{X}(r) - E\left\{\widetilde{X}(r)|\Omega_{\text{trachea}}\right\}}{E\left\{\widetilde{X}(r)|\Omega_{\text{aorta}}\right\} - E\left\{\widetilde{X}(r)|\Omega_{\text{trachea}}\right\}} \tag{9}$$

We show in Fig. 2b the effect of harmonization in the trachea. Note that the linear relationship between the variance of noise and the attenuation level is effectively removed by Eq. (8). Additionally, the intercept is also corrected to the nominal value for air (-1000 HU).

3   Experiments and Results

The PRM study was performed in a set of 48 inspiratory and expiratory scan pairs acquired in the same session from subjects with diagnosed COPD with a range of severity levels. 5 Different devices from 2 different manufacturers were used: GE VCT-64, Siemens Definition Flash, Siemens Definition, Siemens Sensation-64, and Siemens Definition AS+. The doses for the inspiratory and expiratory scans were 200 mAs and 50 mAS respectively in all the acquisitions. Expiratory scans are typically done at a lower dose to reduce total radiation exposure resulting in an increased image noise. The discrepancy in doses implies that different responses in the spatial noise variance and biases (as in Fig. 1).

The assessment of the harmonization technique here proposed was performed by comparing its performance to other reference methods that are commonly used to reduce the effects of noise in medical imaging. We considered the median filter and the non-local means filter as the reference methods for comparison. The median filter has been widely used in the CT imaging community for denoising purposes due to the little assumptions about the underlying noise model [14]. We used two median filters with $3 \times 3 \times 3$ (Median1) and $5 \times 5 \times 5$ (Median2) voxels window respectively. We also chose the non-local means filter (NLM) since it has shown to be an effective filtering technique in multiple modalities [15]. We use the implementation presented in [16] because of its efficiency for 3D volumes. The main parameter of this approach is the noise power. To perform a fair comparison, we estimated the noise power for each case using the same approach that we used in the CT harmonization. After filtering the image with our approach and the reference methods, we computed the percentage of emphysema (Emph%) and FSAD (FSAD%) using the same PRM technique for all the methods (we applied the -950 HU and -856 HU thresholds for inspiratory and expiratory scans as suggested in [5]).

Comparison Between Methods. We performed a population analysis of the difference of emphysema% and FSAD% across the different methods comparing means and concordance between methods. Figure 3a–b show the distributions of emphysema% and FSAD%, where our approach yields a mean score statistically higher to the other methods in pairwise comparisons using Dunn's method for joint ranking (p-value $< 10^{-4}$). The reference methods do not show significant differences among them or even with respect to the original. This discrepancy between the harmonized data with respect to the reference methods and the original image is due to the better detection of emphysema and FSAD. This can be easily confirmed by visual inspection in Fig. 3c–d, where the PRM analysis of a subject with an evident emphysema region is represented for the original and

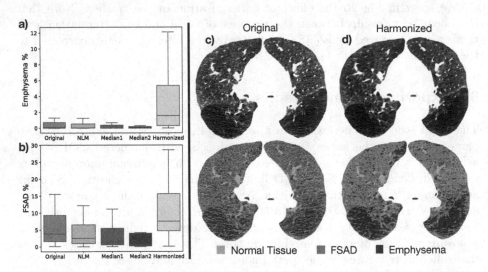

Fig. 3. Left: Distribution of Emph% (a) and FSAD% (b) in the analyzed population across filtering methods. The proposed harmonization approach increased the ability to resolve more emphysema and small airway disease. Right: PRM analysis for the inspiratory scans; original (c) and harmonized (d).

harmonized data. Note that the PRM overestimates the normal tissue because of the noise influence. Conversely, the harmonization mitigates the noise effect in regions of parenchyma and massive emphysema which, in turn, leads to a more accurate measure of emphysema and FSAD. This result suggests that a reduction of noise with the methods available in the literature does not provide a statistically significant difference with the original image when measuring FSAD or emphysema. To confirm this fact, we performed a concordance analysis using the so-called *Concordance Correlation Coefficient* (CCC) proposed by Lin [17], a widely accepted index of agreement in settings with different raters. This measure assumes a positive correlation between raters, is bounded in $[0, 1]$, and considers low concordance for values under 0.9 [18]. In Table 1, we show the concordance results obtained for the emphysema (lower diagonal) and FSAD (upper diagonal). We highlighted values under 0.9 of concordance to enhance the methods that can provide further information compared to the original image. Note that all of the reference methods show an almost exact concordance with the original image and among them. This implies that all the reference methods do not provide further information compared to the original image. The harmonized data, however, shows a lower concordance, suggesting that the emphysema and FSAD description can be improved. Indeed, in the next section, we demonstrate that the harmonized data allows us to distinguish better the interplay between FSAD and emphysema that leads to a better description of functional respiratory outcomes.

Table 1. Concordance correlation coefficients for the PRM metrics: Emphysema% (lower diagonal) and FSAD% (upper diagonal). Low concordance (<0.9) is highlighted with bold letters. The low concordance for emphysema and FSAD of the harmonized image shows that the harmonized data is the only one providing different information about FSAD and emphysema from the one obtained in the original image.

	Original	NLM	Median1	Median2	Harmonized
Original	-	0.99	0.98	0.96	**0.84**
NLM	1.00	-	1.00	0.98	**0.80**
Median1	1.00	1.00	-	1.00	**0.77**
Median2	0.99	1.00	1.00	-	**0.72**
Harmonized	**0.88**	**0.86**	**0.85**	**0.83**	-

Physiological Validation. The common histological references for emphysema and small airway disease are the mean linear intercept and the airway counting approach [1]. However, when histological approaches are not available, indirect functional measures must be used. An indirect validation is usually performed by evaluating the ability of the measurements obtained with each approach to ascertain the physiological response to emphysema and small airway disease. Both processes imply a reduction in lung function due to airway collapse (emphysema) and increase airway resistance (small airway disease) that can be assessed

Table 2. Linear regression analysis for the FEV1% with respect to the amount of emphysema (Emph%) and small airway disease (FSAD%).

	Original $R^2 = 0.51$		NLM $R^2 = 0.50$		Median1 $R^2 = 0.47$		Median2 $R^2 = 0.45$		Harmonized $R^2 = 0.54$	
	Beta	p-value	Beta	p-value	Beta	p-value	Beta	p-value	Beta	p-value
Emph%	0.03	0.95	0.08	0.88	0.03	0.94	0.07	0.89	**-0.72**	<0.001
FSAD%	**-1.93**	<0.001	**-1.88**	<0.001	**-1.73**	<0.001	**-1.63**	<0.001	**-1.19**	<0.001

by the Force Expiratory Volume in 1-second percent predicted (FEV1%). We show in Table 2 the results of the multivariate linear models that relate Emph% and FSAD% to FEV1% for each method. Note that the reference methods obtain the same outcome as the one obtained with the original image: a significant effect of FSAD% in the FEV1%. However, note also that the explained variance is lower for all the reference cases. This result shows that the commonly used noise reduction methods do not provide a better description of FSAD and emphysema interplay. On the other hand, the harmonization improves the explained variance from 51% to 54%, showing that the harmonized data contributes to model the lung function better than the original image and any reference method. Furthermore, with the harmonization, the emphysema becomes statistically significant, showing a negative relationship of the emphysema ratio with the lung function. This result is consistent with the natural progression of COPD: "the function declines as both the emphysema and FSAD ratios increase," and exhibits the importance of the proposed harmonization technique in distinguishing FSAD and emphysema.

4   Conclusion

We have presented a harmonization technique to deal with non-stationary noise and bias in chest CT scans. Our approach rests on a mixture model that describes the local statistics of the CT signal. The model is used to stabilize the noise and generate a stationary process. Then, the spatially varying bias induced by noise is corrected by removing the linear dependence between the signal and the noise variance. Finally, the systematic bias is removed by adjusting with trachea and aorta reference levels. This approach was used in the quantification of both emphysema and small airway disease using the PRM methodology. This is an ideal problem to illustrate our approach as it deals with information from two images acquired at inspiration and expiration with different noise characteristics due to acquisition and lung volume differences. The assessment is performed through a population study of 48 subjects acquired from different scanners and manufacturers. Comparisons with other reference methods show that the CT harmonization provides a significant increase in the detection of both emphysema and airway disease when compared to the original image or the reference methods. This increase results in a better distinction between emphysema and airway disease that cannot be achieved with the PRM analysis in the original image or the image filtered with the reference methods, as the concordance analysis confirmed. Additionally, the better distinction between emphysema and airway disease significantly increases the correlation with functional metrics of airway obstruction suggesting that our approach is better empowered to measure biomarkers that better reflect the disease pathophysiology.

References

1. Hogg, J.C., et al.: The nature of small-airway obstruction in chronic obstructive pulmonary disease. New Engl. J. Med. **350**(26), 2645–2653 (2004)
2. Müller, N.L., Staples, C.A., Miller, R.R., Abboud, R.T.: Density mask. An objective method to quantitate emphysema using computed tomography. Chest **94**(4), 782–787 (1988)
3. Coxson, H.O., Mayo, J., Lam, S., Santyr, G., Parraga, G., Sin, D.D.: New and current clinical imaging techniques to study chronic obstructive pulmonary disease. Am. J. Respir. Crit. Care Med. **180**(7), 588–597 (2009)
4. Matsuoka, S., Kurihara, Y., Yagihashi, K., Hoshino, M., Watanabe, N., Nakajima, Y.: Quantitative assessment of air trapping in chronic obstructive pulmonary disease using inspiratory and expiratory volumetric MDCT. Am. J. Roentgenol. **190**(3), 762–769 (2008)
5. Galbán, C.J., et al.: Computed tomography-based biomarker provides unique signature for diagnosis of COPD phenotypes and disease progression. Nature Med. **18**(11), 1711–5 (2012)
6. Vaishnav, J.Y., Jung, W.C., Popescu, L.M., Zeng, R., Myers, K.J.: Objective assessment of image quality and dose reduction in CT iterative reconstruction. Med. Phys. **41**(7), 071904 (2014)
7. Kim, J.H., Chang, Y., Ra, J.B.: Denoising of polychromatic CT images based on their own noise properties. Med. Phys. **43**(5), 2251–2260 (2016)
8. Vegas-Sánchez-Ferrero, G., Ledesma-Carbayo, M.J., Washko, G.R., San José Estépar, R.: Statistical characterization of noise for spatial standardization of CT scans: enabling comparison with multiple kernels and doses. Med. Image Anal. **40**, 44–59 (2017)
9. Choi, S., Hoffman, E.A., Wenzel, S.E., Castro, M., Lin, C.L.: Improved CT-based estimate of pulmonary gas trapping accounting for scanner and lung-volume variations in a multicenter asthmatic study. J. Appl. Physiol. **117**(6), 593–603 (2014)
10. Kim, S.S., et al.: Improved correlation between CT emphysema quantification and pulmonary function test by density correction of volumetric CT data based on air and aortic density. Eur. J. Radiol. **83**(1), 57–63 (2014)
11. Vegas-Sánchez-Ferrero, G., Ledesma-Carbayo, M.J., Washko, G.R., Estépar, R.S.J.: Autocalibration method for non-stationary CT bias correction. Med. Image Anal. **44**, 115–125 (2018)
12. Chen-Mayer, H.H., et al.: Standardizing CT lung density measure across scanner manufacturers. Med. Phys. **44**(3), 974–985 (2017)
13. Bhatt, S.P.: Association between functional small airway disease and FEV 1 decline in chronic obstructive pulmonary disease. Am. J. Respir. Crit. Care Med. **194**(2), 178–184 (2016)
14. Hilts, M., Duzenli, C.: Image filtering for improved dose resolution in CT polymer gel dosimetry. Med. Phys. **31**(1), 39–49 (2004)

15. Li, Z., et al.: Adaptive nonlocal means filtering based on local noise level for CT denoising. Med. Phys. **41**(1), 011908 (2013)
16. Tristán-Vega, A., García-Pérez, V., Aja-Fernández, S., Westin, C.F.: Efficient and robust nonlocal means denoising of MR data based on salient features matching. Comput. Methods Progr. Biomed. **105**(2), 131–144 (2012)
17. Lin, LIk: A concordance correlation coefficient to evaluate reproducibility. Biometrics **45**(1), 255 (1989)
18. McBride, G.: A proposal for strength-of-agreement criteria for Lin's concordance correlation coefficient. NIWA Client Rep. **45**(1), 307–310 (2005)

Transfer Learning for Segmentation of Injured Lungs Using Coarse-to-Fine Convolutional Neural Networks

Sarah E. Gerard[1], Jacob Herrmann[1,2], David W. Kaczka[1,2,3], and Joseph M. Reinhardt[1,3(✉)]

[1] Department of Biomedical Engineering, The University of Iowa,
Iowa City, IA 52242, USA
sarah-gerard@uiowa.edu
[2] Department of Anesthesia, The University of Iowa, Iowa City, IA 52242, USA
[3] Department of Radiology, The University of Iowa, Iowa City, IA 52242, USA
joe-reinhardt@uiowa.edu

Abstract. Deep learning using convolutional neural networks (ConvNets) achieves high accuracy across many computer vision tasks, with the ability to learn multi-scale features and generalize across a variety of input data. In this work, we propose a deep learning framework that utilizes a coarse-to-fine cascade of 3D ConvNet models for segmentation of lung structures obtained from computed tomographic (CT) images. Deep learning requires a large number of training datasets, which may be challenging in medical imaging, especially for rare diseases. In the present study, transfer learning is utilized for lung segmentation of CT scans in large animal models of the acute respiratory distress syndrome (ARDS) using only 13 subjects. The method was quantitatively evaluated on a human dataset, consisting of 395 3D CT scans from 153 subjects, and an animal dataset consisting of 148 3D CT images from 5 porcine subjects. The human dataset achieved an average Jacaard index of 0.99, and an average symmetric surface distance (ASSD) of 0.29 mm. The animal dataset had an average Jacaard index of 0.94, and an ASSD of 0.99 mm.

Keywords: Segmentation · Computed tomography · Deep learning

1 Introduction

Segmentation of lungs in pulmonary computed tomographic (CT) images is an important precursor for characterizing and quantifying disease patterns, regional functional analysis, and determining treatment interventions. With the increasing resolution and quantity of scans, automatic and reliable lung segmentation is essential to support efficient image analyses. Several methods have been proposed for automatic lung segmentation in thoracic CT images. Intensity-based methods [1,2] are simple and effective for segmentation of healthy lung parenchymal tissue. However, these methods fail to include dense pathological alterations

© Springer Nature Switzerland AG 2018
D. Stoyanov et al. (Eds.): RAMBO 2018/BIA 2018/TIA 2018, LNCS 11040, pp. 191–201, 2018.
https://doi.org/10.1007/978-3-030-00946-5_20

such as fibrosis, edema, or tumors. Additionally, artifacts from pacemakers, stents, central intravenous catheters, or air in the intestines may pose additional challenges for intensity-based methods. More sophisticated methods have incorporated prior shape information in the form of statistical shape models [3] or anatomical atlases [4,5].

More recently, deep learning using convolutional neural network (ConvNet) models has been successfully used for accurate image segmentation across many domains in computer vision [6,7]. A major barrier for deploying deep learning in medical imaging is the high memory demand for the volumetric images and the limited memory in current GPUs that are used for training. Recent studies have investigated the use of ConvNets for lung segmentation in CT images [8,9]. However, these methods involve training ConvNets on 2D slices, which do not incorporate 3D features or other global information. Another major barrier for using deep learning is the availability of labeled training datasets, which may be challenging for medical images as they require expert annotation. Transfer learning is an effective technique in medical imaging of pathologies for which limited labeled training data is available. Here, a learnable model is pre-trained on an extensive dataset from a different problem domain, and then fine-tuned with a limited targeted-domain dataset [10].

In this study, we used a deep learning approach to train a ConvNet model for segmentation of lungs in a large animal model of the acute respiratory distress syndrome (ARDS), using a limited training dataset. ARDS is radiographically characterized by diffuse opacification, producing regions with little or no contrast near the boundary between the lung parenchyma and surrounding mediastinal and chest wall structures [11]. Furthermore, parenchymal consolidation has no distinguishable textural patterns compared to surrounding soft tissue. This makes the segmentation of images depicting ARDS lungs a challenging task, even for manual segmentation by trained operators, resulting in very limited availability of training datasets. We propose a novel coarse-to-fine model consisting of two cascaded 3D ConvNets, which enables learning of both global context and high-resolution features in 3D images. The model is pre-trained on a dataset of human subjects, and then fine-tuned on a small dataset of animal subjects with lung injury mimicking ARDS.

2   Methods

2.1   Image Datasets

A ConvNet model was trained for segmentation of thoracic CT images, using annotated training data from human and animal subjects. The pre-training dataset consisted of 1604 human subjects with chronic obstructive pulmonary disease (COPD), and 152 human subjects with idiopathic pulmonary fibrosis (IPF). Human data were acquired from the COPDGene [12] and SPIROMICS [13] clinical trials. The fine-tuning dataset consisted of 9 canine and 4 porcine subjects with an experimental model of ARDS, each scanned under baseline and injured conditions at various static airway pressures.

We evaluate the performance of the proposed method on human and animal datasets which were not included in training. The human evaluation dataset consisted of 107 subjects with COPD, and 38 subjects with IPF. The animal evaluation dataset consisted of porcine subjects with an experimental lung injury model exhibiting structural derangements similar to ARDS. These subjects were dynamically scanned during mechanical ventilation, producing 4D CT images with high temporal resolution [14]. In total, 148 3D CT images from 5 porcine subjects were included in the animal evaluation dataset.

The ground truth lung segmentations for the human datasets were generated using an intensity-based method [2], followed by manual inspection and correction by an experienced human analyst. The ground truth lung segmentations for the animal datasets were manually delineated by experienced image analysts.

2.2 Convolutional Neural Network

The ConvNet architecture used in this work is a 3D fully convolutional neural network (FCN) [15] called Seg3DNet (Fig. 1) [16]. Seg3DNet consists of an encoder which learns a multi-scale feature representation, and a decoder which combines the multi-scale information through learnable upsampling operations. Seg3DNet has similar properties as U-Net [17]. However, Seg3DNet is extended to 3D and the decoder is less memory-intensive to accommodate 3D convolutions and larger input volumes. The output of Seg3DNet is a probability map with the same resolution as the input image, estimating the probability that a given voxel is contained within the lung.

2.3 Coarse-to-Fine Model

A coarse-to-fine model is used to accommodate learning on large 3D images without having to sacrifice global information for high spatial resolution. Two Seg3DNets are trained in sequence: a low-resolution network (Seg3DNet-LR), and a high-resolution network (Seg3DNet-HR). Seg3DNet-LR is trained with aggressively downsampled images, to facilitate the learning of global lung features. Seg3DNet-HR is trained with high-resolution images to learn precise parenchymal boundary information.

Seg3DNet-LR is trained using images that were downsampled to $64 \times 64 \times 64$ voxels, corresponding to a downsampling factor of approximately 8 along each axis. Seg3DNet-HR was trained using images that were resampled to $1\,\mathrm{mm}^3$ isotropic voxels for the human datasets, and with $0.6\,\mathrm{mm}^3$ isotropic voxels for the animal datasets. The CT images, as well as the coarse probability maps predicted by Seg3DNet-LR were then used as a 2-channel input to Seg3DNet-HR. At this resolution, the memory required to train the network using the entire lung field exceeded available GPU memory. Therefore, axial stacks of size $256 \times 256 \times 32$ were extracted at different axial positions. Without the coarse probability maps provided by Seg3DNet-LR, a model trained exclusively on these stacks would be unable to incorporate global structural features of the lung anatomy. However,

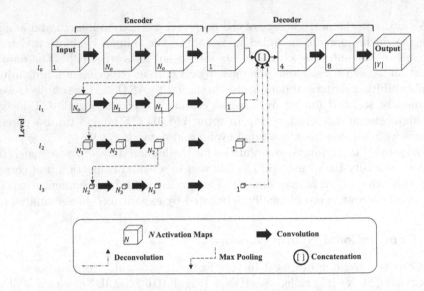

Fig. 1. Seg3DNet architecture. The arrows represent an operation performed by a layer and the cubes represent the intermediate feature representations produced by a layer. For visualization purposes, only the spatial dimensions of the feature representations are illustrated. The number of activation maps (size of channel dimension) is denoted in the lower left corner. For the encoder module, we define $N_i = 2^{i+5}$ so that the number of activation maps increases by a factor of two at each level. The number of kernels used in each convolutional layer can be inferred by the number of activation maps in the layer's output representation, i.e., the first convolutional layer has $N_0 = 2^{0+5} = 32$ kernels. The relative spatial size of the activation maps are drawn to scale. At each level the spatial dimensions of the feature representation gets downsampled by a factor of two. Batch normalization and ReLU nonlinearity are performed after each convolution except the last.

the proposed coarse-to-fine model allows global information to be encoded by using the Seg3DNet-LR prediction.

2.4   Training and Transfer Learning

The coarse-to-fine model was pre-trained using the human training dataset. The ConvNet parameters were randomly initialized using Xavier normal initialization [18]. Transfer learning was used to extend the model to segment lungs in animal models of ARDS, i.e., using the parameters learned from pre-training for initialization, a second coarse-to-fine model was trained by fine-tuning with the animal dataset.

A categorical cross entropy loss function was used for training all networks. Adam optimization [19] was used with a learning rate of 0.0001 for pre-training and 0.00005 for fine-tuning. The implementation used open-source frameworks Theano [20] and Lasagne [21]. Training was performed using a P40 NVIDIA GPU with 24 GB of RAM.

2.5   Post-Processing

The probability map predicted by the Seg3DNet-HR was post-processed using thresholding and connected-component analysis to obtain final binary lung segmentations. The probability map was thresholded at P = 0.5, where P is the probability that a voxel is contained within the lungs. After thresholding, the two largest connected components were selected. If the ratio of volumes of the second largest component to the first largest component was greater than 0.4, the two largest components were identified as the right and left lungs. Otherwise, it was assumed the left and right lungs were connected and only the largest component was selected.

2.6   Experimental Methods

We evaluated the performance of the proposed lung segmentation method on the human and animal evaluation datasets described in Sect. 2.1. The Jacaard index was used to measure volume overlap between the ground truth (GT) and the predicted segmentation (PS). The Jacaard index is defined as

$$J(\text{PS}, \text{GT}) = \frac{|\text{PS} \cap \text{GT}|}{|\text{PS} \cup \text{GT}|}, \tag{1}$$

where $| \cdot |$ is set cardinality. The Jacaard index has values ranging from 0 to 1, with 1 indicating perfect agreement. Additionally, the distance between the predicted lung boundary (B_{PS}) and ground truth lung boundary (B_{GT}) was evaluated. The distance between a voxel x and a set of voxels B is defined as

$$D(x, \text{B}) = \min_{y \in \text{B}} d(x, y), \tag{2}$$

where $d(x, y)$ is the Euclidean distance between voxels x and y. Based on Eq. 2 the average symmetric surface distance (ASSD) between two boundaries is defined as

$$\text{ASSD} = \frac{1}{|\text{B}_{\text{PS}}| + |\text{B}_{\text{GT}}|} \times \left(\sum_{x \in \text{B}_{\text{PS}}} D(x, \text{B}_{\text{GT}}) + \sum_{y \in \text{B}_{\text{GT}}} D(y, \text{B}_{\text{PS}}) \right). \tag{3}$$

3   Results

Jacaard index and ASSD box and whisker plots for the human and animal datasets are displayed in Fig. 2. Overall, the human dataset had an average Jacaard index of 0.99, and an average ASSD of 0.29 mm. The animal dataset had an average Jacaard index of 0.94, and an average ASSD of 0.99 mm. Representative results for the human and animal datasets are displayed in Figs. 3 and 4, respectively. Figure 5 depicts the segmentation result for a porcine subject with severe bilateral dependent consolidation, with maximum and minimum intensity projections included to emphasize the amount of diffuse opacification in the dependent regions of the lung.

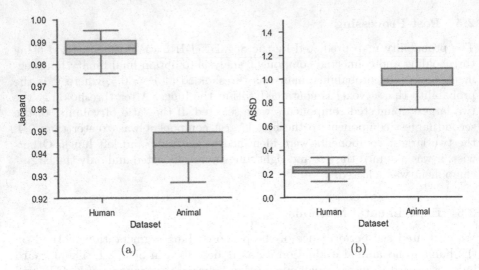

Fig. 2. (a) Jacaard index and (b) average surface distance (ASSD) in mm for the human and animal evaluation datasets. The boxes represent the quartiles and the whiskers represent the range of values.

4   Discussion

We proposed a coarse-to-fine ConvNet model for lung segmentation in human and animal CT images using transfer learning. The pre-trained model accurately segmented lungs in human datasets with severe fibrosis. However, direct application of this model to animals with lung injury similar to ARDS failed to include portions of consolidated lung tissue, and in some instances of normally aerated lung regions. This failure can be attributed to differences in the human and animal datasets (e.g. the lack of consolidated injury in the human images), as well as anatomic variations among the different species. Using 3D CT scans of 9 dog and 4 pig subjects, we were able to fine-tune the model and produce accurate segmentations for 4D CT scans in pigs with ARDS.

The proposed method achieved high segmentation performance on the human and animal datasets, which include challenging cases with dense pathologies. Column (d) in Fig. 3 and Fig. 4 show spatial distributions of discrepancies between the ground truth and predicted lung segmentations. The majority of errors occur within a single-voxel layer at the lung boundary and at the mediastinum where airways and blood vessels enter the lung. The network successfully includes the dense pathologies, such as fibrosis and consolidation.

A limitation of the evaluation is that manual tracing was performed by one observer for each case. Therefore, we were unable to evaluate inter- and intra-observer variability. We would expect there to be a large variability for the injured animal datasets due to the poor contrast between parenchymal tissue and surrounding soft tissue, which could also explain why the performance was

(a)   (b)   (c)   (d)

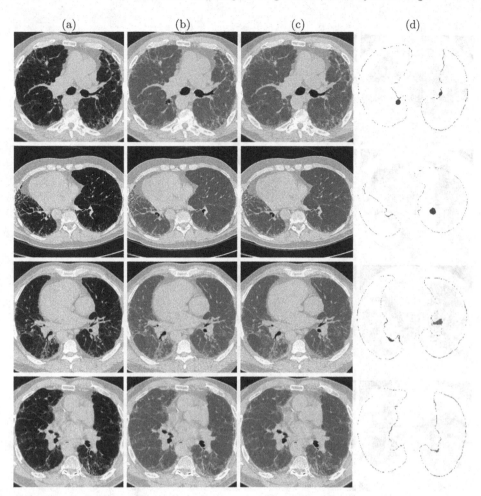

Fig. 3. Segmentation results for 4 human subjects with IPF in rows 1–4. (a) CT image, (b) ground truth lung segmentation, (c) predicted lung segmentation, (d) difference between ground truth and predicted lung segmentations with under- and over-segmented voxels depicted in red and blue, respectively.

worse on the animal datasets. In addition to evaluating inter- and intra-observer variability, in future work we plan to extend the evaluation set to more subjects.

Training all models took approximately 48 h. After training, runtime for segmentation of a new case was approximately 5 s, in contrast to 4–6 h required for manual segmentation of a lung image with ARDS. By automating lung segmentation for this challenging disease case, quantitative clinical assessment of these images can be performed without the time and cost impediments of manual segmentation.

(a)   (b)   (c)   (d)

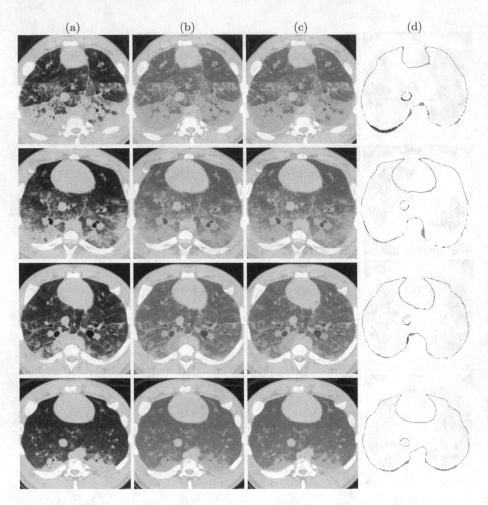

Fig. 4. Segmentation results for 4 porcine subjects with ARDS in rows 1–4. (a) CT image, (b) ground truth lung segmentation, (c) predicted lung segmentation, (d) difference between ground truth and predicted lung segmentations with under- and over-segmented voxels depicted in red and blue, respectively.

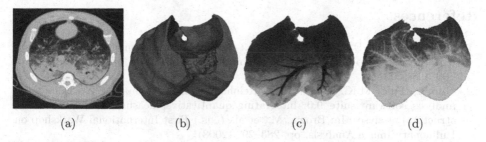

(a)   (b)   (c)   (d)

Fig. 5. Visualization of segmentation result for one phase of a 4D CT scan of porcine subject with ARDS: (a) Axial slice of CT with segmentation contour depicted in magenta; (b) 3D surface rendering of segmentation; (c) and (d) minimum and maximum intensity projections, respectively, of masked CT image. Projection images emphasize the amount of diffuse opacification in the dependent regions of the lung.

5   Conclusion

A deep learning framework was used to train a ConvNet model for segmentation of lungs in human datasets. The model was then able to generalize to a new dataset of 4D porcine scans with ARDS, after fine-tuning the human-trained model with a limited dataset of 3D porcine and canine scans of subjects with ARDS. This approach could be used for parenchymal segmentation in the presence of other pathophysiologic processes, such as pulmonary edema, atelectasis, or pneumonia - conditions for which limited training datasets are available, and manual segmentation is prohibitively tedious and difficult.

Acknowledgments. This work was supported in part by NIH grant CA166703 (J. M. Reinhardt and S. E. Gerard), the National Heart, Lung, and Blood Institute Grants R01-HL-112986, and R01-HL-126838 (D. W. Kaczka), the University of Iowa, Department of Anesthesia (D. W. Kaczka and J. Herrmann), and by the Office of the Assistant Secretary of Defense for Health Affairs through the Peer Reviewed Medical Research Program under Award no. W81XWH-16-1-0434 (D. W. Kaczka).

S.E. Gerard received support from a Presidential Fellowship through the University of Iowa Graduate College and from a NASA Iowa Space Grant Consortium Fellowship.

The authors thank Dr. Eric Hoffman and Dr. Junfeng Guo from the University of Iowa for providing the CT image data and ground truth segmentations for the IPF cases.

Disclosure: Opinions, interpretations, conclusions, and recommendations are those of the authors and are not necessarily endorsed by the U.S. Department of Defense. J. M. Reinhardt is a shareholder in VIDA Diagnostics, Inc.

References

1. Hu, S., Hoffman, E.A., Reinhardt, J.M.: Automatic lung segmentation for accurate quantitation of volumetric X-ray CT images. IEEE Trans. Med. Imaging **20**(6), 490–498 (2001)
2. Guo, J., Fuld, M.K., Alford, S.K., Reinhardt, J.M., Hoffman, E.A.: Pulmonary analysis software suite 9.0: integrating quantitative measures of function with structural analyses. In: Brown, M., et al., (eds.) First International Workshop on Pulmonary Image Analysis, pp. 283–292 (2008)
3. Sun, S., Bauer, C., Beichel, R.: Automated 3-D segmentation of lungs with lung cancer in CT data using a novel robust active shape model approach. IEEE Trans. Med. Imaging **31**(2), 449–460 (2012)
4. Sluimer, I., Prokop, M., Van Ginneken, B.: Toward automated segmentation of the pathological lung in CT. IEEE Trans. Med. Imaging **24**(8), 1025–1038 (2005)
5. Van Rikxoort, E.M., de Hoop, B., van de Vorst, S., Prokop, M., van Ginneken, B.: Automatic segmentation of pulmonary segments from volumetric chest CT scans. IEEE Trans. Med. Imaging **28**(4), 621–630 (2009)
6. LeCun, Y., Bottou, L., Bengio, Y., Haffner, P.: Gradient-based learning applied to document recognition. Proc. IEEE **86**(11), 2278–2324 (1998)
7. Krizhevsky, A., Sutskever, I., Hinton, G.E.: Imagenet classification with deep convolutional neural networks. In: Advances in Neural Information Processing Systems, pp. 1097–1105 (2012)
8. Harrison, A.P., Xu, Z., George, K., Lu, L., Summers, R.M., Mollura, D.J.: Progressive and multi-path holistically nested neural networks for pathological lung segmentation from CT images. In: Descoteaux, M., Maier-Hein, L., Franz, A., Jannin, P., Collins, D.L., Duchesne, S. (eds.) MICCAI 2017. LNCS, vol. 10435, pp. 621–629. Springer, Cham (2017). https://doi.org/10.1007/978-3-319-66179-7_71
9. Anthimopoulos, M., Christodoulidis, S., Ebner, L., Geiser, T., Christe, A., Mougiakakou, S.: Semantic segmentation of pathological lung tissue with dilated fully convolutional networks. arXiv preprint arXiv:1803.06167 (2018)
10. Tajbakhsh, N., et al.: Convolutional neural networks for medical image analysis: full training or fine tuning? IEEE Trans. Med. Imaging **35**(5), 1299–1312 (2016)
11. Kaczka, D.W., Cao, K., Christensen, G.E., Bates, J.H., Simon, B.A.: Analysis of regional mechanics in canine lung injury using forced oscillations and 3D image registration. Ann. Biomed. Eng. **39**(3), 1112–1124 (2011)
12. Regan, E.A.: Genetic epidemiology of COPD (COPDGene) study design. COPD J. Chronic Obstructive Pulm. Dis. **7**(1), 32–43 (2011)
13. Sieren, J.P., et al.: SPIROMICS protocol for multicenter quantitative computed tomography to phenotype the lungs. Am. J. Respir. Crit. Care Med. **194**(7), 794–806 (2016)
14. Herrmann, J., Hoffman, E.A., Kaczka, D.W.: Frequency-selective computed tomography: Applications during periodic thoracic motion. IEEE Trans. Med. Imaging **36**(8), 1722–1732 (2017)
15. Shelhamer, E., Long, J., Darrell, T.: Fully convolutional networks for semantic segmentation. IEEE Trans. Patt. Anal. Mach. Intell. **39**(4), 640–651 (2017)
16. Gerard, S.E., Patton, T.J., Christensen, G.E., Bayouth, J.E., Reinhardt, J.M.: FissureNet: A deep learning approach for pulmonary fissure detection in CT images. IEEE Trans. Med. Imaging (2018)

17. Ronneberger, O., Fischer, P., Brox, T.: U-Net: convolutional networks for biomedical image segmentation. In: Navab, N., Hornegger, J., Wells, W.M., Frangi, A.F. (eds.) MICCAI 2015. LNCS, vol. 9351, pp. 234–241. Springer, Cham (2015). https://doi.org/10.1007/978-3-319-24574-4_28
18. Glorot, X., Bengio, Y.: Understanding the difficulty of training deep feedforward neural networks. In: Proceedings of the Thirteenth International Conference on Artificial Intelligence and Statistics, pp. 249–256 (2010)
19. Kingma, D., Ba, J.: Adam: A method for stochastic optimization. arXiv preprint arXiv:1412.6980 (2014)
20. Theano Development Team: Theano: A Python framework for fast computation of mathematical expressions. arXiv e-prints abs/1605.02688, May 2016
21. Dieleman, S., et al.: Lasagne: First Release, vol. 3. Zenodo, Geneva (2015)

High Throughput Lung and Lobar Segmentation by 2D and 3D CNN on Chest CT with Diffuse Lung Disease

Xiaoyong Wang[1,2], Pangyu Teng[1,2], Pechin Lo[1,2], Ashley Banola[1,2], Grace Kim[1,2], Fereidoun Abtin[1,2], Jonathan Goldin[1,2], and Matthew Brown[1,2(✉)]

[1] Center for Computer Vision and Imaging Biomarkers, University of California, Los Angeles, 924 Westwood Blvd., Suite 615, Los Angeles, CA, USA
xiaoyongw@ucla.edu, mbrown@mednet.ucla.edu
[2] Department of Radiological Sciences, University of California, Los Angeles, Los Angeles, CA, USA

Abstract. Deep learning methods have been widely and successfully applied to the medical imaging field. Specifically, fully convolutional neural networks have become the state-of-the-art supervised segmentation method in a variety of biomedical segmentation problems. Two fully convolutional networks were proposed to sequentially achieve accurate lobar segmentation. Firstly, a 2D ResNet-101 based network is proposed for lung segmentation and 575 chest CT scans from multicenter clinical trials were used with radiologist approved lung segmentation. Secondly, a 3D DenseNet based network is applied to segment the 5 lobes and a total of 1280 different CT scans were used with radiologist approved lobar segmentation as ground truth. The dataset includes various pathological lung diseases and stratified sampling was used to form training and test sets following a ratio of 4:1 to ensure a balanced number and type of abnormality present. A 3D CNN segmentation model was also built for lung segmentation to investigate the feasibility using current hardware. Using 5-fold cross validation a mean Dice coefficient of 0.988 ± 0.012 and Average Surface Distance of 0.562 ± 0.49 mm was achieved by the proposed 2D CNN on lung segmentation. 3D DenseNet on lobar segmentation achieved Dice score of 0.959 ± 0.087 and Average surface distance of 0.873 ± 0.61 mm.

Keywords: CT · Lung segmentation · Lobar segmentation · CNN

1 Introduction

1.1 Conventional Lung and Lobar Segmentation

Segmentation of pathologic lungs on CT images has been investigated in a number of studies. Voxel classification utilizing local texture features has been used to segment abnormal lung regions [1]. Applying anatomical model constraint was another strategy to overcome the challenge of pathological lung segmentation [2]. For example, curvature of ribs [3] was used to assist the selection of optimal thresholds to segment the

© Springer Nature Switzerland AG 2018
D. Stoyanov et al. (Eds.): RAMBO 2018/BIA 2018/TIA 2018, LNCS 11040, pp. 202–214, 2018.
https://doi.org/10.1007/978-3-030-00946-5_21

lung. A modified convex hull algorithm [4] was introduced to extract coarse lung regions present with diffuse lung disease followed by morphological analysis as post-processing. Traditional lobar segmentation is usually achieved by fissure detection/segmentation and a variety of methods have been proposed to accomplish this task, such as watershed, level set, and SVM based. Occasionally, segmentation of airway and vessels are used to assist. However, most of the methods were evaluated on a relatively small datasets and their efficiency is not ideal for high throughput processing. More importantly, they still struggle when confronted with pathological lungs which are common in clinical practice.

1.2 Deep Learning in Medical Image Segmentation

Deep learning methods have been successfully applied to various medical image analysis problems [5–7]. More specifically, fully convolutional neural networks (FCN) [8] have become the state-of-the-art approach for segmentation on many imaging modalities. U-Net [9] has demonstrated success in many biomedical image segmentation problems, including cell segmentation in microscopic images. SegNet [10], which is a deep Encoder-Decoder neural network, showed promising results regarding lung segmentation in chest radiographs. Volumetric image based methods were also introduced, such as 3D U-Net [11] and V-Net [12], to segment prostate and kidney in MR. As for FCN application on chest CT, Harrison et al. [13] proposed a progressive and multi-path holistically nested 2D network (P-HNN) for lung segmentation. The method was evaluated on a large dataset including many pathological lungs. A V-Net [14] like architecture was proposed by IBM research aimed at volumetrically segmenting the lung with more spatial context. It demonstrated promising results using a 3D CNN. A relatively small input size was used to compromise the memory constraints and this actually caused noticeable under-segmentation near the boundary. George et al. [15] applied the same P-HNN method on lobar segmentation using 2D axial slices, and the crude segmentation from CNN was followed by a 3D random walker to refine it. Presumably, it is difficult to segment different lobes based on 2D slices without spatial context and a 3D volume based method has the potential to overcome this obstacle.

1.3 ResNet and DenseNet

The Residual Network (ResNet [16]) has been the state-of-the-art image recognition architecture and won first place on the ILSVRC-2015 classification task. Due to its much deeper network with residual learning it demonstrated exceptional performance, surpassing previous models such as VGG [17] and GoogleNet [18]. More recently, DenseNet [19] was introduced in which each layer is connected to every other layer in a feed-forward fashion. It is easier to train due to the improved flow of gradients throughout the network and able to achieve better performance using fewer parameters.

In this paper, we will introduce two fully convolutional networks applied sequentially achieve accurate lobar segmentation. In the first stage, a 2D ResNet-101 based model is used for lung segmentation. Thereafter, a 3D DenseNet based network is applied to perform lobar segmentation based on the initial lung segmentation.

2   Materials

The chest CT images used in this study were collected retrospectively from 6 multi-center clinical trials. This provides image acquisition at different sites with variations in slice thickness, reconstruction kernel, scanner, etc. The slice thickness range is [0.625 mm, 3 mm], in-plane (x-y) spacing range is [0.467 mm, 1 mm], tube current range is [80 mA, 644 mA] and reconstruction kernels include a range from smooth to sharp. In total, 575 chest CT scans from different subjects were used, each with radiologist-approved lung segmentation. 143 scans are from subjects enrolled in Chronic Obstructive Pulmonary Disease (COPD) clinical trials and 432 are from interstitial pulmonary fibrosis (IPF) trials. These cases contain common lung parenchymal abnormalities including emphysema, ground glass, fibrosis, nodule, and honeycombing. Sample axial images of these disease patterns are shown in Fig. 1.

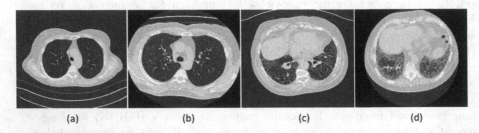

(a)   (b)   (c)   (d)

Fig. 1. Sample axial chest CT of cases with different lung disease in our dataset, including (a) emphysema, (b) ground glass, (c) honeycombing, and (d) fibrosis.

The ground truth reference lung segmentations of these scans were derived using an independent semi-automated segmentation. Specifically, the scans were segmented using a threshold-based anatomical model technique [20, 21], followed by manual editing by lab technologists. Finally, radiologists performed review, editing as needed, and approved the final segmentation. Two thoracic radiologists were involved, both with more than 20 years experience.

Balanced sampling, rather than random sampling, was used to form training and test sets that were balanced in terms of the number and type of abnormalities present. The whole image set was sorted based on the mean Hounsfield Unit (HU) within the lung in ascending order. As a consequence, scans with lower and higher mean lung intensity are likely corresponding to cases with emphysema and IPF, respectively. For every 5 scans of the sorted image set, they were split into training, and test following a ratio of 4:1. 5-fold cross validation with balanced distribution was used and each scan was used for testing exactly once. At each fold, the training set consisted of 460 scans, and the test set was composed of 115 scans. Using this approach similar to stratified cross validation [22], the composition distributions of training, and test set are similar to the original dataset. For a specific scan, only slices (axial images) with lung segmentation (i.e., containing lung) were used.

For lobar segmentation, 705 more scans were used to increase the size of data set with a total number of 1280 scans and all of them have corresponding radiologist approved lobar segmentations. The resolution (z spacing) limit is <= 3 mm since our method is 3D volume based. Similar to the previous 575 scans used in lung segmentation, the additional 705 scans also include different types of lung abnormalities. In terms of breath-hold type, 1193 scans were acquired at Total Lung Capacity (TLC) and 87 at Residual Volume (RV). The same data sorting and splitting strategy was used to form training and test set.

3   Methods

3.1   Network Architectures

Figure 2 shows the general structure of ResNet-101 based segmentation architecture with input and output size of 256 × 256. The original input image was progressively scaled down 5 times (from 256 × 256 to 8 × 8). Each down-sampling stage includes a residual block, stride of 2 convolution to downsize feature maps. In the de-convolution section, corresponding 5 times up-sampling was used to recover the same resolution as the input image, i.e., from 8 × 8 back to 256 × 256. Each up-sampling stage includes transposed convolution, concatenation and a residual block. Following the same strategy suggested by Szegedy et al. [23], the number of feature maps in the de-convolutional layer was cut by half every time the image size doubles. Also, skip-connections were used in the up-sampling process to incorporate finer details from the lower layers as well as abstract and sematic information from higher layers.

The 3D DenseNet based network is shown in Fig. 3. The down-sampling path includes 4 Transitions Down and 4 Dense Block. Corresponding up-sampling path includes 4 Transitions Up and 4 Dense Block. Transitions Down modules include [Convolution3D, Dropout and Max-pooling]. Transitions Up modules include [Transposed Convolution3D and Dropout]. The Dense Block includes 4 densely connected layers. This architecture was used both in 3D lung segmentation (to compare with 2D CNN) and lobar segmentation. In the case of lung segmentation, the input was a raw image and a sigmoid is used in the final layer. For the lobar segmentation, the input is raw image plus lung mask and softmax is used. To mitigate memory constraints, we decided to perform lobar segmentation on the left and right lung separately. A previous anatomical model based method [21] was used for left and right lung separation.

3.2   Pre-processing, Data Augmentation, and Training

Preprocessing of each CT scan prior to inputting to the CNN involved normalization and rescaling. Image intensity was clipped to range from −1000 HU to +1000 HU and then normalized to [0.0, 1.0]. For 2D model, each slice was resized to 256 × 256.

Similarly, each scan was resized to 128 × 128 × 128 as the input for 3D model. The model was trained from scratch, rather than applying transfer learning using pretrained weights. Real-time data augmentation was applied using rotation and

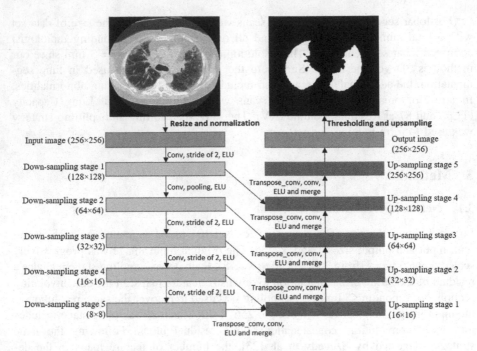

Fig. 2. ResNet-101 based lung segmentation architecture.

translation, with the CPU responsible for generating new samples and the GPU for the computation to improve the uniqueness of the augmented data. Dice loss was used as the loss function since it has been shown to be more robust in segmentation problems.

Training of the model was performed using a NVIDIA TITAN X with 12 GB of memory. The Keras deep learning package [24] was used for implementation. Dice Similarity Coefficient and Average Surface Distance were used as evaluation metric.

4   Results

4.1   Lung Segmentation

During testing, the whole scan was fed into the segmentation network to generate a 3D lung segmentation for both the 2D and 3D CNN model. For a single test scan with 200 slices, it takes about 5 s to segment the whole lung.

Table 1 illustrates the segmentation results by the proposed 2D CNN model, 3D CNN model and also previous threshold and anatomical based method [20, 21] developed by our group. Specifically, only 3 out of the total 575 scans from 2D CNN segmentation and 9 scans from 3D CNN segmentation had a Dice coefficient below 0.95. While for our previous method, there were 111 cases with a Dice score below 0.95 from.

Figure 4 shows three example segmentations with different amount of fibrosis present (from mild to severe) by the proposed 2D based CNN, 3D based CNN and

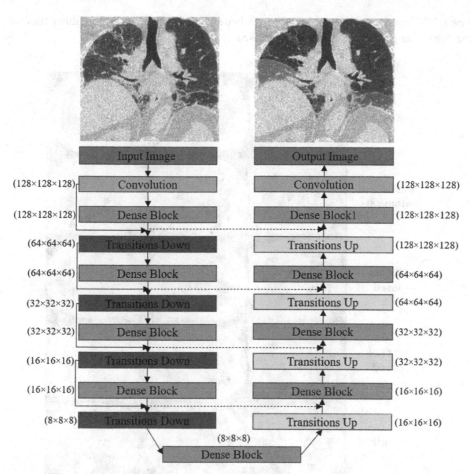

Fig. 3. 3D DenseNet architecture used for lobar segmentation. Dashed lines indicate skip connection from down-sampling to up-sampling.

Table 1. Lung segmentation results comparison between the CNN based and previous threshold and anatomical model based methods

	Dice coefficient	ASD (mm)
2D CNN based	0.988 ± 0.012	0.562 ± 0.49
3D CNN based	0.980 ± 0.017	0.581 ± 0.52
Threshold and anatomical model	0.965 ± 0.023	0.599 ± 0.47

previous threshold anatomical model based methods. The second row corresponds to Dice scores of (0.954, 0.931, 0.847) and ASD of (0.575 mm, 1.689 mm, 4.51 mm) by the threshold and anatomical model based method. 2D CNN achieved Dice scores of (0.989, 0.980, 0.976) and ASD of (0.36 mm, 0.505 mm, 1.18 mm). 3D CNN achieved Dice scores of (0.979, 0.969, 0.970) and ASD of (0.484 mm, 0.677 mm, 1.653 mm).

The CNN based methods achieved much better segmentation when the attenuation of the lung changed significantly due to disease.

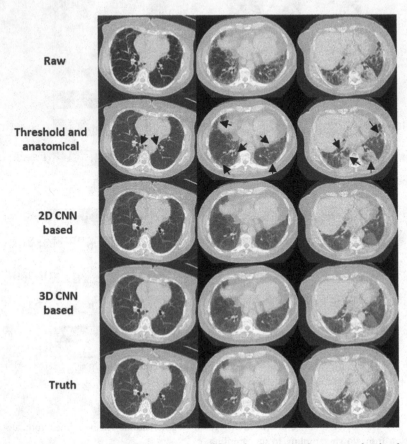

Fig. 4. Three examples with differing degrees of fibrosis. Segmentations errors by the threshold and anatomical model based method in the second row are highlighted with red arrows. (Color figure online)

Figure 5 shows example segmentations of emphysema, ground glass and honeycombing by the proposed the CNN methods as well as our previous threshold and anatomical model based method for comparison. In these examples, there are no major attenuation changes in the lung and all three methods were able to achieve good segmentation relative to the ground truth. The Dice scores of these 3 cases (from left to right) are (0.992, 0.973, 0.974) by the threshold and anatomical based method, (0.991, 0.984, 0.976) by 2D CNN, (0.989, 0.981, 0.972) by 3D CNN. Comparable ASD were achieved by the 3 segmentation methods: (0.355 mm, 0.55 mm, 0.503 mm) vs. (0.352 mm, 0.327 mm, 0.479) vs. (0.356 mm, 0.374 mm, 0.488 mm). One minor difference is the successful exclusion of airway by CNN in this honeycombing case.

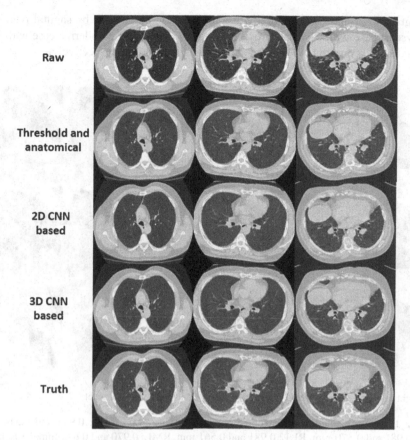

Fig. 5. Example segmentations on emphysema, ground glass and honeycombing cases.

4.2   Lobar Segmentation

The overall Dice score across 5 lobes is 0.959 ± 0.087 and Average surface distance is 0.873 ± 0.61 mm. More specific performance on each lobe is shown in Table 2.

Table 2. Segmentation results of 5 different lobes by 3D DenseNet

	Dice coefficient	ASD (mm)
RUL	0.971 ± 0.078	0.699 ± 0.432
RML	0.923 ± 0.114	1.542 ± 1.164
RLL	0.970 ± 0.126	0.783 ± 0.372
LUL	0.972 ± 0.083	0.807 ± 0.594
LLL	0.962 ± 0.105	0.861 ± 0.753

Figures 6, 7, and 8 show three lobar segmentation examples by sagittal plane: an emphysema case with TLC, a fibrosis case with TLC and a scleroderma case with RV. Detailed Dice score and ASD were shown in their captions respectively.

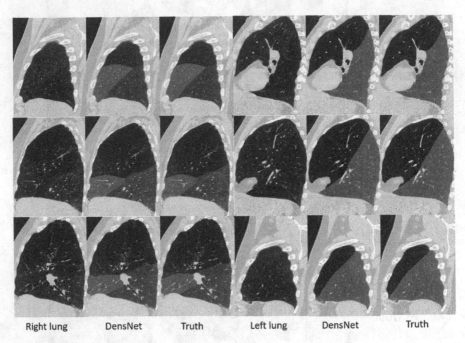

Right lung   DensNet   Truth   Left lung   DensNet   Truth

Fig. 6. Lobar segmentation on an emphysema case with TLC. [LUL: 0.983 and 0.514 mm, LLL: 0.981 and 0.570 mm, RUL: 0.981 and 0.561 mm, RML: 0.970 and 0.673 mm, RLL: 0.977 and 0.635 mm].

5   Discussion

The CNN based method achieved highly accurate lung segmentation based on Dice score and Average surface distance. The 2D based CNN model has been successfully applied to segment over 5000 chest CT scans in clinical practice. Our method showed substantial advantages when large amounts of fibrosis are present, especially in peripheral areas close to other soft tissue. Another strength of the CNN based method is its ability to consistently exclude airway trees regardless of the disease patterns and many other methods occasionally require post-processing. In comparison with P-HNN, our work differs in terms of using a radiologist edited and approved reference segmentation for training and testing, as well as the use of a simpler single channel architecture (train from scratch) and no post-processing (such as 3D hole filling).

Using current hardware in clinical practice, the 2D slice based CNN slightly outperformed the 3D volume based CNN. Although 3D based model is able to incorporate more contextual information, this is actually not surprising considering following. Firstly, the variation of slice spacing along the z direction is much larger than in the

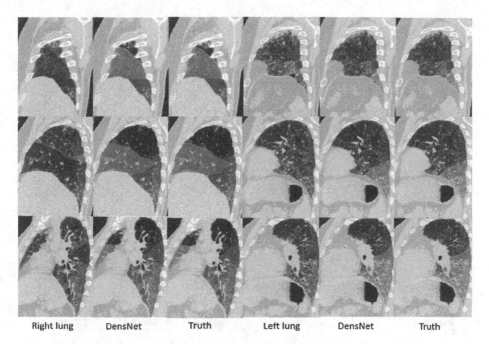

Right lung   DensNet   Truth   Left lung   DensNet   Truth

Fig. 7. Lobar segmentation on a fibrosis case with TLC. [LUL: 0.978 and 0.427 mm, LLL: 0.960 and 0.538 mm, RUL: 0.975 and 0.496 mm, RML: 0.967 and 0.585 mm, RLL: 0.965 and 0.583 mm].

x-y plane. One strategy would be to resample all the scans to the same resolution but this is computationally expensive. Secondly, the number of training samples is also much smaller when a 3D scan is used instead of individual 2D slices. As such, the 2D model was built with more diverse dataset. Lastly, the image was down-sampled more aggressively in the scenario of 3D CNN (512 to 128 vs. 512 to 256). This would inevitably cause more information loss especially fine details near boundary and this is also observed in the work by IBM research [14].

Using the initial lung segmentation from ResNet-101, the 3D DenseNet model successfully segmented the five lobes correctly on pathological lungs. Conventional fissure detection based methods often fail when fissures are incomplete or impacted by lung abnormalities, such as emphysema, fibrosis. However, our 3D CNN model demonstrated robustness in those challenging cases. One deficiency of our current model is the assumption that five lobes are present which may not be true when a lobe collapses, for example. In the future, we will include these highly abnormal cases in training and also expand our evaluation to include public data sets.

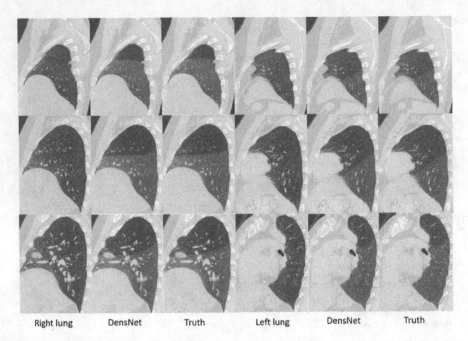

Right lung   DensNet   Truth   Left lung   DensNet   Truth

Fig. 8. Lobar segmentation on a scleroderma case with RV. [LUL: 0.977 and 0.453 mm, LLL: 0.973 and 0.544 mm, RUL: 0.979 and 0.444 mm, RML: 0.947 and 0.584 mm, RLL: 0.974 and 0.496 mm]

6 Conclusion

We developed two fully convolutional neural network to segment lung and lobes sequentially. The 2D ResNet-101 based segmentation architecture was successfully applied to lung segmentation on chest CT without the need for any additional post-processing. It achieved high accuracy even in the presence of challenging diffuse lung diseases. The 3D DenseNet based network demonstrated competitive lobar segmentation performance on various pathological lungs.

References

1. Mansoor, A., et al.: A generic approach to pathological lung segmentation. IEEE Trans. Med. Imaging **33**(12), 2293–2310 (2014)
2. Birkbeck, N., et al.: Lung Segmentation from CT with Severe Pathologies Using Anatomical Constraints. In: Golland, P., Hata, N., Barillot, C., Hornegger, J., Howe, R. (eds.) MICCAI 2014. LNCS, vol. 8673, pp. 804–811. Springer, Cham (2014). https://doi.org/10.1007/978-3-319-10404-1_100
3. Prasad, M.N., et al.: Automatic segmentation of lung parenchyma in the presence of diseases based on curvature of ribs. Acad. Radiol. **15**(9), 1173–1180 (2008)

4. Pulagam, A.R., Kande, G.B., Ede, V.K.R., Inampudi, R.B.: Automated lung segmentation from HRCT scans with diffuse parenchymal lung diseases. J. Digit. Imaging 29(4), 507–519 (2016)
5. Antony, J., McGuinness, K., Connor, N.E.O., Moran, K.: Quantifying radiographic knee osteoarthritis severity using deep convolutional neural networks, arXiv cs.CV, vol. 9, p. 02469 (2016)
6. Kim, E., Corte-Real, M., Baloch, Z.: A deep semantic mobile application for thyroid cytopathology. In: Proceedings of SPIE, vol. 9789, pp. 97890A–97890A-9 (2016)
7. Suk, H.-I., Shen, D.: Deep learning-based feature representation for AD/MCI classification. In: Mori, K., Sakuma, I., Sato, Y., Barillot, C., Navab, N. (eds.) MICCAI 2013. LNCS, vol. 8150, pp. 583–590. Springer, Heidelberg (2013). https://doi.org/10.1007/978-3-642-40763-5_72
8. Long, J., Shelhamer, E., Darrell, T.: Fully convolutional networks for semantic segmentation. In: Proceedings of the IEEE Computer Society Conference on Computer Vision and Pattern Recognition, 12 June 2015, vol. 07, pp. 3431–3440 (2015)
9. Ronneberger, O., Fischer, P., Brox, T.: U-Net: convolutional networks for biomedical image segmentation. In: Navab, N., Hornegger, J., Wells, W.M., Frangi, A.F. (eds.) MICCAI 2015. LNCS, vol. 9351, pp. 234–241. Springer, Cham (2015). https://doi.org/10.1007/978-3-319-24574-4_28
10. Kalinovsky, A., Kalinovsky, A., Kovalev, V.: Lung image segmentation using deep learning methods and convolutional neural networks lung image segmentation using deep learning methods and convolutional neural networks, October 2016
11. Çiçek, Ö., Abdulkadir, A., Lienkamp, S.S., Ronneberger, O.: 3D U-Net: learning dense volumetric segmentation from sparse annotation, arXiv Prepr. arXiv:1606.06650 (2016)
12. Milletari, F., Navab, N., Ahmadi, S.-A.: V-Net: fully convolutional neural networks for volumetric medical image segmentation, arXiv Prepr. arXiv:1606.04797, pp. 1–11 (2016)
13. Harrison, A.P., Xu, Z., George, K., Lu, L., Summers, R.M., Mollura, D.J.: Progressive and multi-path holistically nested neural networks for pathological lung segmentation from CT images, CoRR, vol. abs/1706.0 (2017)
14. Negahdar, M., Beymer, D.: Automated volumetric lung segmentation of thoracic CT images using fully convolutional neural network, February 2018
15. George, K., Harrison, A.P., Jin, D., Xu, Z., Mollura, D.J.: Pathological pulmonary lobe segmentation from CT images using progressive holistically nested neural networks and random walker, ArXiv e-prints, August 2017
16. He, K., Zhang, X., Ren, S., Sun, J.: Deep residual learning for image recognition, CoRR, vol. abs/1512.0 (2015)
17. Simonyan, K., Zisserman, A.: Very deep convolutional networks for large-scale image recognition. In: ImageNet Challenge, pp. 1–10 (2014)
18. Szegedy, C., Vanhoucke, V., Ioffe, S., Shlens, J., Wojna, Z.: Rethinking the Inception Architecture for Computer Vision (2015)
19. Huang, G., Liu, Z., Van Der Maaten, L., Weinberger, K.Q.: Densely connected convolutional networks. In: Proceedings - 30th IEEE Conference Computer Vision Pattern Recognition, CVPR 2017, January, vol. 2017, pp. 2261–2269 (2017)
20. Brown, M.S., et al.: Method for segmenting chest CT image data using an anatomical model: preliminary results. IEEE Trans. Med. Imaging 16(6), 828–839 (1997)
21. Brown, M.S., et al.: Reproducibility of lung and lobar volume measurements using computed tomography. Acad. Radiol. 17(3), 316–322 (2010)

22. Kohavi, R.: A study of cross-validation and bootstrap for accuracy estimation and model selection, pp. 1137–1143 (1995)
23. Szegedy, C., et al.: Going deeper with convolutions. In: Computer Vision and Pattern Recognition (CVPR) (2015)
24. Chollet, F.: "Keras." GitHub (2015)

Multi-structure Segmentation from Partially Labeled Datasets. Application to Body Composition Measurements on CT Scans

Germán González[1]([✉]) [iD], George R. Washko[2], and Raúl San José Estépar[3] [iD]

[1] Sierra Research S.L., Alicante, Spain
ggonzale@sierra-research.com
[2] Division of Pulmonary and Critical Care Medicine, Department of Medicine, Brigham and Womens Hospital, Harvard Medical School, Boston, MA, USA
gwashko@bwh.harvard.edu
[3] Applied Chest Imaging Laboratory, Department of Radiology, Brigham and Women's Hospital, Harvard Medical School, Boston, MA, USA
rjosest@bwh.harvard.edu

Abstract. Labeled data is the current bottleneck of medical image research. Substantial efforts are made to generate segmentation masks to characterize a given organ. The community ends up with multiple label maps of individual structures in different cases, not suitable for current multi-organ segmentation frameworks. Our objective is to leverage segmentations from multiple organs in different cases to generate a robust multi-organ deep learning segmentation network. We propose a modified cost-function that takes into account only the voxels labeled in the image, ignoring unlabeled structures. We evaluate the proposed methodology in the context of pectoralis muscle and subcutaneous fat segmentation on chest CT scans. Six different structures are segmented from an axial slice centered on the transversal aorta. We compare the performance of a network trained on 3,000 images where only one structure has been annotated (PUNet) against six UNets (one per structure) and a multi-class UNet trained on 500 completely annotated images, showing equivalence between the three methods (Dice coefficients of 0.909, 0.906 and 0.909 respectively). We further propose a modification of the architecture by adding convolutions to the skip connections (CUNet). When trained with partially labeled images, it outperforms statistically significantly the other three methods (Dice 0.916, $p < 0.0001$). We, therefore, show that (a) when keeping the number of organ annotation constant, training with partially labeled images is equivalent to training with wholly labeled data and (b) adding convolutions in the skip connections improves performance.

This study was supported by the NHLBI awards R01HL116931, R01HL116473, and R21HL140422. We gratefully acknowledge the support of NVIDIA Corporation with the donation of the Titan Xp GPU used for this research.

D. Stoyanov et al. (Eds.): RAMBO 2018/BIA 2018/TIA 2018, LNCS 11040, pp. 215–224, 2018.
https://doi.org/10.1007/978-3-030-00946-5_22

Keywords: Deep learning · Multi-organ · Segmentation · Unet Pectoralis

1   Introduction

Segmentation of structures of interest is one of the main tasks of medical image analysis, serving as a prior step to biomarker quantification. Deep learning has been used to solve many segmentation problems [1] in images ranging from computed tomography [2] to MRI [3] or even in multi-modality images with the same network, [4] for one or multiple-organs [5].

Current deep-learning segmentation algorithms are trained on a dataset where the structures of interest are annotated, producing a complete mask per case. Every voxel is given a label, as being either a structure or background. This enables to optimize cost functions such as the normalized cross entropy or the dice coefficient [6, 7].

While this learning methodology has achieved great performance in single and multi-structure detection, it is not scalable to complete multi-organ segmentation, since it would require an extensive dataset where all the voxels are annotated. The expenses incurred in the generation of such dataset are beyond the scope of the effort that the community can afford. However, through the organization of challenges and public datasets, a great wealth of annotated cases with one or few structures of interest are currently available. What if we could leverage these single-organ databases for the generation of multiple-organ segmentation algorithms?

In this manuscript, we address this issue and propose a principled methodology to train a multi-class deep-learning segmentation algorithm from partially labeled datasets. The proposed method encodes the labels in a one-hot schema and optimizes the average per-structure dice coefficient. The proposed custom loss function adapts to the labels being provided. One of the most popular segmentation network architectures is the UNet [8], consisting of an encoding path, a decoding path and a set of skip connections [9]. We will, therefore, perform our experiments with UNet-based networks. We further such architecture by adding convolutions in the skip connections. Such is done to allow for flexibility between the information used in the encoding and decoding paths of the UNet. Such UNet, labeled CUNet, shows statistically significant improved performance over the baseline UNet.

We illustrate the proposed methodology in the problem of pectoralis and subcutaneous fat segmentation. Those structures have been shown to be of clinical relevance in different diseases like Chronic Obstructive Pulmonary Disease and Lung Cancer [10, 11]. Prior work has attempted to segment this structures using atlas-based techniques [12] and standard UNets [13].

This work is closely related to the work of [14], where the authors use few 2D annotated axial slices to train networks able to segment the whole 3D structures using a weighted softmax cost function. In their work, unlabeled voxels are given a zero weight and therefore do not contribute to the computation of the error.

Our works differs from [14] in the sense that we use a weighted cost function on the per-structure dice score. Our proposed cost function penalizes pixels that are not assigned to the right structure, even if the precise right structure of such pixel is unknown.

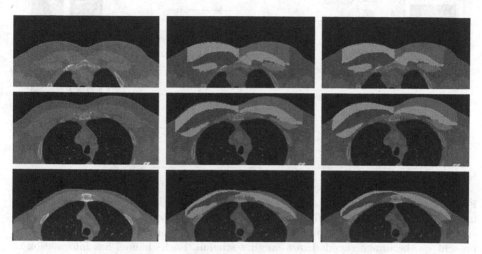

Fig. 1. Left: Axial slice at the level of the transversal aorta zoomed at the pectoralis region. Middle: Reference standard. Right: Segmentation obtained with the proposed method. Color code: blue: right pectoralis major, green: right pectoralis minor, yellow: right subcutaneous fat, light blue: left pectoralis minor, magenta: left pectoralis minor, red: left subcutaneous fat. (Color figure online)

2   Materials and Methods

2.1   Data

CT scans were acquired from a large retrospective COPD observational study [15]. An expert identified the axial slice where pectoralis muscles were most visible at the level of the transversal aorta and segmented six different structures: left pectoralis major, left pectoralis minor, right pectoralis major, right pectoralis minor, left pectoralis subcutaneous fat and right pectoralis subcutaneous fat. The annotations were generated by applying intensity thresholds to the image and manually in-painting the structures of interest. Subcutaneous fat was defined as the layer of fat between lying between the margins of the major pectoralis muscle and the skin. Complete annotations (for the six structures) were generated for 2,000 cases, forming the completely annotated dataset. Partial annotations (only one structure per case) were generated for 3,000 cases, forming the partially annotated dataset.

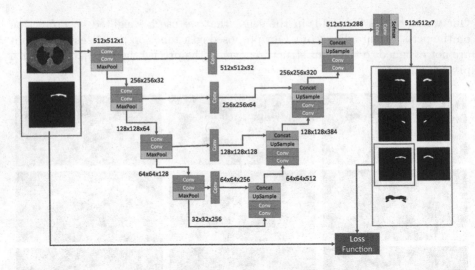

Fig. 2. Schema of the proposed training methodology. The input to the network is an image, the segmentation mask where only one of the structures is segmented and the structure identifier. The output of the network is a segmentation of all the structures present on the image encoded in a one-hot schema. Each channel has information of only one structure or the background. Only the channel corresponding to the labeled structure is used to compute the loss metric. The structure of the network is, in this case, the proposed CUNet - a UNet with convolutions in the skip connections.

2.2 Algorithm

Network: The network structure of the proposed algorithm is the same as the UNet [8], but allowing for multi-class segmentation by adding a one-hot coding schema in the last layer, which has a softmax activation. We name such network a partial-UNet (PUNet). The output of the network is an image of the same dimensions as the original, but with N+1 channels, one per each of the N structures and an extra one for the background. We further modify such architecture by adding convolutions in the skip connections (CUNet). The schema of the modified network is depicted in Fig. 2. The input to the networks is the 512×512 pixels CT axial slice, where the Hounsfield units (HU) have been clipped to the range $[-300, 500]$ and then normalized to the range $[-0.5, 0.5]$. The training set is formed by $\{X_i, (Y_i, id_i)\}$, where X_i is the image, and Y_i is the segmentation mask associated with the structure identifier id_i. The final per-pixel class is computed in a maximum likelihood fashion.

Cost Function: We use a cost-function that is the sum of the per-structure soft dice score for the structures that are present in the mini-batch. Thus, the loss function for a training point can be written as:

$$f(Y_i, \hat{Y}_i) = \frac{\sum_{i=1}^{n} \delta(id_i = i) dice(Y_i, \hat{Y}_i)}{\sum_{i=1}^{n} \delta(id_i = i)} \quad (1)$$

where δ is a function equal to one if the structure is present in the masks of the minibatch and zero otherwise, *dice* stands for the Dice coefficient, $\hat{Y}$ is the output of the softmax layer of the network, and n stands for the number of structures in the problem. Please note that $\hat{Y}$ is a real-valued scored over all the voxels of the image. Therefore the cost function is an approximation of the real dice coefficient.

Baseline Algorithms: We compare the results of the UNet trained on with partial labels (PUNet) and the modified architecture trained with partial labels (CUNet) against (a) a multi-class u-net trained completely annotated images (UNet) using as cost function the per-class normalized dice score and (b) six per-organ u-nets (6xUNet) trained on the partially labeled dataset.

Training: 500 cases with complete annotations were used to train the baseline UNet, 3,000 cases with partial annotations were used to train the CUNet, the PUNet and six the per-structure UNets; 500 cases with complete annotations were used to validate the training, perform model selection and optimize meta-parameters and 1,000 cases with complete annotations were used only for testing and to report the results. We use the well-known ADAM optimizer to train the network with a learning rate fixed to 0.00005. The training is performed for a maximum of 30 epochs, and the validation loss is monitored. Training is stopped if the validation loss does not improve or decreases for five consecutive epochs.

2.3   Statistical Analysis

We use the Kruskal-Wallis statistical method to test if the per-method Dice score samples are coming from the same distributions. Upon rejection of the null hypothesis, we perform a non-parametric comparison for all pairs of methods using the Dunn method for joint ranking. Statistical analysis was performed with JMP Statistical Software (SAS Institute Inc.).

3   Results

The UNet trained with partial labels (PUNet) obtained a Dice score of 0.909, similar to that of the six per-class UNets (0.907) and the UNet trained with complete annotation (0.909). The modified architecture, (CUNet) achieved an overall average dice score of 0.916, improving over the other methods. The per-structure analysis can be found in Table 1. The Kruskal-Wallis test showed differences between the CUNet and the other methods for the average dice ($p < 0.0001$). PUNet, 6xUNets and UNet average dice scores did not reach significance between them, indicating an equivalent behavior between such methods.

Figure 3 displays box-plots of the performance of the method per structure. There is an evident presence of outliers for all the structures. Some selected outliers are displayed in Fig. 4. We performed a post-hoc difference analysis

Table 1. Average dice score and standard deviation per structure and global for the proposed method and the alternative algorithms. UNet: multi-class unet trained in 500 annotated cases. 6xUNet: six UNets trained, one for each structure, in 500 cases with partial labels. PUNet: unet multiclass trained in the partially labeled dataset with the loss function of Eq. 1. CUNet: the proposed: the architecture of Fig. 2 trained on the partially labeled dataset.

	UNet	6xUNets	PUNet	CUNet
Left minor pectoralis	0.877 (0.087)	0.888 (0.091)	0.884 (0.084)	0.878 (0.100)
Left major pectoralis	0.915 (0.063)	0.923 (0.064)	0.918 (0.060)	0.922 (0.058)
Left subcutaneous fat	0.931 (0.068)	0.942 (0.070)	0.935 (0.066)	0.940 (0.064)
Right minor pectoralis	0.878 (0.082)	0.884 (0.091)	0.872 (0.087)	0.890 (0.078)
Right major pectoralis	0.921 (0.055)	0.914 (0.061)	0.919 (0.057)	0.928 (0.051)
Right subcutaneous fat	0.933 (0.068)	0.896 (0.109)	0.932 (0.067)	0.940 (0.063)
Mean per-case dice score	0.909 (0.049)	0.908 (0.056)	0.910 (0.050)	0.916 (0.048)

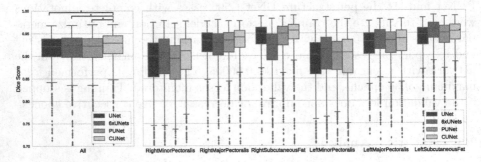

Fig. 3. Boxplots of the dice scores obtained with the different methdos. Left: all dice scores per method. Horizontal bars with stars denote statistical significance. Only the CUNet is statistically significantly different to the other methods. Right: per structure boxplot. Statsitical significance bars have been removed for clarity.

between each method pair for each structure using the Dunn's non-parametric test. The modified architecture, CUNet, mean dice score was greater than the traditional UNet for all structures analyzed ($p < 0.0001$). The CUNet did not show significant differences with the 6xUNets for the left major and right minor pectoralis and performed worse for the left subcutaneous fat and left minor pectoralis structures ($p < 0.01$). However, CUNet performed on average better than 6xUNets ($p < 0.0001$).

Training time ranged from ≈ 3 min/epoch for the UNet trained with complete labels to ≈ 18 min/epoch for the other methods, since they need to circle through six times the number of raw training images. At test time, all methods analyzed an image in $\approx 1s$, while the 6xUNet needed $6s$. All times measured in a 1080Ti GPU.

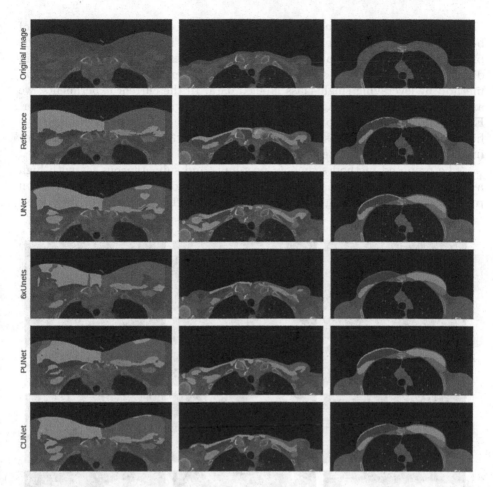

Fig. 4. Some challenging cases of the database. Each column is a different case. From top to bottom: reference standard, jointly trained UNet, individually trained UNet, UNet trained with partial labels (PUNet) and the UNet with convolutions in the skip connections trained with partial labels (CUNet). We use the same color schema as in Fig. 1. (Color figure online)

4 Discussion

We have presented a training methodology and a cost-function that enable the generation of multi-class deep learning segmentation algorithms from partially labeled images. We further the results by proposing a modification of the network architecture. Our method has shown improvement over a UNet trained on wholly annotated datasets and over six UNets trained for each organ individually, improving statistically significantly over the overall Dice score. The proposed CUNet improves the segmentation with respect to a traditional UNet when keeping the rest of parameters constant.

We have tested training with partially labeled datasets in the context of body composition measurements from axial images in CT scans. However, the proposed method is generalizable to any other context where multiple labels in different cases are present and could be used to train multi-organ segmentation method by leveraging single-class labeled data. In the current experiments, we are assuming that each image has only been labeled with a single organ. However, Eq. 1 could enable a variable number of classes to be present in each image. We have focused on 2D images. However, extensions to 3D are straightforward, for instance using a v-net instead of a u-net [14, 16].

The proposed method segments pectoralis and subcutaneous fat with high average dice coefficients, enabling its use for large cohort research. However, when presented with images with poor quality, cases with thin pectoralis or with dense

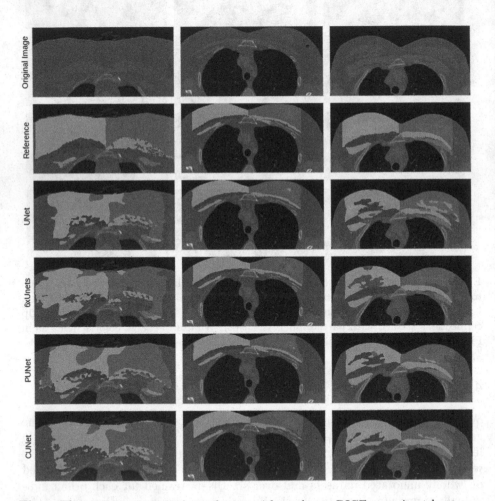

Fig. 5. Three extra segmentations of cases with moderate DICE score in at least one structure. The color conventions follows that of Fig. 4. Best viewed in color.

breasts, the segmentation can be mislead, as shown in Fig. 5. Further analysis of such outliers, and an importance sampling strategy that over-represents such fringe cases, could be used to improve the performance of the algorithm.

We have chosen as cost function the average of the per-structure dice coefficient, which is independent of the size of the structure being segmented. This might pose problems with structures that are small or too difficult to segment. An extension of the proposed method would be to modulate the cost function with weights that take into account such structural properties. Such analysis is left for future work. We have trained with a balanced dataset, in the sense that each structure had the same number of annotated images in the partial database. Modifications of Eq. 1 and data augmentation strategies can be made to compensate for unbalanced datasets.

Deep learning segmentation methods have conquered most of single organ segmentation problems. The next challenge in medical image segmentation would be to segment complex images, such as CT scans entirely. With this work, we have demonstrated that we can create multi-organ segmentation algorithms from partially labeled datasets that are equivalent or better than algorithms trained with wholly labeled datasets. This could be extrapolated to the creation of multi-organ segmentation networks from the already existing per-organ segmentation databases.n.

References

1. Kayalibay, B., Jensen, G., van der Smagt, P.: CNN-based segmentation of medical imaging data. arXiv preprint arXiv:1701.03056 (2017)
2. Cai, J., Lu, L., Xie, Y., Xing, F., Yang, L.: Improving deep pancreas segmentation in CT and MRI images via recurrent neural contextual learning and direct loss function. arXiv preprint arXiv:1707.04912 (2017)
3. Fidon, L., et al.: Scalable multimodal convolutional networks for brain tumour segmentation. In: Descoteaux, M., Maier-Hein, L., Franz, A., Jannin, P., Collins, D.L., Duchesne, S. (eds.) MICCAI 2017. LNCS, vol. 10435, pp. 285–293. Springer, Cham (2017). https://doi.org/10.1007/978-3-319-66179-7_33
4. Drozdzal, M., Chartrand, G., Vorontsov, E.: Learning normalized inputs for iterative estimation in medical image segmentation. Med. Image Anal. **44**, 1–13 (2018)
5. Roth, H.R., et al.: Hierarchical 3D fully convolutional networks for multi-organ segmentation. arXiv preprint arXiv:1704.06382 (2017)
6. Fidon, L., et al.: Generalised wasserstein dice score for imbalanced multi-class segmentation using holistic convolutional networks. arXiv preprint arXiv:1707.00478 (2017)
7. Sudre, C.H., Li, W., Vercauteren, T., Ourselin, S., Jorge Cardoso, M.: Generalised dice overlap as a deep learning loss function for highly unbalanced segmentations. In: Cardoso, M.J., et al. (eds.) DLMIA/ML-CDS -2017. LNCS, vol. 10553, pp. 240–248. Springer, Cham (2017). https://doi.org/10.1007/978-3-319-67558-9_28
8. Ronneberger, O., Fischer, P., Brox, T.: U-net: convolutional networks for biomedical image segmentation. In: Navab, N., Hornegger, J., Wells, W.M., Frangi, A.F. (eds.) MICCAI 2015. LNCS, vol. 9351, pp. 234–241. Springer, Cham (2015). https://doi.org/10.1007/978-3-319-24574-4_28

9. Drozdzal, M., Vorontsov, E., Chartrand, G., Kadoury, S., Pal, C.: The importance of skip connections in biomedical image segmentation. In: Carneiro, G., et al. (eds.) LABELS/DLMIA -2016. LNCS, vol. 10008, pp. 179–187. Springer, Cham (2016). https://doi.org/10.1007/978-3-319-46976-8_19

10. McDonald, M.L.N., et al.: Quantitative computed tomography measures of pectoralis muscle area and disease severity in chronic obstructive pulmonary disease. A cross-sectional study. Ann. Am. Thorac. Soc. **11**(3), 326–334 (2014)

11. Kinsey, C.M., San Josée Estéepar, R., Van der Velden, J., Cole, B.F., Christiani, D.C., Washko, G.R.: Lower pectoralis muscle area is associated with a worse overall survival in non- small cell lung cancer. Cancer Epidemiol., Biomark. Prev.: Publ. Am. Assoc. Cancer Res., Cosponsored Am. Soc. Prev. Oncol. **26**(1), 38–43 (2017)

12. Harmouche, R., Ross, J.C., Washko, G.R., San José Estépar, R.: Pectoralis muscle segmentation on CT images based on bayesian graph cuts with a subject-tailored atlas. In: Menze, B., et al. (eds.) MCV 2014. LNCS, vol. 8848, pp. 34–44. Springer, Cham (2014). https://doi.org/10.1007/978-3-319-13972-2_4

13. Moreta-Martinez, R., Onieva-Onieva, J., Pascau, J., San Jose Estépar, R.: Pectoralis muscle and subcutaneous adipose tissue segmentation on CT images based on convolutional networks. In: Computer Assisted Radiology and Surgery. Springer (2017)

14. Çiçek, Ö., Abdulkadir, A., Lienkamp, S.S., Brox, T., Ronneberger, O.: 3D u-net: learning dense volumetric segmentation from sparse annotation. In: Ourselin, S., Joskowicz, L., Sabuncu, M.R., Unal, G., Wells, W. (eds.) MICCAI 2016. LNCS, vol. 9901, pp. 424–432. Springer, Cham (2016). https://doi.org/10.1007/978-3-319-46723-8_49

15. Regan, E.A., et al.: Genetic epidemiology of copd (copdgene) study design. COPD **7**(1), 32–43 (2010)

16. Milletari, F., Navab, N., Ahmadi, S.A.: V-net: fully convolutional neural networks for volumetric medical image segmentation. In: 2016 Fourth International Conference on 3D Vision (3DV), pp. 565–571. IEEE (2016)

3D Pulmonary Artery Segmentation from CTA Scans Using Deep Learning with Realistic Data Augmentation

Karen López-Linares Román[1,2,4](✉), Isaac de La Bruere[3], Jorge Onieva[4],
Lasse Andresen[4], Jakob Qvortrup Holsting[4], Farbod N. Rahaghi[3],
Iván Macía[1], Miguel A. González Ballester[2,5], and Raúl San José Estepar[4]

[1] Vicomtech Foundation and Biodonostia, San Sebastián, Spain
klopez@vicomtech.org
[2] BCN Medtech, Universitat Pompeu Fabra, Barcelona, Spain
[3] Division of Pulmonary and Critical Care Medicine,
Brigham and Women's Hospital, Harvard Medical School, Boston, USA
[4] Applied Chest Imaging Laboratory, Department of Radiology,
Brigham and Women's Hospital, Harvard Medical School, Boston, USA
[5] ICREA, Barcelona, Spain

Abstract. The characterization of the vasculature in the mediastinum, more specifically the pulmonary artery, is of vital importance for the evaluation of several pulmonary vascular diseases. Thus, the goal of this study is to automatically segment the pulmonary artery (PA) from computed tomography angiography images, which opens up the opportunity for more complex analysis of the evolution of the PA geometry in health and disease and can be used in complex fluid mechanics models or individualized medicine. For that purpose, a new 3D convolutional neural network architecture is proposed, which is trained on images coming from different patient cohorts. The network makes use a strong data augmentation paradigm based on realistic deformations generated by applying principal component analysis to the deformation fields obtained from the affine registration of several datasets. The network is validated on 91 datasets by comparing the automatic segmentations with semi-automatically delineated ground truths in terms of mean Dice and Jaccard coefficients and mean distance between surfaces, which yields values of 0.89, 0.80 and 1.25 mm, respectively. Finally, a comparison against a Unet architecture is also included.

Keywords: Pulmonary artery · Deep learning · CTA
Convolutional neural network · Segmentation

This study was supported by the NHLBI awards R01HL116931 and R01HL116473.
The Titan Xp used for this research was donated by the NVIDIA Corporation.

D. Stoyanov et al. (Eds.): RAMBO 2018/BIA 2018/TIA 2018, LNCS 11040, pp. 225–237, 2018.
https://doi.org/10.1007/978-3-030-00946-5_23

1   Introduction

The morphological assessment of the Pulmonary Artery (PA) is essential to evaluate several Pulmonary Vascular Diseases (PVD). Most patients with Pulmonary
Hypertension (PH), present a remodeled main PA with a diameter considerably
larger than that of a control subject and thus, being an important biomarker for
predicting and detecting hypertension. In the Chronic Obstructive Pulmonary
Disease (COPD), a widening of the PA is associated with increased risks of exacerbation and decreased survival rates. Pulmonary Embolism (PE) refers to the
blockage of one of the pulmonary arteries, mostly caused by blood clots. Thus,
it is essential to monitor the arterial obstruction to evaluate the severity of PE.

Computed tomography (CT) and CT angiography (CTA) play a crucial role
in the diagnosis and management of PVD since they allow to assess macroscopic
pulmonary vascular morphology quantitatively. In this study, we aim at leveraging CTA images of several patient cohorts to segment the PA with a new 3D
Convolutional Neural Network (CNN) architecture. Deep learning has already
been applied to segment other vascular structures from CT images with promising results [3,7,10], which encouraged us to use it for PA segmentation.

2   Literature Review

The segmentation of PA can be challenging due to its complicated and variable shape, motion artifacts, and proximity to other blood vessels such as the
pulmonary vein that may hamper the correct segmentation. Even if there are
many studies in the literature about pulmonary vascular tree segmentation, they
usually focus on vessel segmentation within the lungs or pulmonary emboli and
nodule detection, without specifically analyzing the PA.

Regarding the segmentation of the PA outside the lung, which is our goal,
only a few studies have been proposed. In [2] a Hessian matrix based preprocessing followed by a region growing method is proposed, which relies on a previous
extraction of the lungs and the heart. The method in [14] also requires a priori knowledge of the artery morphology followed by a fast-marching algorithm
and a registration to a target reference volume, which did not fully address
the variability in PA sizes and shapes. In [6] a semi-automated tool which uses
level sets and geodesic active contours to segment the main PA is presented,
with the goal of measuring the PA diameters in patients with PH. From the
obtained segmentations, the authors extract the artery centerline and measure
the diameter, reporting a mean error up to 6 mm. A similar study to measure
PA cross-sectional area is proposed in [9], where the artery is segmented using
dilation and erosion operations on 14 normal patient CTA scans.

Compared to previous works in the literature, our method combines images
from PE cohorts, PH cohorts, and control patients and is tested on many volumes. Additionally, it is fully automatic, it does not include any shape prior and
it yields a mean error when measuring PA diameters of 2.5 mm.

3   Materials

A total of 51 CTA volumes of different patients are employed to train our CNN. Among these datasets, 39 patients have PE, 8 of them are control subjects who were thought to have PH, and the remaining 4 have hypertension. The mean intensity in the PA is higher than 550 HU in all the CTA volumes, and motion-related artifacts are present in most of the images. Figure 1 shows sample CTA slices of three patients coming from different cohorts.

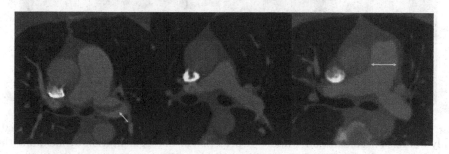

Fig. 1. Sample CTA slices of 3 patients from different cohorts. Left - Pulmonary embolism dataset, where the arrow points towards a clot; Middle - Control subject; Right - Pulmonary hypertension case, where the arrows show a dilated artery.

To test the network, an additional 91 CTA volumes are used, all of them corresponding to patients with PE, being it our largest cohort. The mean intensity in the PA in these cases ranges between 350 HU and 550 HU.

3.1   Fuzzy Ground Truth Generation

For the 142 patients, ground truth labels are obtained semi-automatically using ITK-Snap [16]. The first step consists of selecting a region of interest around the PA, extracting a sub-volume that starts at the aortic valve and expands until the main PA is not observed.

Then, an initial segmentation is extracted with the region competition snake approach, using a thresholded version of the image as the feature image that drives the evolution and forces the snake to fit the boundary of the artery. The minimum and maximum thresholds employed to create the feature image for the training datasets are set to 500 HU and 900 HU, respectively, whereas for the test images, the employed thresholds are 300 HU and 900 HU. A seed point is placed within the main PA to initialize the evolution of the snake, which is manually stopped when an approximate segmentation is obtained. The parameters that control the evolution of the front, i.e. the region competition force and the smoothing or curvature force, are set to 1 and 0.5, respectively.

Finally, the output segmentation from the region competition snake approach is manually refined, as shown in Fig. 2. Two main corrections are applied:

- Removal of veins and other structures incorrectly labeled as arteries
- Inclusion of clots in the segmentation to ensure a natural artery shape

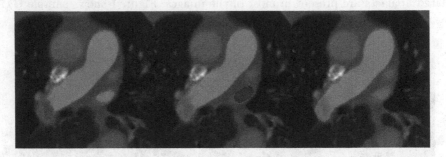

Fig. 2. Correction of the automatically generated ground truth labels. Left - Automatically obtained segmentation; Middle - Correction of the segmentation by including the clot (green) and removing the vein (blue); Right - Final fuzzy ground truth used for the CNN. (Color figure online)

The resulting ground truth segmentations are considered fuzzy, since it is difficult to have a precise delimitation of the artery contour when there is a large clot in the artery. Additionally, small artery branches have not been consistently labeled across the different datasets.

4   Methods

Hereby, we propose a new 3D convolutional neural network for the segmentation of the PA from CTA volumes. The proposed network, fully described in Sect. 4.3, is inspired by the 3D V-net [8] with modifications introduced from the 2D Fully Convolutional DenseNet (FC-DenseNet) [5] and the 2D Efficient neural network (ENet) [11]. We employ a training strategy that relies on a strong use of data augmentation, mostly generated with realistic deformations, as explained in Sect. 4.1. Finally, we validate our network with the test set by comparing the semi-automatically generated ground truths with the network predictions in terms of Dice and Jaccard scores. Since the final clinical goal is to characterize the aortic morphology, we also measure the distance at each point between the two surfaces, i.e., the ground truth and the output from the network.

4.1   Data Augmentation Using Realistic Deformations

Data augmentation have been largely used in deep learning in the biomedical field due to the limited number of annotated datasets. In particular, for the case of 3D datasets, it is difficult and time-consuming to obtain a corpus of annotated images that are large enough to account for the anatomical variability between subjects. Thus, researchers usually apply data augmentation techniques, mostly in the form of rotations and translations to generate new volumes. In [12] a new data augmentation approach was proposed, based on applying random elastic deformations to the original volumes. The use of these synthetically generated volumes seemed to be the key to train a segmentation network with very few annotated samples.

Inspired by this work, we efficiently augment our dataset using realistic elastic deformations as well as traditional rotations and translations. Unlike in [12], where the applied deformations were random, we propose to generate realistic deformation vectors from the Principal Component Analysis (PCA) of a subset of deformation fields extracted directly from the affine registration of several volumes. The steps are the following:

1. Register 10 CTA volumes to a reference volume of a control subject using 3D Slicer [1] and extract the 3D deformation fields corresponding only to the affine transformation
2. Extract the mean deformation and the eigenvectors and eigenvalues of the ten deformation fields using two PCA models:
   - PCA1-Model: considers the correlation between the components of the deformation fields, i.e., x, y, and z
   - PCA2 Model: considers each component of the fields independently
3. Generate new deformation fields by randomly weighing the first six eigenvectors (which account for most of the variability) with values from 0 to the square root of the corresponding eigenvalue
   - For PCA1-Model the three components are weighted equally
   - For PCA2-Model we weight x, y and z independently
4. Generate new synthetic volumes by applying these deformation fields to each original CTA volume in the training set, as shown in Eq. 1 for PCA1-Model and in Eq. 2 for PCA2-Model.

$$\tilde{I}_j : \sum_{i=1}^{6} < w_i * B_i > + \mu \tag{1}$$

$$\tilde{I}_j : \sum_{i=1}^{6} < w_{x_i} * B_{x_i} > + \mu_x + \sum_{i=1}^{6} < w_{y_i} * B_{y_i} > + \mu_y + \sum_{i=1}^{6} < w_{z_i} * B_{z_i} > + \mu_z \tag{2}$$

where $\tilde{I}_j$ is the generated synthetic image, w_i are the weights generated from the eigenvalues, B_i are the eigenvectors, and μ is the mean image extracted from the 10 original deformation fields.

Following this procedure, we create 50 new volumes per each original input CTA. 30 of them are extracted with PCA1-Model, whereas another 20 are generated with PCA2-Model. This allows the network to learn invariance to deformations without the need to see these transformations in the annotated image corpus. This is particularly important in biomedical segmentation since deformation is the most common variation in tissue and realistic deformations can be simulated efficiently with the proposed approach. Examples of the generated volumes in 2D and 3D are shown in Figs. 3 and 4, respectively.

4.2 Related Networks Served as Inspiration

The **V-Net** [8] network is one of the few architectures in the literature specifically designed to work with 3D images. It is composed of convolution, deconvolution and pooling layers arranged in an encoding and a decoding path. Every couple of layers in the encoding path a down-convolution is performed, and for every pooling the number of feature maps is doubled to allow the network to distribute the information from the previous layer throughout the maps, instead of losing it when reducing the spatial resolution. Before each down-convolution, a skip-connection is introduced to pass higher resolution maps to the decoding path. In the decoding path, an up-convolution is performed every couple

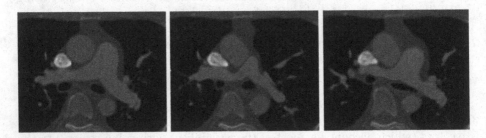

Fig. 3. Sample axial slices of volumes generated using the realistic deformation based data augmentation technique. Right: original axial slice; Middle: corresponding slice generated using PCA2-Model; Left: corresponding slice generated using PCA1-Model.

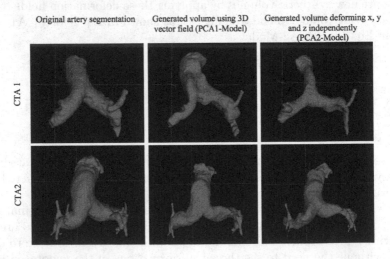

Fig. 4. Sample volumes generated using the realistic deformation based data augmentation technique.

of layers and feature fusion with the skip connections is applied, improving the convergence time and the quality of the segmentation.

FC-DenseNet [5] is one of the most recent networks for 2D semantic segmentation. As the V-Net, FC-DenseNet also uses an encoding and a decoding pathway to obtain global features, incorporating feature fusion. However, opposed to the idea in V-Net, this architecture uses many convolutional layers but each of them with few channels, whereas in V-net there are fewer convolutional layers and the information is distributed in more filters. Each layer is directly connected to every other layer in a feed-forward fashion and batch normalization is implemented before all convolutional layers, which helps to control over-fitting.

Finally, in [11] the **ENet** is proposed, which aims at providing real-time semantic segmentation by using a low amount of parameters, squeezing in as much information as possible in every parameter. A critical contribution of ENet is the introduction of a down-sampling block that combines max pooling and strided convolution to avoid representational bottlenecks.

4.3 Proposed Convolutional Neural Network

Figure 5 shows the main building blocks of our proposed network, displayed in Fig. 6. It has an encoding and a decoding path as the V-Net and the FC-DenseNet. As in FC-DenseNet, the input is propagated through the network via dense connections and channels are appended throughout. The structure of the encoder is also changed to an ENet style block. We also remove some layers as compared to FC-DenseNet, but increase the width. The number of filters in each

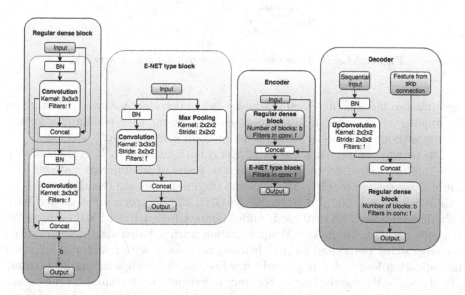

Fig. 5. The several blocks that compose the proposed convolutional neural network.

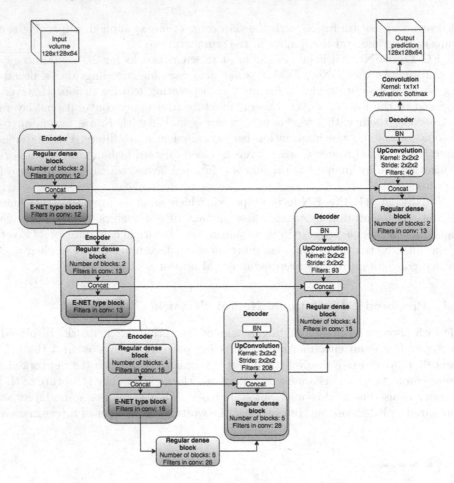

Fig. 6. Scheme of the proposed convolutional neural network.

regular dense block is increased gradually. In the decoding pathway, we decrease the number of channels steadily to reach an amount that is computationally feasible without performing extreme information compression.

The network is implemented using Keras with tensorflow. It is trained with 3468 volumes extracted by augmenting the scans of 91 different patients. All volumes are resized to $128 \times 128 \times 64$ and the intensities are rescaled to 0–1.

The model is built in a Xeon E7 3.6 GHz, 62 GB processor equipped with a Nvidia GeForce GTX1080 card, under Linux Ubuntu 16.04 SMP 64 bits. We train the network using ADAM optimization with a batch size of 1, an initial learning rate of 1e−03 and plateau learning rate decay with a factor of 0.2 when the validation loss is not improved after five epochs, with a minimum learning rate of 1e−05. We use the binary accuracy metric and try to minimize the binary cross entropy loss function. Early stopping is also applied to avoid overfitting, thus, stopping the learning process after 20 epochs, as shown in Fig. 7.

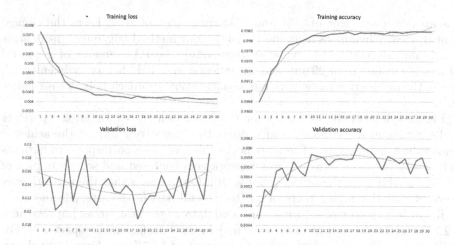

Fig. 7. Training and validation loss and accuracy curves and fitted polynomial trendline as a function of epochs. Over-fitting is observed after epoch 20.

Finally, the model is tested on the 91 less contrasted CTA scans described in Sect. 3. The predictions are 3D probability maps where the intensity of each pixel is the probability of it being PA. We apply gaussian smoothing to the output grayscale image, followed by Otsu's thresholding that aims at selecting an optimal case-specific threshold when the image contains two classes following bi-modal histogram and voting binary hole filling to obtain the final binary segmentation.

4.4   Validation Approach

To evaluate the performance of our network, we compare the automatically obtained segmentation with the fuzzy ground truths in terms of Dice and Jaccard scores for the 91 test cases, and we calculate the mean and standard deviation.

Since the final clinical goal is to characterize PA morphology, i.e. its diameter, we generate the 3D surfaces of both segmentations using VTK [13] to calculate the mean distance between them. First, we use the Discrete Marching Cubes method to extract the surfaces and the normals at every point. Then, we create a Kd-tree spatial decomposition of the set of points of each surface. Finally, we use a point locator to find the closest point in the ground truth surface for every point in our segmentation, and we measure the Euclidean distance between them. The distance between surfaces is the mean distance of all the points in the surface, which corresponds to the mean error when measuring the PA radius.

5   Results

Table 1 summarizes the results for the proposed network using realistic deformation-based data augmentation and without using it. Our method yields a mean Dice coefficient of 89% and a Jaccard score of 80%. From the clinical point of view, when measuring the PA radius our method falls into a mean error of 1.25 mm. According to several studies [4,15], the PA diameter of a control subject is smaller than 29 mm and in patients with PH the artery is enlarged. Hence, the mean error made with our segmentation approach falls at least below 8.6%.

Figure 8 depicts the box plots for the validation scores for all the patients used for testing, where some clear outliers that negatively impact the achieved mean values are observed. The most noticeable two cases correspond to patients with a very big liver, in which the network gets confused and segments part of the liver as if it were the artery (see Fig. 10). Our guess is that the network may interpret that this region corresponds to the end part of the artery branch.

Regarding the use of deformation-based data augmentation, an improvement of 2.3% and 3.9% is obtained for Dice and Jaccard coefficients, respectively. For the distance between surfaces, an improvement of 1.57% is achieved. As shown in Fig. 8, the Dice and Jaccard score's improvement is statistically significant according to the Wilcoxon test but it is not for the distance between surfaces.

Finally, we also trained and tested the V-net in [8] to compare the results, which are shown in Table 2. Even if the Dice and Jaccard scores are very similar for both architectures, the distance between surfaces is much larger in the case of the Unet and the statistical significance is notable, with a p-value of $1.73e-09$ for the case of the distance according to the Wilkoxon test (Fig. 9). This suggest that our architecture enables better quantification of mean pulmonary artery diameters.

Table 1. Evaluation metrics for the proposed network when including realistic deformable registration based data augmentation and without it.

	Mean Dice Score	Mean Jaccard Score	Mean distance between surfaces (mm)
Without augmentation	0.87 ± 0.07	0.77 ± 0.09	1.27 ± 0.98
With data augmentation	0.89 ± 0.07	0.80 ± 0.09	1.25 ± 1.17

Table 2. Evaluation metrics for the proposed method as compared to a traditional Unet when using the deformation-based data augmentation.

	Mean Dice Score	Mean Jaccard Score	Mean distance between surfaces (mm)
Unet	0.89 ± 0.04	0.80 ± 0.05	1.66 ± 1.03
Proposed architecture	0.89 ± 0.07	0.80 ± 0.09	1.25 ± 1.17

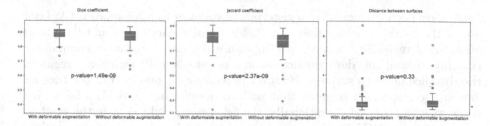

Fig. 8. Plots showing the Dice and Jaccard scores and the mean distance between surfaces for all the test volumes when using the proposed data augmentation technique, and without it. The p-values corresponding to the Wilkoxon test are also displayed.

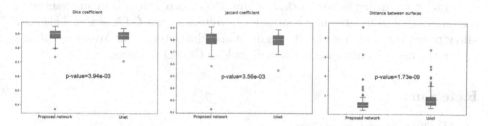

Fig. 9. Plots showing the Dice and Jaccard scores and the mean distance between surfaces for the proposed architecture and a Unet. The p-values corresponding to the Wilkoxon test are also displayed.

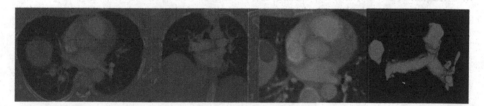

Fig. 10. Outlier test case of a patient with a very big liver, which the network segments as artery.

6 Conclusions

Hereby, we proposed a new CNN to PA segmentation from CTA images, which opens up the opportunity for more complex analysis of the evolution of the PA geometry (i.e. going beyond just measuring the diameter). The network is based on an encoder-decoder scheme similar to the V-net [8], but by including Dense blocks and Enet blocks, we are able to improve the segmentation results, mostly in terms of distance between surfaces. Adding bootstrapping to the loss function could further increase the accuracy of our model.

Additionally, a novel data augmentation approach has been described, which relies on a PCA analysis of deformation fields extracted from the affine registration of several volumes. For the current work, 10 different base deformation fields have been extracted by registering 10 volumes to a reference CTA. Looking at the results, it seems that more fields are necessary to account for a larger anatomical variability between patients since the improvement as compared to training without this data augmentation is not statistically significant regarding the distance between surfaces. However, a tendency is observed in the Dice and Jaccard scores, which suggests that with more deformation fields a better outcome may be achieved. Additionally, the fields generated to create the synthetic images after the PCA analysis are obtained by varying the weight of each eigenvector with the square root of the corresponding eigenvalue, which limits the range of deviation from the mean deformation. Weighting each eigenvector with a wider value range could also account for more variability in the input data.

Finally, regarding future work, our aim is to incorporate a data augmentation technique that simulates non-contrast CT volumes from CTA scans. This may allow to use the same network to segment and characterize the artery in cohorts where the use of contrast is not usual, such as COPD patients.

References

1. 3D Slicer. https://www.slicer.org/
2. Ebrahimdoost, Y., Qanadli, S.D., Nikravanshalmani, A., Ellis, T.J., Shojaee, Z.F., Dehmeshki, J.: Automatic segmentation of pulmonary artery (PA) in 3D pulmonary CTA images. In: Proceedings of the DSP, pp. 1–5 (2011)
3. Ibragimov, B., Toesca, D., Chang, D., Koong, A., Xing, L.: Combining deep learning with anatomical analysis for segmentation of the portal vein for liver SBRT planning. Phys. Med. Biol. **62**(23), 8943–8958 (2017)
4. Collins, J., Stern, E.J.: Chest Radiology, the Essentials. Lippincott Williams & Wilkins, Philadelphia (2007)
5. Jégou, S., Drozdzal, M., Vázquez, D., Romero, A., Bengio, Y.: The one hundred layers tiramisu: fully convolutional densenets for semantic segmentation. CoRR abs/1611.09326 (2016)
6. Linguraru, M.G., Pura, J.A., Uitert, R.L.V., Mukherjee, N., Summers, R.M.: Segmentation and quantification of pulmonary artery for noninvasive CT assessment of sickle cell secondary pulmonary hypertension. Med. Phys. **37**(4), 1522–1532 (2010)
7. Meijs, M., Manniesing, R.: Artery and vein segmentation of the cerebral vasculature in 4D CT using a 3D fully convolutional neural network. In: Proceedings of the SPIE, vol. 10575, p. 6 (2018)
8. Milletari, F., Navab, N., Ahmadi, S.: V-Net: fully convolutional neural networks for volumetric medical image segmentation. In: Proceedings of the 3DV, pp. 565–571 (2016)
9. Moses, D., Sammut, C., Zrimec, T.: Automatic segmentation and analysis of the main pulmonary artery on standard post-contrast CT studies using iterative erosion and dilation. Int. J. Comput. Assist. Radiol. Surg. **11**(3), 381–395 (2016)
10. Nardelli, P., Jimenez-Carretero, D., Bermejo-Peláez, D., Ledesma-Carbayo, M.J., Rahaghi, F.N., Estépar, R.S.J.: Deep-learning strategy for pulmonary artery-vein classification of non-contrast ct images. In: Proceedings of the ISBI, pp. 384–387 (2017)
11. Paszke, A., Chaurasia, A., Kim, S., Culurciello, E.: ENet: a deep neural network architecture for real-time semantic segmentation. CoRR abs/1606.02147 (2016)

12. Ronneberger, O., Fischer, P., Brox, T.: U-Net: convolutional networks for biomedical image segmentation. CoRR abs/1505.04597 (2015)
13. Schroeder, W., Martin, K., Lorensen, B.: The Visualization Toolkit–An Object-Oriented Approach to 3D Graphics, 4th edn. Kitware Inc., Clifton Park (2006)
14. Sebbe, R., Gosselin, B., Coche, E.: Segmentation of opacified thorax vessels using model-driven active contour. In: Proceedings of the IEEE EMBS, vol. 3, pp. 2535–2538 (2005)
15. Truong, Q.A., et al.: Reference values for normal pulmonary artery dimensions by noncontrast cardiac computed tomography: the Framingham heart study. Circ. Cardiovasc. Imaging 5(1), 147–154 (2012)
16. Yushkevich, P.A., et al.: User-guided 3D active contour segmentation of anatomical structures: significantly improved efficiency and reliability. Neuroimage 31(3), 1116–1128 (2006)

Automatic Airway Segmentation in Chest CT Using Convolutional Neural Networks

A. Garcia-Uceda Juarez[1,2(✉)], H. A. W. M. Tiddens[2,3], and M. de Bruijne[1,4(✉)]

[1] Biomedical Imaging Group Rotterdam, Departments of Medical Informatics
and Radiology, Erasmus MC, 3015 CE Rotterdam, The Netherlands
{a.garciauceda,debruijne}@erasmusmc.nl
[2] Department of Pediatric Pulmonology, Erasmus MC-Sophia Children Hospital,
3015 CE Rotterdam, The Netherlands
[3] Department of Radiology and Nuclear Medicine,
Erasmus MC-Sophia Children Hospital, 3015 CE Rotterdam, The Netherlands
[4] Department of Computer Science, University of Copenhagen,
2100 Copenhagen, Denmark

Abstract. Segmentation of the airway tree from chest computed tomography (CT) images is critical for quantitative assessment of airway diseases including bronchiectasis and chronic obstructive pulmonary disease (COPD). However, obtaining an accurate segmentation of airways from CT scans is difficult due to the high complexity of airway structures. Recently, deep convolutional neural networks (CNNs) have become the state-of-the-art for many segmentation tasks, and in particular the so-called Unet architecture for biomedical images. However, its application to the segmentation of airways still remains a challenging task. This work presents a simple but robust approach based on a 3D Unet to perform segmentation of airways from chest CTs. The method is trained on a dataset composed of 12 CTs, and tested on another 6 CTs. We evaluate the influence of different loss functions and data augmentation techniques, and reach an average dice coefficient of 0.8 between the ground-truth and our automated segmentations.

Keywords: Airway segmentation · Convolutional neural networks
Data augmentation · Bronchiectasis · CT

1 Introduction

Segmentation of airways in chest computed tomography (CT) images is critical to obtain reliable biomarkers to assess the presence and extent of airway diseases. Biomarkers such as airway lumen diameter, airway wall thickness, airway tapering and airway-artery diameter ratio help in detection of early signs of disease and quantification of its severity. However, the segmentation of airways is a difficult task due to the complex tree-like structure of airways, with a large number of branches of very different sizes and orientations.

© Springer Nature Switzerland AG 2018
D. Stoyanov et al. (Eds.): RAMBO 2018/BIA 2018/TIA 2018, LNCS 11040, pp. 238–250, 2018.
https://doi.org/10.1007/978-3-030-00946-5_24

There are several methods proposed for automatic extraction/segmentation of the airway tree in chest CTs. Conventional methods such as region growing can successfully capture the main bronchi, but systematically fail at extracting the peripheral bronchi of smaller size. Other more sophisticated techniques are: [1], based on a region growing approach using an airway probability map computed by a voxel classifier, together with an airway/vessel orientation similarity term; [2], based on a tube-likeness shape detector computed from the Gradient Vector Flow field properties; or [3,4], based on optimal surface graph-cut methods which find a globally optimal solution accounting for both airway lumen and outer wall surfaces with a wide range of tailored geometric constraints. These and other airway segmentation methods were evaluated by Lo et al. in the EXACT09 challenge [5].

Since recently, the state-of-the-art methods for many image segmentation tasks are based on convolutional neural networks (CNNs) [6]. In particular, the so-called Unet network proposed by Ronneberger et al. [7] has become popular in segmentation tasks of biomedical images. With regards to airway segmentation, a number of CNNs-based methods [8–11] have been proposed which have outperformed the classical methods compared in [5]. In particular, [8–10] use the 3D Unet network to analyse volumetric images. Another novel method for airway extraction is proposed by Selvan et al. [12], by formulating it as a mean field approximation based graph refinement task that resembles feed forward neural networks.

In this paper, we propose a robust fully automatic end-to-end method based on 3D Unets to perform airway segmentation in chest CT images. Other Unet-based approaches are more complex, such as [8] which relies on a tracking algorithm of the connected structure of the airway tree, and uses a local volume of interest (VOI) around single tracked branches. In contrast, our method is simpler and end-to-end optimised, whose only input are large images patches containing various branches at once. This makes it more robust.

2 Methodology

The processing pipeline for airway segmentation proposed in this work is described in the next subsections, including pre- and postprocessing techniques.

2.1 Network Architecture

The 3D Unet is adopted for volumetric image analysis by replacing the operators of the original 2D U-Net proposed in [7]: (i) convolution; (ii) pooling; (iii) upsampling; with their analogous 3D operator. The Unet method consists of an encoder/downsampling path followed by a decoder/upsampling path, each with 5 levels of resolution. Each level in the downsampling path is composed of two $3 \times 3 \times 3$ convolutional layers followed by a $2 \times 2 \times 2$ pooling layer. At each level the number of feature channels is doubled, with a number of channels in the first level of 16. In the upsampling path, only one $3 \times 3 \times 3$ convolutional layer is used before an $2 \times 2 \times 2$ upsample layer. This is in order to reduce memory requirements of the network, since convolutions in the upsampling path can be less relevant, as mentioned in [13]. Each convolution operator is followed by a rectified linear unit (ReLU). At each level the number of feature channels is halved. The final layer consists of a $1 \times 1 \times 1$ convolutional layer followed by a sigmoid activation function. This way the network output is a voxelwise probability map of the sought airways, of the same size as input images. The total number of convolutional layers in the network is 15.

In the convolution operations, an adequate zero-padding is used to obtain an output of the same size as the input. This is for sake of simplicity in designing the same network for arbitrary sizes of input image. Moreover, due to size constraints of the input images, we disable the convolution/pooling operators applied in axial direction in the deepest level of the network, i.e. we use $1 \times 3 \times 3$ convolutions and $1 \times 2 \times 2$ pooling.

As regularisation, we use exclusively on-the-fly data augmentation during training, explained in Sect. 2.3. No dropout has been used. The reason for this is twofold: (i) our experiments showed that data augmentation was more efficient for regularisation, and (ii) the use of dropout in Keras incurs in a large increase in memory footprint, since the feature maps input to the dropout layers are duplicated. Indeed, the main challenge of our experiments is the maximum size of the network that fits in GPU memory, more important than computational speed. And while the inclusion dropout layers requires a significant reduction of size, data augmentation is generated on the fly with no memory overhead and a negligible increase in computational time.

2.2   Choice of Loss Function

Two different loss functions for training the network have been tested in our experiments, namely: (i) weighted binary cross-entropy (wBCE) (Eq. 1), and (ii) Dice coefficient (dice) loss (Eq. 2).

$$\mathcal{L}_1 = w_B \sum_{x \in N_B \cap N_L} \log(1 - p(x)) + w_A \sum_{x \in N_A \cap N_L} \log(p(x)) \tag{1}$$

$$\mathcal{L}_2 = \frac{2 \sum_{x \in N_L} p(x) g(x)}{\sum_{x \in N_L} p(x) + \sum_{x \in N_L} g(x) + \epsilon} \tag{2}$$

where $p(x), g(x)$ are the voxelwise airway probability maps and airway ground-truth, respectively. The subindexes B, A refer to the ground-truth classes background/airways, respectively, and L corresponds to the region of interest (ROI): the lungs. N_k is the group of voxels for each class. ϵ is a tolerance needed when there are no ground-truth voxels found in the (sub)image.

We force the training of the network to the ROI: the lungs fields, so that only voxels within this region contribute to the loss. This is achieved by masking the probability maps and ground-truth with a lung segmentation. This is indicated by the intersection $N_B \cap N_L$ in Eqs. 1–2. This approach forces the voxelwise classification to focus only on discriminating between airways and lung parenchyma (background), ignoring other non-relevant structures including ribs, adipose tissue, and skin. The lung segmentation needed in this approach is easily computed by a region-growing method [1].

In the wBCE function (Eq. 1), the weights w_B, w_A are used to compensate for a large interclass imbalance of lung parenchyma (background)/airways voxels. The weights are computed on the fly, for a given input image patch, as the ratio of the opposite class voxels with respect to the total voxels, or analogously: $w_B = 1, w_A = N_B/N_A$.

2.3 Preprocessing

The main challenge of our experiments is that chest CT images have a size much larger than the maximum input to the network that fits in GPU memory. We apply several preprocessing steps to adapt the input images and reduce the memory footprint.

Cropping Images. The CTs are cropped to the region of interest: the lungs. The bounding-box is of fixed size in x, y dimensions: 352×240 pixels, and centered in each lung. The axial dimension is different for each CT. The box is enlarged by 30 voxels in each direction to account for border effects.

Sliding-Window. A sliding-window approach is used to extract smaller image patches from the input CTs that fit to the size requirements of the network, similar to the method in [6]. The sliding is undertaken only in axial direction with a stride of 104 pixels, while the x, y dimensions are fixed and equal to the network input size: 352×240 pixels. This is schematically shown in Fig. 1. The sliding stride is set to have 75% overlap in between the extracted patches, in order to prevent border effects. The sliding-window is used for all CTs of training and validation sets. The resulting image patches are generated on the fly during training, to prevent any memory overhead, and are randomly shuffled at the beginning of each epoch.

Data Augmentation. Data augmentation is applied systematically to the input images during training, by means of (i) rigid transformations, and/or (ii) elastic deformations. The former operations consist of random flipping and rotations with a maximum value of 10 degrees, in the three dimensions. The elastic deformations consist of smooth voxel displacements computed using bicubic interpolation from random displacement vectors on a coarse grid of 3×3, which are sampled from a Gaussian distribution with 25 voxels standard deviation. This methodology is similar to the one used in [7]. This is schematically shown in Fig. 1. The data augmentation is applied over the 3D images patches extracted by the sliding-window method, on both the training and validations sets. The resulting images are generated on the fly during training, and these are the input to the network.

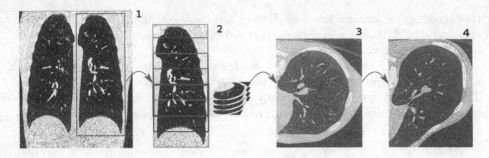

Fig. 1. Preprocessing pipeline of input images to the network. 1: crop CTs. 2: Extract 3D images patches by sliding-window. 3, 4: Apply data augmentation (elastic deformations) to the input patch, which is fed to the network.

2.4   Post-processing

Zero-padding in convolution operations in the network is used for simplicity, but the results suffer from border effects where the probability maps are less reliable towards the image boundaries. Instead, a network composed of valid convolutions ensures a fully reliable output, but its size is strongly reduced to roughly 25–50% of input size. This is an issue in our experiments where the axial dimension of input patches is rather small.

The technique implemented to prevent border effects is schematically shown in Fig. 2 and works as follows: the output probability maps are multiplied with a function that is: (i) "1" within a window corresponding to the output of a similar network with valid convolutions, (ii) elsewhere, a quadratic polynomial decreasing towards the output borders. The function in 1D corresponds to Eq. 3, with x_l, x_r the limits of the output in (i), and image dimensions $x \in [0, x_m]$.

$$f(x) = \begin{cases} (x/x_l)^2 & \text{if } x < x_l \\ 1 & \text{if } x_l \leq x \leq x_r \\ ((x_m - x)/(x_m - x_r))^2 & \text{if } x > x_r \end{cases} \tag{3}$$

The full size output is reconstructed by placing together output patches following the structure generated for input images, and normalizing for patches overlap. Finally, the output outside the lung ROI is discarded by masking the probability maps with the binary mask of lungs. The final airway tree is obtained by thresholding the resulting airway probability maps.

3   Dataset and Experiments Set-Up

The dataset used to conduct the experiments consists of 24 inspiratory chest CT scans from pediatric subjects, 12 controls and 12 with respiratory disease: 11 with Cystic fibrosis (CF) and 1 with Common Variable Inmune Deficiency (CVID). Both groups were gender and age matched: range 6 to 17 years old, 5 females, per group. Scanning was undertaken using spirometry-guidance in

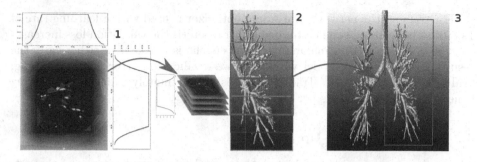

Fig. 2. Postprocessing of output probability maps. 1: diminish output near image boundaries to prevent border effects. 2, 3: Reconstruct full size probability maps, and apply thresholding to obtain airway tree.

a Siemens SOMATOM Definition Flash scanner. Similar kernel reconstructions were used for all scans: I70f/3, B75f, and B70f. This dataset has been prepared in the works of [14, 15].

Each CT scan consists of a number of cross-sectional slices, from 265 to 971 slices, with varying thickness in the range 0.75–1.0 mm, and slice spacing from 0.3 to 1.0 mm. Each slice is of fixed size equal to 512×512 pixels, with a pixel size in the range 0.44–0.71 mm.

The 12 CTs for control and disease patients are randomly split in three categories: training, validation and testing, with proportion 50/25/25%, respectively. The final data groups are then: 12 CTs for training, 6 CTs for validation and 6 CTs for testing.

The ground-truth used to train the network are reference segmentations of the airways outer wall obtained from an accurate airway segmentation method [4] applied on manual annotations of centrelines. These are manually extracted for the entire airway tree using specialised software in the work of [14]. A coarse segmentation is generated from the centrelines, and then the surface graph-cut method [4] is applied to refine this and obtain an accurate segmentation of both airway lumen and outer wall.

The experiments are conducted in a GPU NVIDIA GeForce GTX 1080 Ti with 11 GB memory. The network architecture has been implemented in Keras framework[1].

3.1 Network Optimisation

The network is designed to accommodate the largest input images possible that fit the GPU memory during training. This corresponds to input images of size $104 \times 352 \times 240$ with a batch containing only one image. It has been observed that this is advantageous over increasing the batch size using smaller input images.

---

[1] https://keras.io/.

For training the network, the Adam optimizer is used with a learning rate of 1.0e-05. The training time is stopped either when (i) the validation loss increases over 15 epochs, or (ii) a maximum of 300 epochs is reached. In either case, the results consists of the model with the lowest validation error during training, evaluated on the test set. Training time is approximately 1 day, while testing time is only a few seconds per CT scan.

3.2 Experiments Set-Up

The various experiments conducted correspond to different set-ups of the network, namely: (i) use of (a) dice or (b) wBCE loss function, and (ii) use of (a) rigid transformations or (b) elastic deformations as data augmentation. All the experiments are displayed in Table 1.

4   Results and Discussion

The free ROC (FROC) curves for all models in Table 1 are displayed in Fig. 3. This shows the sensitivity and number of false positives for the segmentations

Table 1. List of set-ups of experiments conducted

	Loss function	Data augmentation	Name
1	wBCE	None	wBCE-None
2	wBCE	Rigid	wBCE-Rigid
3	dice	None	dice-None
4	dice	Rigid	dice-Rigid
5	dice	Elastic	dice-Elastic

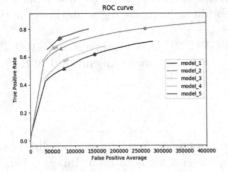 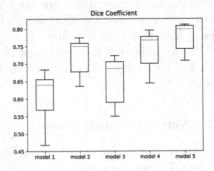

Fig. 3. Left: FROC curve computed on the test set, by varying the thresholding in the probability maps, for all models in Table 1. The circle/triangle corresponds to a threshold of 0.5/optimal value, respectively. The optimal thresholds are: with dice loss: 0.5; with wBCE loss: around 0.9. Right: average Dice coefficient on the test set. The results correspond to the optimal threshold for each model.

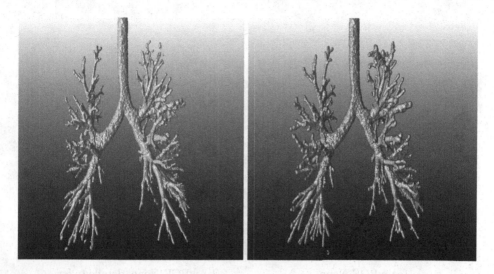

Fig. 4. Left: visualization of the segmented airway tree, obtained for one of test CTs with the model "dice-Elastic" and optimal threshold. Right: ground-truth

obtained when varying the threshold level in the probability maps. An optimal threshold value for each case is estimated as the point on the FROC curve closest to the upper-left corner. The accuracy measured as the Dice coefficient averaged over the test set is also shown in Fig. 3. The trachea and main bronchi are excluded from this calculation. For visualization, the segmented airway tree for one of test CTs obtained with the model "dice-Elastic" in Table 1 is displayed in Fig. 4, together with the ground-truth. Furthermore, the false positives and false negatives voxels for the segmentations obtained with all models tested (Table 1) on the same CT are displayed in Fig. 5. These results correspond to the optimal threshold for each model.

The most accurate segmentations are obtained when using the dice loss function, and elastic deformations as data augmentation. The average Dice coefficient on the test set is 0.80, excluding the trachea and main bronchi. This accuracy is similar to the results reported in [8] on a larger dataset.

In Fig. 5 it is seen that the largest errors are false negatives located in the tip of peripheral airways, which indicates that the method captures slightly shorter branches than the ground-truth. Also false positives are important in this region. Nevertheless, some of these errors might be due to missing smaller airways in the ground-truth, explained by the fact that some terminal branches were missed in the centrelines annotations. Other false positives are present in the form of small disconnected blobs. To reduce these errors, one could select the largest connected component or apply post-processing techniques such as Conditional Random Fields (CRF) [16]. Furthermore, when using wBCE loss, one could further reduce the number of misclassifications by locally increasing the weights at the peripheral airways.

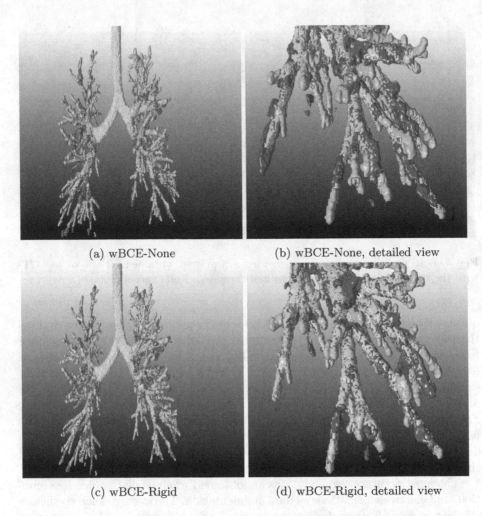

(a) wBCE-None   (b) wBCE-None, detailed view

(c) wBCE-Rigid   (d) wBCE-Rigid, detailed view

Fig. 5. Left: visualization of false positives (red) and false negatives (blue) voxels, together with true positives (yellow), for the airway segmentations obtained for one of test CTs and all models tested (Table 1). The results correspond to the optimal threshold for each model. Left: view of full airways tree. Right: detailed view around the peripheral branches in the lower-right section of the tree.

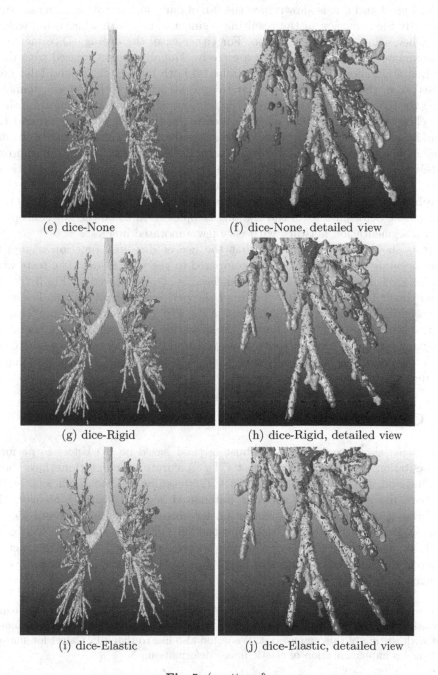

(e) dice-None

(f) dice-None, detailed view

(g) dice-Rigid

(h) dice-Rigid, detailed view

(i) dice-Elastic

(j) dice-Elastic, detailed view

Fig. 5. (*continued*)

In Figs. 3 and 5 it is shown how the use of data augmentation increases substantially the accuracy in the resulting segmentations, both when using wBCE and when using dice loss function. For either case, the average Dice increases approximately by 0.1 and 0.05, respectively. The airways segmented with data augmentation show a much lower number of both false positives and false negatives. Also, they show more regular tubular structure, with uniform diameter along the branches. On the contrary, the results without data augmentation show branches with irregular blob shape, observed by the false positives around the branches. In particular, elastic deformation as data augmentation has been very efficient in our experiments, resulting in an increase of average Dice of approximately 0.05 when compared to the same set-up but using rigid transformations. Also, it is seen in Fig. 5 that it leads to further decrease in false negatives in peripheral branches. This agrees with the observation in [7] that "especially random elastic deformations of the training samples seem to be the key concept to train a segmentation network with very few annotated images".

It is shown in Figs. 3 and 5 that the use of dice loss function results in more accurate segmentation when compared to the wBCE loss. The tests with wBCE loss show over-segmented branches, as it is observed in Fig. 5 by the larger amount of false positives around the peripheral airways. This is due to the weighting for the airways class used in the wBCE formula. This compensates for the intraclass imbalance, but on the downside causes an over-segmentation of airways. In order to reduce this issue, one could adopt an approach where the ratio between the airways and background weights is reduced as the training of the network proceeds.

5   Conclusions

This paper shows a simple but robust method based on 3D Unets to perform segmentation of airways from chest CTs. Accurate segmentations have been obtained on a dataset containing 24 CTs, reaching a Dice coefficient of 0.8 between the ground-truth and our automated segmentations. Moreover, the importance of using data augmentation for our experiments has been demonstrated, in particular elastic deformations. In contrast to other CNNs-based methods, our approach is simpler and end-to-end optimised, and extracts a coherent and accurate airway tree based on voxelwise airway probabilities, with no need to input any prior knowledge of the connected tree structure.

Acknowledgments. This work has been funded by the EU Innovative Medicines Initiative (IMI). We would like to thank F. Dubost for his help with the experiments and with writing of this manuscript. We would also like to thank F. Calvet for sharing with us his implementation of elastic image deformation.

References

1. Lo, P., Sporring, J., Ashraf, H., Pedersen, J.H., de Bruijne, M.: Vessel-guided airway tree segmentation: a voxel classification approach. Med. Image Anal. **14**(4), 527–538 (2010)
2. Bauer, C., Bischof, H., Beichel, R.: Segmentation of airways based on gradient vector flow. In: Proceedings of 2nd International Workshop Pulmonary Image Analysis, pp. 191–201 (2009)
3. Liu, X., Chen, D.Z., Tawhai, M., Wu, X., Hoffman, E., Sonka, M.: Optimal graph search based segmentation of airway tree double surfaces across bifurcations. IEEE Trans. Med. Imag. **32**, 493–510 (2012)
4. Petersen, J., et al.: Optimal surface segmentation using flow lines to quantify airway abnormalities in chronic obstructive pulmonary disease. Med. Image Anal. **18**, 531–541 (2014)
5. Lo, P.: Extraction of airways from CT (EXACT09). IEEE Trans. Med. Imaging **31**(11), 2093–2107 (2012)
6. Long, J., Shelhamer, E., Darrell, T.: Fully convolutional networks for semantic segmentation. In: IEEE Conference on Computer Vision and Pattern Recognition (CVPR) (2015)
7. Ronneberger, O., Fischer, P., Brox, T.: U-Net: convolutional networks for biomedical image segmentation. In: Navab, N., Hornegger, J., Wells, W.M., Frangi, A.F. (eds.) MICCAI 2015. LNCS, vol. 9351, pp. 234–241. Springer, Cham (2015). https://doi.org/10.1007/978-3-319-24574-4_28
8. Meng, Q., Roth, H.R., Kitasaka, T., Oda, M., Ueno, J., Mori, K.: Tracking and segmentation of the airways in chest CT using a fully convolutional network. In: Medical Image Computing and Computer-Assisted Intervention MICCAI 2017, pp. 198–207 (2017)
9. Çiçek, Ö., Abdulkadir, A., Lienkamp, S.S., Brox, T., Ronneberger, O.: 3D U-Net: learning dense volumetric segmentation from sparse annotation. In: Ourselin, S., Joskowicz, L., Sabuncu, M.R., Unal, G., Wells, W. (eds.) MICCAI 2016. LNCS, vol. 9901, pp. 424–432. Springer, Cham (2016). https://doi.org/10.1007/978-3-319-46723-8_49
10. Milletari, F., Navab, N., Ahmadi, S.A.: V-Net: fully convolutional neural networks for volumetric medical image segmentation. In: 4th International Conference on 3D Vision (3DV) (2016)
11. Charbonnier, J.P., van Rikxoort, E.M., Setio, A.A.A., Schaefer-Prokop, C.M., van Ginneken, B., Ciompi, F.: Improving airway segmentation in computed tomography using leak detection with convolutional networks. Med. Image Anal. **36**, 52–60 (2017)
12. Selvan, R., Welling, M., Pedersen, J.H., Petersen, J., de Bruijne, M.: Mean field network based graph refinement with application to airway tree extraction. arXiv preprint arXiv:1804.03348 (2018)
13. Baumgartner, C.F., Koch, L.M., Pollefeys, M., Konukoglu, E.: An exploration of 2D and 3D deep learning techniques for cardiac MR image segmentation. In: Pop, M., Sermesant, M., Jodoin, P.-M., Lalande, A., Zhuang, X., Yang, G., Young, A., Bernard, O. (eds.) STACOM 2017. LNCS, vol. 10663, pp. 111–119. Springer, Cham (2018). https://doi.org/10.1007/978-3-319-75541-0_12
14. Kuo, W., et al.: Diagnosis of bronchiectasis and airway wall thickening in children with cystic fibrosis: objective airway-artery quantification. Eur. Radiol. **27**(11), 4680–4689 (2017)

15. Perez-Rovira, A., Kuo, W., Petersen, J., Tiddens, H.A.W.M., de Bruijne, M.: Automatic airway-artery analysis on lung CT to quantify airway wall thickening and bronchiectasis. Med. Phys. **43**(10), 5736–5744 (2016)
16. Krhenbhl, P., Koltun, V.: Efficient inference in Fully connected CRFs with Gaussian edge potentials. Adv. Neural Inf. Process. Syst. **24**, 109–117 (2011)

Detecting Out-of-Phase Ventilation Using 4DCT to Improve Radiation Therapy for Lung Cancer

Wei Shao[1(✉)], Taylor J. Patton[2], Sarah E. Gerard[3], Yue Pan[1],
Joseph M. Reinhardt[3], John E. Bayouth[4], Oguz C. Durumeric[5],
and Gary E. Christensen[1,6]

[1] Department of Electrical and Computer Engineering,
University of Iowa, Iowa City, USA
wei-shao@uiowa.edu
[2] Department of Medical Physics, University of Wisconsin-Madison, Madison, USA
[3] Department of Biomedical Engineering, University of Iowa, Iowa City, USA
[4] Department of Human Oncology, University of Wisconsin-Madison, Madison, USA
[5] Department of Mathematics, University of Iowa, Iowa City, USA
[6] Department of Radiation Oncology, University of Iowa, Iowa City, USA

Abstract. Functional avoidance radiation therapy (RT) uses lung function images to identify and minimize irradiation of high-function lung tissue. Lung function can be estimated by local expansion ratio (LER) of the lung, which we define in this paper as the ratio of the maximum to the minimum local lung volume in a breathing cycle. LER is computed using deformable image registration. The end exhale (0EX) and the end inhale (100IN) phases of four-dimensional computed tomography (4DCT) are often used to estimate LER, which we refer to as LER3D. However, the lung may have out-of-phase ventilation, i.e., local lung volume change is out of phase with respect to global lung expansion and contraction. We propose the LER4D measure which estimates the LER measure using all phases of 4DCT. The purpose of this paper is to quantify the amount of out-of-phase ventilation of the lung. Out-of-phase ventilation is defined to occur when the LER4D measure is 5% or more than the LER3D measure. 4DCT scans of 14 human subjects were used in this study. Low-function (high-function) regions are defined as regions that have less (greater) than 10% expansion. Our results show that on average 19.3% of the lung had out-of-phase ventilation; 3.8% of the lung had out-of-phase ventilation and is labeled as low-function by both LER3D and LER4D; 9.6% of the lung is labeled as low-function by LER3D while high-function by LER4D; and 5.9% of the lung had out-of-phase ventilation and is labeled as high-function by both LER3D and LER4D. We conclude that out-of-phase ventilation is common in all 14 human subjects we have investigated.

Keywords: Out-of-phase ventilation · Ventilation imaging
Radiation therapy · Lung cancer

© Springer Nature Switzerland AG 2018
D. Stoyanov et al. (Eds.): RAMBO 2018/BIA 2018/TIA 2018, LNCS 11040, pp. 251–259, 2018.
https://doi.org/10.1007/978-3-030-00946-5_25

1   Introduction

Lung cancer is the leading cause of cancer death (25.9% of all cancer deaths) in the United States [11]. Approximately 50% of the patients receive radiation therapy (RT) during the course of lung cancer [4]. The goal of RT is to deliver high-energy radiation beams to the tumors to kill cancer cells. However, irradiation of the surrounding healthy lung tissue during RT causes lung toxicity to about 5% to 20% of lung cancer patients [10]. To reduce this radiation-induced lung injury, functional avoidance RT has been proposed to minimize irradiation of high-function lung regions [3,8,9,13–17,19].

In functional avoidance RT planning, the high-function lung regions can be identified by imaging of lung function. In this paper, we use ventilation as a synonym for lung function since the main function of lung is for gas exchange. Clinical standard ventilation modalities such as single photon emission computed tomography (SPECT) and positron emission tomography (PET) have been used in functional RT planning [3,9,13,14]. Although studies have shown the possibility of reducing dose to high-function tissue in RT using SPECT and PET, these techniques are often limited by low spatial resolution, high cost, long scan time, and/or low accessibility to patients [18]. Recently, ventilation images derived from four-dimensional computed tomography (4DCT) data have been used in functional avoidance RT [5,8,15,17,19]. One advantage of CT ventilation imaging is that it only requires processing of 4DCT data and acquisition of a 4DCT scan is often included in the treatment planning for lung cancer. Therefore, CT ventilation imaging is less expensive and more accessible to patients than clinical standard ventilation imaging techniques. Moreover, 4DCT has a shorter scan time and can be used to generate CT ventilation images with a higher spatial resolution than clinical standard lung function modalities.

CT ventilation images may be estimated by local expansion ratio (LER) of the lung [6,12]. We define the LER at each voxel as the ratio of the maximum to the minimum local lung volume in a breathing cycle. Most CT ventilation imaging algorithms use pairwise image registration to find a one-to-one correspondence map between the end exhale (0EX) CT image and the end inhale (100IN) CT image. Pulmonary ventilation at each voxel can then be estimated by the Jacobian determinant of the correspondence map at that voxel [12], which we refer to as LER3D.

However, the lung may have out-of-phase ventilation, i.e., local lung volume change is out of phase with respect to global lung expansion and contraction. In such a situation, the LER3D measure which only uses the 0EX and 100IN phases may underestimate the LER quantity. In this paper, we proposed a new measure of LER by all phases of 4DCT, which we refer to as LER4D. Note that both LER3D and LER4D provide voxel-wise measurement of lung function. The purpose of this paper is to quantify the amount of out-of-phase ventilation of the lung.

2   Methods

2.1   Image Acquisition

This study evaluated fourteen human subjects undergoing radiation therapy and was approved by the University of Wisconsin-Madison institutional review board. Two 4DCT scans were acquired for each subject before radiation treatment, with a 5-min break between two scans. The 4DCT scans were acquired on a Siemens EDGE CT scanner using 120 kV, 100 mAs per rotation, 0.5 s tube rotation period, 0.09 pitch, 76.8 mm beam collimation, 128 detector rows, and reconstructed slice thicknesses ranging between 0.6 and 3 mm. Musical melody and voice instruction guidance were played throughout the scan to improve the repeatability of the respiratory pattern. Each 4DCT data set was reconstructed into 10 breathing phases, with 20% (20IN), 40% (40IN), 60% (60IN), 80% (80IN) and 100% (100IN) inspiration phases and 80% (80EX), 60% (60EX), 40% (40EX), 20% (20EX) and 0% (0EX) expiration phases.

2.2   Tissue-Volume Preserving Deformable Image Registration

Given a fixed image and a moving image, the goal of image registration is to find a one-to-one correspondence map between the two images. Image registration is an optimization problem whose objective function is a combination of the difference between the fixed image and the deformed image, and the smoothness of the correspondence map. In this paper, we focus on pairwise registration of volumetric CT images.

We denote the fixed and moving CT lung images by $I_0 : \Omega \to \mathbb{R}$ and $I_1 : \Omega \to \mathbb{R}$, respectively, where the closed and bounded set $\Omega \subset \mathbb{R}^3$ is the image domain. The CT images in Housfield unit (HU) can be converted into tissue ratio images by

$$\frac{HU - HU_{air}}{HU_{tissue} - HU_{air}} = \frac{HU + 1000}{1000} \tag{1}$$

where the HUs of the tissue and the air are approximately $HU_{tissue} = 0$ and $HU_{air} = -1000$.

We denote the tissue ratio images associated with I_0 and I_1 by R_0 and R_1, respectively, i.e., $R_0 = \frac{I_0 + 1000}{1000}$ and $R_1 = \frac{I_1 + 1000}{1000}$. The HU of CT lung image varies with tissue density change during breathing (see Eq. 1). To take into account this variation of CT intensity, we use the sum of squared tissue volume difference (SSTVD) similarity metric [1,7,20].

The input to the registration algorithm are the tissue ratio images R_0 and R_1. The moving image R_1 is deformed by the transformation $\phi : \Omega \to \Omega$ by the operation of ϕ acting on R_1 denoted by $\phi \cdot R_1$. This action is defined as follows: $\phi \cdot R_1 \triangleq |J_\phi| \times R_1 \circ \phi$, where $|J_\phi|$ is the Jacobian determinant of ϕ. It can be shown that this definition is a group action. The SSTVD similarity metric is then given by

$$C_{SSTVD} = \int_\Omega \left(R_0(x) - |J_\phi|(x) \times R_1(\phi(x)) \right)^2 dx \tag{2}$$

The regularization constraint is given by

$$Reg(\phi) = \int_{\Omega} \Big(c_1 (\nabla \cdot \nabla) u(x) + c_2 \nabla (\nabla \cdot u(x)) \Big) dx \qquad (3)$$

where $\nabla = [\frac{\partial}{\partial x_1}, \frac{\partial}{\partial x_2}, \frac{\partial}{\partial x_3}]^T$, $\nabla \cdot$ is the divergence operator, $u = \phi - \mathrm{Id}$ is the associated displacement vector field, and c_1 and c_2 are constants.

We choose $c_1 = 0.75$ and $c_2 = 0.25$ in this paper. The objective function is given by

$$C_{total} = C_{SSTVD} + \lambda \cdot Reg(\phi) \qquad (4)$$

where the variable λ is used to balance the weights put on similarity cost and regularization cost.

The image registration algorithm used in this paper has been shown to have sub-voxel accuracy [2].

2.3   Local Expansion Ratio by Two 4DCT Phases (LER3D)

The SSTVD deformable image registration algorithm is used to find a plausible correspondence map (transformation) ϕ from the 0EX CT image to the 100IN CT image. The Jacobian matrix J_ϕ of the transformation ϕ is given by

$$J_\phi \triangleq \begin{bmatrix} \frac{\partial \phi_1}{\partial x_1} & \frac{\partial \phi_1}{\partial x_2} & \frac{\partial \phi_1}{\partial x_3} \\ \frac{\partial \phi_2}{\partial x_1} & \frac{\partial \phi_2}{\partial x_2} & \frac{\partial \phi_2}{\partial x_3} \\ \frac{\partial \phi_3}{\partial x_1} & \frac{\partial \phi_3}{\partial x_2} & \frac{\partial \phi_3}{\partial x_3} \end{bmatrix} = \mathbb{I}_3 + J_u. \qquad (5)$$

where $\mathbb{I}_3$ is the 3×3 identity matrix and J_u is the Jacobian of the displacement field $u = \phi - \mathrm{Id}$.

Reinhardt et al. [12] proposed to estimate local expansion ratio of the lung at each voxel x by the Jacobian determinant of ϕ (LER3D), i.e.,

$$LER3D(x) \triangleq |J_\phi(x)| \qquad (6)$$

2.4   Local Expansion Ratio by All 4DCT Phases (LER4D)

The LER3D measure may underestimate LER when out-of-phase ventilation happens. To solve this problem, we propose to estimate LER by all 4DCT phases, which we refer to as LER4D. We perform a nonrigid registration from each breathing phase to the 0EX phase and denote the resulting Jacobian determinant images by $\mathbb{J}_1, \cdots, \mathbb{J}_N$, where N is number of breathing phases of a 4DCT scan. The LER4D measure at each point $x \in \Omega$ is given by the ratio of the maximum to the minimum local lung volume:

$$LER4D(x) = \max_{i \in \{1, \cdots, N\}} \mathbb{J}_i(x) \Big/ \min_{i \in \{1, \cdots, N\}} \mathbb{J}_i(x) \qquad (7)$$

By definition, the LER4D measure is always greater or equal to the LER3D measure, and we hypothesize that it may provide a more accurate estimate of local lung expansion ratio.

2.5   Out-of-Phase Ventilation

The lung has out-of-phase ventilation when local lung volume change is out of phase with respect to global lung volume change. By definition, out-of-phase ventilation occurs whenever the LER4D measure is greater than the LER3D measure. We define the lung to have out-of-phase ventilation if $LER4D \geq T \times LER3D$, where $T > 1$ a threshold value. The threshold T is used to reduce the effect of noise. We choose the out-of-phase threshold T to be 1.05, i.e., the LER4D measure is greater than or equal to 5% of the LER3D measure. We chose 1.05 as the threshold value since the standard deviation of the ratio of two LER3Ds for repeated 4DCT scans is about 0.05.

3   Results

For each of the 14 human subjects, we compute the LER3D measure and the LER4D measure by Eqs. 6 and 7, respectively. Figure 1 shows the cumulative 2D histogram of LER3D image versus LER4D image for all 14 subjects. A logarithmic scale is used for visualization. Overlaid on this histogram are the functions $y = x$ and $y = 1.05x$. Notice all points lie above the $y = x$ solid line since $LER4D \geq LER3D$ by our definition. Points that lie above the $y = 1.05x$ dashed line are defined to be out-of-phase ventilation and points that lie between the two lines are defined to be in-phase ventilation.

We divide the 2D plane in Fig. 1 into four regions: A, B, C and D, where region A corresponds to in-phase ventilation, and regions B, C and D correspond to out-of-phase ventilation. Low-function (high-function) regions are defined as regions that have less (greater) than 10% expansion and are denoted by the dashed lines at 1.1. On average for all 14 subjects, 80.7% of all voxels are in region A, i.e., 80.7% of the lung has in-phase ventilation. Conversely, 19.3% of the lung has out-of-phase ventilation. 3.8% of all voxels are in region B, i.e., on average 3.8% of the lung volume is labeled as low-function by both of the LER3D and LER4D measures and at the same time has out-of-phase ventilation. 9.6% of all voxels are in region C, i.e., on average 9.6% of the lung volume is labeled as low-function by the LER3D measure while high-function by the LER4D measure. 5.9% of all voxels are in region D, i.e., on average 5.9% of the lung volume is labeled as high-function by both of the LER3D and LER4D measures and at the same time has out-of-phase ventilation.

Table 1 summarizes the percentages of the lung volume for regions A, B, C and D for each of the 14 subjects. This table shows that every subject has out-of-phase ventilation in more than 10% of the lung volume. The last row of Table 1 shows the mean (± standard deviation) over all 14 subjects for all regions.

Figure 2 shows the location of the tumor and the spatial distribution of regions A, B, C and D of two subjects. Both subject 1 and subject 8 have less out-of-phase ventilation than the average. Note that for subject 1, large regions near the tumor have out-of-phase ventilation. This means it is possible that some of the tissue that was classified as low-functioning by LER3D should have been classified as high-functioning when using LER4D due to out-of-phase

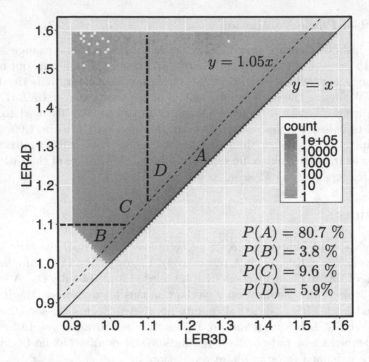

Fig. 1. Cumulative 2D histogram of LER3D images versus LER4D images for 14 subjects. A logarithmic scale is used for visualization. Low-function (high-function) regions are defined as regions that have less (greater) than 10% expansion and are denoted by the dashed lines at 1.1. Region A is where the lung has in-phase ventilation, region B, C and D are regions where the lung has out-of-phase ventilation. The lung is considered as low-function by both LER3D and LER4D in region B, the lung is considered as low-function by LER3D while high-function by LER4D in region C, the lung is considered as high-function by both LER3D and LER4D in region D. We use $P(A)$, $P(B)$, $P(C)$, and $P(D)$ to denote the percentages of the voxels in regions A, B, C and D, respectively.

ventilation. For this subject, using the LER4D measure instead of the LER3D measure will make a difference to the functional avoidance treatment plan. However, for subject 8, out-of-phase regions are far from the tumor and using the LER4D measure will not make much difference to functional avoidance plan derived from LER3D.

4   Discussion and Conclusions

We are conducting a clinical trial at UW-Madison (NCT02843568) that uses both conventional and functional avoidance treatment plans to treat patients with lung cancer. In this trial, the LER3D method is used in functional avoidance RT to minimize radiation delivered to the regions of high-function. The goal of this trial is to show functional avoidance RT can reduce damage to healthy

Table 1. Percentages of the lung volume for Regions A, B, C and D.

Subject	Region			
	A	B	C	D
1	82.9%	2.0%	6.9%	8.2%
2	84.5%	2.2%	9.8%	3.5%
3	80.7%	1.5%	9.4%	8.4%
4	76.0%	4.6%	14.2%	5.2%
5	89.6%	0.4%	2.8%	7.2%
6	77.3%	7.1%	12.8%	2.8%
7	89.9%	0.7%	4.9%	4.5%
8	87.8%	1.4%	3.4%	7.4%
9	2.9%	5.1%	6.0%	.0%
10	69.3%	3.9%	18.9%	7.9%
11	77.6%	4.9%	15.5%	2.0%
12	77.8%	2.9%	11.0%	8.3%
13	73.6%	12.4%	12.1%	1.9%
14	79.8%	3.4%	7.1%	9.7%
Average	80.7% ± 6.02%	3.8% ± 3.13%	9.6% ± 4.76%	5.9% ± 2.61%

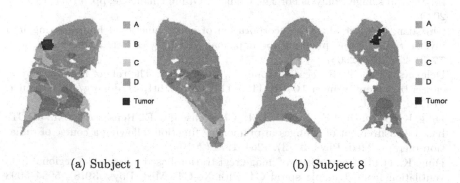

(a) Subject 1   (b) Subject 8

Fig. 2. Spatial distribution of regions A, B, C and D of two subjects. Region A is where the lung has in-phase ventilation; region B is where the lung has out-of-phase ventilation and is labeled as low-function by both LER3D and LER4D; region C is where the lung is labeled as high-function by LER4D while low-function by LER3D; region D is where the lung has out-of-phase ventilation and is labeled as high-function by both LER3D and LER4D.

lung tissue compared to conventional treatment. In total, 120 patients will be recruited in this clinical trial; half will be treated with conventional RT and the other half will be treated with functional avoidance RT. In this paper, we have shown that out-of-phase ventilation was common in all 14 human subjects that we investigated. When large difference between LER4D and LER3D happens near the tumor (e.g. subject 1), then using the LER4D measure may preserve more healthy lung tissue than the LER3D measure in functional avoidance RT.

In conclusion, we investigated the out-of-phase ventilation of 14 human subjects. Our study shows that all subjects had out-of-phase ventilation in more than 10% of the lung volume. Our results show that on average 19.3% of the lung has out-of-phase ventilation; 3.8% of the lung has out-of-phase ventilation and is labeled as low-function by both of LER3D and LER4D; 9.6% of the lung is labeled as low-function by LER3D while high-function by LER4D; and 5.9% of the lung has out-of-phase ventilation and is labeled as high-function by both LER3D and LER4D.

Acknowledgments. This work is supported in part by National Cancer Institute of the National Institute of Health (NIH) under award numbers CA166703 and CA166119.

References

1. Cao, K., Ding, K., Christense, G.E., Reinhardt, J.M.: Tissue volume and vesselness measure preserving nonrigid registration of lung CT images. Proc. SPIE **7623**, 762309 (2010)
2. Cao, K., Du, K., Ding, K., Reinhardt, J., Christensen, G.: Regularized nonrigid registration of lung CT images by preserving tissue volume and vesselness measure. In: Medical Image Analysis For The Clinic: A Grand Challenge, pp. 43–54, January 2010
3. Christian, J.A., et al.: The incorporation of spect functional lung imaging into inverse radiotherapy planning for non-small cell lung cancer. Radiother. Oncol. **77**(3), 271–277 (2005)
4. Delaney, G., Jacob, S., Featherstone, C., Barton, M.: The role of radiotherapy in cancer treatment. Cancer **104**(6), 1129–1137 (2005). https://doi.org/10.1002/cncr.21324
5. Ding, K., Bayouth, J.E., Buatti, J.M., Christensen, G.E., Reinhardt, J.M.: 4DCT-based measurement of changes in pulmonary function following a course of radiation therapy. Med. Phys. **37**(3), 1261–1272 (2010)
6. Ding, K., et al.: Comparison of image registration based measures of regional lung ventilation from dynamic spiral CT with Xe-CT. Med. Phys. **39**(8), 5084–5098 (2012)
7. Gorbunova, V., Lo, P., Ashraf, H., Dirksen, A., Nielsen, M., de Bruijne, M.: Weight preserving image registration for monitoring disease progression in lung CT. In: Metaxas, D., Axel, L., Fichtinger, G., Székely, G. (eds.) MICCAI 2008. LNCS, vol. 5242, pp. 863–870. Springer, Heidelberg (2008). https://doi.org/10.1007/978-3-540-85990-1_104
8. Huang, T.C., Hsiao, C.Y., Chien, C.R., Liang, J.A., Shih, T.C., Zhang, G.G.: IMRT treatment plans and functional planning with functional lung imaging from 4D-CT for thoracic cancer patients. Radiat. Oncol. **8**(1), 3 (2013)
9. Lavrenkov, K., et al.: A potential to reduce pulmonary toxicity: the use of perfusion spect with imrt for functional lung avoidance in radiotherapy of non-small cell lung cancer. Radiother. Oncol. **83**(2), 156–162 (2007)
10. Marks, L.B., Yu, X., Vujaskovic, Z., Small, W., Folz, R., Anscher, M.S.: Radiation-induced lung injury. Semin. Radiat. Oncol. **13**(3), 333–345 (2003)

11. National Cancer Institute, Bethesda, MD.: Cancer Stat Facts: Lung and bronchus cancer. Hypertext Document, January 2018. https://seer.cancer.gov/statfacts/html/lungb.html
12. Reinhardt, J.M., Ding, K., Cao, K., Christensen, G.E., Hoffman, E.A., Bodas, S.V.: Registration-based estimates of local lung tissue expansion compared to xenon ct measures of specific ventilation. Med. Image Anal. **12**(6), 752–763 (2008)
13. Siva, S., et al.: Ga-68 MAA perfusion 4d-PET/CT scanning allows for functional lung avoidance using conformal radiation therapy planning. Technol. Cancer Res. Treat. **15**(1), 114–121 (2016)
14. Siva, S., et al.: High-resolution pulmonary ventilation and perfusion PET/CT allows for functionally adapted intensity modulated radiotherapy in lung cancer. Radiother. Oncol. **115**(2), 157–162 (2015)
15. Vinogradskiy, Y., et al.: Regional lung function profiles of stage i and iii lung cancer patients: an evaluation for functional avoidance radiation therapy. Int. J. Radiat. Oncol. Biol. Phys. **95**(4), 1273–1280 (2016)
16. Yamamoto, T., et al.: Changes in regional ventilation during treatment and dosimetric advantages of ct ventilation image-guided radiotherapy for locally advanced lung cancer. Int. J. Radiat. Oncol. Biol. Phys. (2018)
17. Yamamoto, T., Kabus, S., Bal, M., Keall, P., Benedict, S., Daly, M.: The first patient treatment of computed tomography ventilation functional image-guided radiotherapy for lung cancer. Radiother. Oncol. **118**(2), 227–231 (2016)
18. Yamamoto, T., Kabus, S., Von Berg, J., Lorenz, C., Keall, P.J.: Impact of four-dimensional computed tomography pulmonary ventilation imaging-based functional avoidance for lung cancer radiotherapy. Int. J. Radiat. Oncol. Biol. Phys. **79**(1), 279–288 (2011)
19. Yaremko, B.P.: Reduction of normal lung irradiation in locally advanced non-small-cell lung cancer patients, using ventilation images for functional avoidance. Int. J. Radiat. Oncol. Biol. Phys. **68**(2), 562–571 (2007). https://doi.org/10.1016/j.ijrobp.2007.01.044. http://www.sciencedirect.com/science/article/B6T7X-4NCKJT4-P/2/f6e5dac7bef5f8ef7b954ccb8ed11972
20. Yin, Y., Hoffman, E.A., Lin, C.L.: Mass preserving non-rigid registration of CT lung images using cubic B-spline. Med. Phys. **36**(9), 4213–4222 (2009)

XeMRI to CT Lung Image Registration Enhanced with Personalized 4DCT-Derived Motion Model

Adam Szmul[1(✉)], Tahreema Matin[2], Fergus V. Gleeson[2,3],
Julia A. Schnabel[1,4], Vicente Grau[1], and Bartłomiej W. Papież[1,5]

[1] Institute of Biomedical Engineering, Department of Engineering Science,
University of Oxford, Oxford, UK
adam.szmul@eng.ox.ac.uk
[2] Department of Oncology, University of Oxford, Oxford, UK
[3] Department of Radiology, Oxford University Hospitals NHS FT, Oxford, UK
[4] Department of Biomedical Engineering, School of Biomedical Engineering
and Imaging Sciences, King's College London, London, UK
[5] Big Data Institute, Li Ka Shing Centre for Health Information and Discovery,
University of Oxford, Oxford, UK

Abstract. This paper presents a novel method for multi-modal lung image registration constrained by a motion model derived from lung 4DCT. The motion model is estimated based on the results of intra-patient image registration using Principal Component Analysis. The approach with a prior motion model is particularly important for regions where there is not enough information to reliably drive the registration process, as in the case of hyperpolarized Xenon MRI and proton density MRI to CT registration. Simultaneously, the method addresses local variations between images in the supervoxel-based motion model parameters optimization step. We compare our results in terms of the plausibility of the estimated deformations and correlation coefficient with 4DCT-based estimated ventilation maps using state-of-the-art multi-modal image registration methods. Our method achieves higher average correlation scores, showing that the application of Principal Component Analysis-based motion model in the deformable registration, helps to drive the registration for the regions of the lungs with insufficient amount of information.

Keywords: Lung 4D CT · XeMRI · Multi-modal image registration
Lung motion model · Ventilation estimation

1 Introduction

Medical images acquired at different time points, or originating from different scanners, need to be brought into spatial alignment to assess complementary structural and/or functional information. This process is called image registration and is one of the fundamental medical image analysis procedures [23].

© Springer Nature Switzerland AG 2018
D. Stoyanov et al. (Eds.): RAMBO 2018/BIA 2018/TIA 2018, LNCS 11040, pp. 260–271, 2018.
https://doi.org/10.1007/978-3-030-00946-5_26

Deformable image registration is particularly important for lung applications where, for example, the different breath-hold levels need to be compensated in the acquired images. Single-modality lung registration, especially Computed Tomography (CT)-CT registration, has been widely studied [4,17] and dedicated image registration methods have been proposed [7,10,11,25,28].

While CT-CT lung image registration is a non-trivial task, mainly because of sliding motion between the surfaces of the lungs, the ribcage, and diaphragm [18,22], multi-modal lung image registration is even more challenging due to more complex deformations and directly incomparable intensities between the acquired scans. Registration between proton density Magnetic Resonance Imaging (pMRI) and CT is one such example, where the difficulty stems from the low proton density in the lungs and susceptibility to acquisition artifacts caused by the interfaces between air and lung tissue. Such registration, however, plays an important role in the analysis of hyperpolarized Xenon MRI (XeMRI) [2]. XeMRI, due to its non-ionizing nature, has received substantial attention in the field for imaging ventilation, perfusion, and gas transfer in the lungs [16]. As XeMRI does not provide structural information, its correspondences to the patient anatomy rely on pMRI, which is acquired during the same imaging session but not within the same breath-hold. Even though patients are provided with bags containing 1l of gas for both image acquisitions, due to different properties of air and xenon, as well as individual breathing patterns, the images might be acquired at different levels of lung inflation. It is not, therefore, straightforward to directly map XeMRI to diagnostic lung CT, for instance in the case of patients undergoing radiotherapy treatment. An intermediate registration between pMRI and CT is needed to find this mapping, as shown in Fig. 1. This registration becomes particularly challenging for a number of reasons, including the lower spatial resolution of pMRI compared with CT, the limited information from lung tissue in pMRI due to its low proton density, and the presence of susceptibility artifacts. For these reasons, the registration can easily result in under or over-estimation of deformations inside the lungs.

An alternative approach for this problem might be the application of lung motion models [15]. For instance, a statistical motion model based on deformations estimated from 4DCT was proposed in [5]. The individual motion models estimated for each subject from the dataset have been co-registered to an average shape and intensity model was generated from reference frames from 4DCT. This resulted in a development of an average inter-subject model. In [13], after estimating the deformations from 4DCT, the surface point distribution model of the shape of the lungs was constructed. After applying Principal Component Analysis (PCA) to reduce the dimensionality, the statistical model between the estimated deformations and point-based shape variations was calculated. Similar approach has been presented in [29], with the diaphragm position used as a surrogate of the motion to control the model. To create a lung motion model, Finite Element Analysis (FEA) could be also used, such as in [9], where a patient-specific bio-mechanical model has been proposed for lung CT registration. However, to achieve satisfying accuracy the FEA model-based method requires an

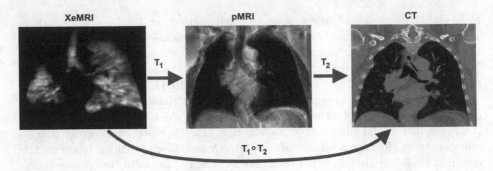

Fig. 1. To bring XeMRI into alignment with CT, we compose two transformations: transformation T_1 that compensates for a possible initial misalignment between XeMRI and pMRI, and transformation T_2 estimated based on registration between pMRI and CT. The dedicated framework addressing this problem is the main contribution of this work.

additional registration. All of the aforementioned methods have been applied to CT-to-CT registration problem. In the case of pMRI-to-CT registration, the task may be even more challenging due to the low out-of-plane spatial resolution of pMRI and lack of direct intensity correspondences.

In this work, we address the issue of insufficient amount of information inside the lungs in pMRI, by proposing a personalized 4D-CT statistical motion model for a supervoxel-based graphical image registration [11,25]. The main contribution is a dedicated framework, which addresses the challenges of XeMRI to CT deformable registration in the form of supervoxel-based motion model enhanced method. The evaluation has been performed on a clinical dataset and compared with state-of-the-art image registration methods, showing higher correlation of XeMRI with ventilation maps estimated from 4DCT.

2   Methods

The proposed method consists of three main steps: (1) creation of a personalized lung motion model from 4DCT, (2) lung image clustering and (3) graph-based pMRI-to-CT registration. We introduce these steps in detail in this section. An overview of the proposed method is presented in Fig. 2.

2.1   Personalized Lung Motion Model from 4DCT

In our work, to create a personalized motion model we use displacements resulting from 4DCT registration to a reference volume. We apply an image registration method dedicated to lung applications [25], which has the potential to more accurately estimate abnormal lung motion. The method has shown good performance in terms of accuracy, plausibility of the resulting deformations for lung CT registration, and the ability to address the sliding motion problem.

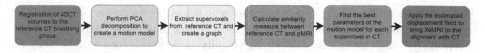

Fig. 2. Diagram presenting the workflow of the proposed method. We start from registering all the 4DCT volumes for each of the patients to the chosen reference frame. Over the estimated deformation fields we apply PCA decomposition to create a motion model. Subsequently, we extract supervoxels from the lungs in the reference CT volume. We create a graph, where every supervoxel is represented by a node an all adjacent supervoxels are connected by an edge. For every supervoxel we find the best set of motion model parameters to bring pMRI into alignment with CT using graph cuts optimization. We apply the estimated deformation field to XeMRI as the ultimate goal of the registration framework.

Subsequently, we perform PCA to the estimated deformations to obtain major motion patterns for each patient.

In the proposed method, for each patient, all breathing phases from 4DCT are co-registered to a reference volume, which is chosen as the peak inhale breathing phase volume. Our 4DCT data consists of 10 volumes; therefore as a result of the alignment we acquired 9 displacement fields. After the registration, we create for the reference volume vectors comprising all the estimated deformation fields:

$$R^p(\mathbf{x}) = [V_1^p(\mathbf{x}), V_2^p(\mathbf{x}), ..., V_n^p(\mathbf{x})], \tag{1}$$

where p is the direction the deformations (anterior-posterior, left-to-right, up-to-down), n is the number of volumes co-registered to the reference volume, and $\mathbf{x}$ is a voxel location.

After applying PCA, we can reformulate Eq. 1 in terms of eigenvalues and eigenvectors:

$$R^p(\mathbf{x}) \simeq \mu_d^p + \sum_{i=1}^{n} \lambda_i^p \nu_i^p(\mathbf{x}), \tag{2}$$

where μ_d^p is the mean displacement, $\nu_i^p(\mathbf{x})$ is i-th eigenvector and λ_i^p is corresponding eigenvalue for direction p (anterior-posterior, left-to-right, up-to-down) for voxel's spatial location $\mathbf{x}$. We restricted the motion model to use the first eigenvector, as it covers the main motion pattern observed during the registration (in anterior-posterior - 83%, left-to-right - 82% and up-to-down - 95% directions on average for our dataset). The restriction to the use of first eigenvector makes the optimization more efficient, while taking advantage of the personalized motion model application. Regional variations from the motion pattern are compensated by applying supervoxel-based motion model parameters optimization registration step.

2.2 Lung Clustering

Image clustering provides a compact image representation, which has the potential to represent anatomically consistent regions in the form of larger structures.

The peak inhale breathing phase volume, which has been chosen as a reference frame, is clustered using the well-established Simple Linear Iterative Clustering method [1], which groups spatially and visually close voxels into supervoxels. In this method, a fixed number of seeds for the expected number of supervoxels is uniformly located in the image. Their initial position is corrected by moving the seeds to a position of the lowest gradient in a $3 \times 3 \times 3$ neighborhood. This step is performed to avoid placing them on an edge or a noisy voxel. Following that, every voxel in the image is assigned to the closest supervoxel, based on the distance measure: $D = \sqrt{(d_e)^2 + (d_I/S)^2 m^2}$, where d_e is the Euclidean distance of a particular voxel to the supervoxel center, d_I is a voxel's intensity distance from the supervoxel average intensity, and m is a compactness parameter. The resultant clustering of a CT image is shown in Fig. 3.

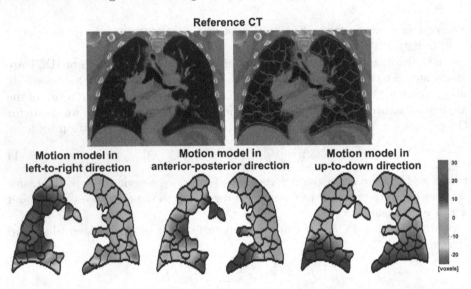

Fig. 3. The reference CT image in the coronal view and superpixels estimated for the lungs imposed on the image are shown in the upper row. Below, the estimated motion model for the reference CT volume frame left-to-right, anterior-posterior and up-to-down directions shown in coronal view with propagated superpixels from the CT image. For illustrative purposes, we show superpixels extracted from a 2D image, whereas in our method we use supervoxels extracted from 3D volumes.

2.3   Graph-Based Lung Image Registration

Image registration, as a problem of finding the optimal transformation between two images, can be stated using an Markov Random Fields-based optimization and posed on a graph. Graphical methods for deformable image registration [6,10,11,19,25] have achieved state-of-the-art accuracy and good performance in addressing sliding motion. Therefore, following image clustering, we create a graph where every supervoxel is represented by a node and all nodes corresponding to adjacent supervoxels are connected by an edge. The edge values are uniformly set to 1.

We apply a similar approach to [25], with graph cuts [3] as an optimization scheme. In the proposed method, we create a predefined set of labels $l \in L$, where every label l is a set of parameters of the motion model in form of a vector $[l_x l_y l_z]$. This is one of the main differences compared with the majority of other methods in the field, where labels usually directly represent displacements. The label is applied to the corresponding patch of the motion model, and therefore, even if the algorithm assigns the same labels to neighboring supervoxels, they may potentially still have different displacements. The displacement inside the patch is not uniform and should mimic the motion of its tissue. Such an approach restricts the possible displacements of the patches to those which have been estimated for the particular regions of the lungs, and therefore results in more anatomically plausible estimated displacements. At the same time, the method still allows for local adjustments to the model by the estimated parameters. The estimation of the motion model parameters in a form of l_x, l_y and l_z is one advantage of our application, as it compensates for the residual differences, when ideal rigid alignment of pMRI and CT is difficult to achieve. This alignment is challenging mainly because of the multi-modal nature of the images, differences in position inside the scanner, as well as possible variations in the patient anatomy, for instance due to tumor appearance. The model was created from 4DCT, based on co-registration of images acquired with the patient remaining at the same position in a scanner. Therefore our approach gives more degrees of freedom than a classic model based-approaches to compensate for the misalignments, while at the same time taking the advantage of the main motion patterns represented by the motion model.

As a similarity measure to find the optimal parameters of the motion model for every supervoxel we have applied the local correlation coefficient (LCC) [12], which is a well established approach for measuring image similarity in medical image registration. The general formulation of the energy to be minimized during the optimization process is:

$$E(l) = \underbrace{\sum_p \overline{LCC(I_{fix}(\mathbf{x}_p), I_{mov}(\mathbf{x}_p + l_p * R(\mathbf{x}_p))}}_{data\ term} + \alpha \underbrace{\sum_{p,q \in N} \|l_p - l_q\|^2}_{smoothness\ term}, \quad (3)$$

where the data term is formulated as a mean error calculated for all voxels $\mathbf{x}$ in the fixed image I_{fix} and moving image I_{mov} clustered in a certain supervoxel represented by a node p, for the applied motion model R with the parameters represented by a label l_p. The piecewise smoothness term represents quadratic distance between the labels. The influence of the piecewise smoothness term on the energy is controlled by a weighting parameter α. Since no XeMRI ventilation signal is expected to be present outside of the lung, our registration framework is therefore restricted to estimating deformations inside the volume of the lungs. The lungs are segmented from CT and registration is done only inside the masks.

Akin to [11], we use a single resolution level with multiple layers of supervoxels, slightly varying their size and initial location. The estimated deformations are averaged across all layers.

The displacements estimated for the pMRI-to-CT registration are propagated to XeMRI, just as shown in Fig. 1, resulting in their alignment. Visual assessment of the framework are presented in Fig. 4, where we also display the estimated displacement fields for all the methods.

3   Experiments and Results

Our experiments have been performed on a dataset of three patients undergoing radiotherapy at Churchill Hospital in Oxford. For each patient, imaging data consisting of 4DCT, pMRI and XeMRI have been acquired, with the resolution of $0.98 \times 0.98 \times 2.5 \, [\text{mm}^3]$. Each 4DCT consisted of 10 3D volumes of CTs acquired in axial plane. A mixture of 129Xe gas (80%) and air was polarized on-site to between 4% and 12%, by using a commercial polarizer operating on the rubidium vapor spin-exchange optical pumping basis. The hyperpolarized gas has been delivered to patients during the imaging in 1.0-L bags [14]. The pMRI and XeMRI have been performed at 1.5 T MR scanner as 3D volumes from coronal acquisition the resolution of $1.56 \times 20 \times 1.56 \, [\text{mm}^3]$.

Following [26], pMRI volumes and reference volume from 4DCT were carefully aligned initially using rigid registration with mutual information as a similarity measure. In our application it is important to achieve good alignments at the apex and upper parts of the lungs. The resulting transformation was propagated to the corresponding XeMRI volumes, bringing them into rigid alignment with the reference CT volume.

We subsequently performed deformable registration of pMRI-to-CT and compared results of our registration method with the results of the deeds deformable image registration [10] and free form deformation-based registration using B-splines [21]. The deeds method originally proposed for lung CT registration shows good performance in multi-modal image registration application due to its image descriptor-based similarity measure, while FFDs on B-splines with mutual information as a similarity measure is one of the most established approaches for multi-modal image registration.

For the proposed method we have extracted supervoxels consisting of approximately 500 voxels each, with the compactness parameter set to 0.1, and used 20 layers of supervoxels. The range of motion model parameters l_x, l_y and l_z is set between -0.6 and 0.6, at the intervals of 0.1. The weighting parameter α is 0.2 and local cross correlation was calculated for a $7 \times 7 \times 7$ voxels patch size. Our method has been implemented in Matlab environment and its running time with the chosen parameters setting is approximately 45 min on a i7 laptop machine. The running times for the deeds and B-splines were approximately 13 min and 25 min, respectively, with C++ implementation. Our method is capable of further optimization and parallelization, which should result in significant running time reduction.

Visual inspection from Fig. 4 of the results reveals that the displacements estimated by the proposed method are anatomically more consistent. We decided to compare the XeMRI ventilation images with ventilation maps estimated from 4DCT, which is obtained using image registration of the dynamic sequence to a reference CT volume. To estimate ventilation maps, we have used a method based on the changes of the lung intensity expressed in Hounsfield units between peak inhale and peak exhale breathing phases [27]. An alternative approaches

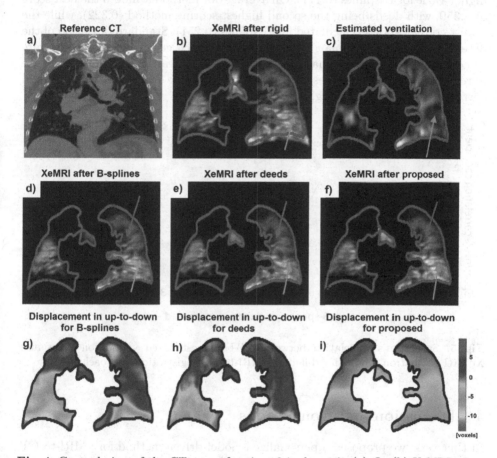

Fig. 4. Coronal view of the CT scan of patient 2 is shown in (a). In (b) XeMRI after applying rigid registration (T_1 from Fig. 1) and in (c) ventilation estimated from 4DCT are presented. The remaining figures show XeMRI ventilation images for the corresponding to CT slices. The lung border from CT is super-imposed on the ventilation images. The results of the XeMRI ventilation after applying deformable registration are shown only inside of the lung mask in the middle row. The possible under-estimation of the motion for B-splines [21] (d) and deeds [10] (e) are pointed by green arrows, and implausible deformations by blue arrows. The results for the proposed method are shown in (f). In the bottom row we show displacements in up-to-down direction for the corresponding slices for all the methods in (g), (h) and (i). (Color figure online)

could estimate the ventilation from 4D CT based on determinant of Jacobian [8,20] or with the use of supervoxel tracking [24]. We calculate Spearman's correlation coefficient of the registered XeMRI ventilation images with the estimated 4DCT-based ventilation maps. Our method resulted in higher correlation coefficient for patient 1 and patient 2 (0.344 and 0.572) compared to both other image registration methods (0.217 and 0.367 for B-splines and 0.299 and 0.5 for deeds). For patient 3 all methods achieved comparable results, with a slightly higher value for B-splines (0.171). On average our method achieved the best score of 0.359, with deeds being the second highest-scoring method (0.322), while the lowest correlation was calculated for B-splines (0.251). Standard deviation of the determinant of the Jacobian of deformations, which can be seen as a measure of complexity of the deformations, for our method was on average 0.35, compared with 1.15 for B-splines and 0.63 for deeds. The results of the calculated correlations are shown in Fig. 5.

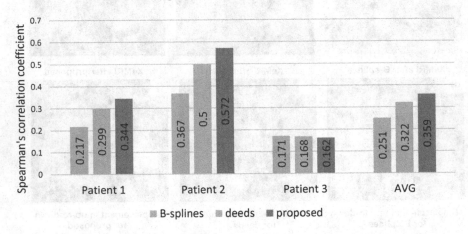

Fig. 5. Spearman's correlation between CT-based estimated ventilation maps and XeMRI ventilation images for different pMRI-to-CT registration approaches.

4 Discussion and Conclusions

In this work, we proposed a personalized model-driven method for pMRI-to-CT lung image registration. The method was evaluated on three datasets of patients undergoing radiation treatment for lung cancer. The visual results presented in Fig. 4, where we show the estimated deformations, might suggest that the proposed method better mimic the motion of the lungs. The sudden changes in the direction of the motion estimated by B-splines and deeds, especially for the left lung, are unlikely to be present during breathing. We calculated correlation between CT-based estimated ventilations and XeMRI brought into alignment with CT by our method. On average, our method outperformed other image registration approaches in terms of the correlation with ventilation maps estimated from 4DCT. The slightly lower score for patient 3 was possibly caused by the fact that the difference in the lung volume between pMRI/XeMRI and CT was the lowest in this case. This observation seems to be supported by the fact that all the methods achieved comparable results.

Our motion model-based method requires an accurate initial rigid registration. The upper parts of the lungs and apexes should be well aligned initially, or else the motion model-based registration might result in suboptimal performance. Such behavior is imposed by the lung physiology and should not be considered as a limitation of the method.

One of the challenges in our work is the lack of ground truth or landmarks set in both modality images. Low out-of-plane resolution of pMRI and XeMRI (20 mm) is another factor and, hence, the registration problem is not a trivial one to address. The correlation of XeMRI with 4DCT-based estimated ventilation maps resulted in the overall moderate correlation. The reason for that might be different breathing patterns in 4DCT compared to XeMRI/pMRI, related to physical properties of xenon gas, which is much heavier than air. Ventilation maps based on 4DCT are estimated based on the changes of the tissue density, which should correspond to the lungs filling with air, however in practice they might provide complementary information. Another limitation is that we had access to only one 4DCT scan of each patient. Therefore our method might be prone to intra breathing cycle variations. This issue could potentially be eliminated by including more scans, such as diagnostic CT, of the same patient in the breathing motion creation step.

The presented method shows promising results for the challenging application of XeMRI to CT registration. The application of the Principal Component Analysis-based motion model in the deformable registration step of the framework, seems to have the potential to help drive the registration for the regions of the lungs with insufficient amount of information.

Acknowledgments. AS and BWP would like to acknowledge funding from the CRUK and EPSRC Cancer Imaging Centre in Oxford. BWP acknowledges Oxford NIHR Biomedical Research Centre (Rutherford Fund Fellowship at HDR UK). JAS was supported by EP/P023509/1 and Wellcome Trust/EPSRC Centre for Medical Engineering.

References

1. Achanta, R., Shaji, A., Smith, K., Lucchi, A., Fua, P., Süsstrunk, S.: SLIC superpixels compared to state-of-the-art superpixel methods. IEEE Trans. Pattern Anal. Mach. Intell. **34**, 2274–2282 (2012)
2. Albert, M.S., et al.: Biological magnetic resonance imaging using laser-polarized ^{129}Xe. Nature **370**(6486), 199–201 (1994)
3. Boykov, Y., Veksler, O., Zabih, R.: Fast approximate energy minimization via graph cuts. IEEE Trans. Pattern Anal. Mach. Intell. **23**(11), 1222–1239 (2001)
4. Castillo, R., et al.: A framework for evaluation of deformable image registration spatial accuracy using large landmark point sets. Phys. Med. Biol. **54**(7), 1849–1870 (2009)

5. Ehrhardt, J., Werner, R., Schmidt-Richberg, A., Handels, H.: Statistical modeling of 4D respiratory lung motion using diffeomorphic image registration. IEEE Trans. Med. Imaging **30**, 251–265 (2011)
6. Glocker, B., Sotiras, A., Komodakis, N., Paragios, N.: Deformable medical image registration: Setting the state of the art with discrete methods. Ann. Rev. Biomed. Eng. **13**(1), 219–244 (2011)
7. Gorbunova, V., et al.: Mass preserving image registration for lung CT. Med. Image Anal. **16**(4), 786–795 (2012)
8. Guerrero, T., et al.: Quantification of regional ventilation from treatment planning CT. Int. J. Radiat. Oncol.*Biol.*Phys. **62**(3), 630–634 (2005)
9. Han, L., Dong, H., McClelland, J.R., Han, L., Hawkes, D.J., Barratt, D.C.: A hybrid patient-specific biomechanical model based image registration method for the motion estimation of lungs. Med. Image Anal. **39**, 87–100 (2017)
10. Heinrich, M.P., Jenkinson, M., Brady, M., Schnabel, J.A.: MRF-based deformable registration and ventilation estimation of lung CT. IEEE Trans. Med. Imag. **32**(7), 1239–1248 (2013)
11. Heinrich, M.P., Simpson, I.J., Papież, B.W., Brady, S.M., Schnabel, J.A.: Deformable image registration by combining uncertainty estimates from super-voxel belief propagation. Med. Image Anal. **27**, 57–71 (2016)
12. Hermosillo, G., Chefd'Hotel, C., Faugeras, O.: Variational methods for multimodal image matching. Int. J. Comput. Vis. **50**(3), 329–343 (2002)
13. Liu, X., Oguz, I., Pizer, S.M., Mageras, G.S.: Shape-correlated deformation statistics for respiratory motion prediction in 4D lung (2010)
14. Matin, T.N., et al.: Chronic obstructive pulmonary disease: lobar analysis with hyperpolarized 129 Xe MR imaging. Radiology **282**, 857–868 (2016)
15. McClelland, J.R., Hawkes, D.J., Schaeffter, T., King, A.P.: Respiratory motion models: a review. Med. Image Anal. **17**(1), 19–42 (2013)
16. Mugler, J.P., Altes, T.A.: Hyperpolarized ^{129}Xe MRI of the human lung. J. Magn. Reson. Imaging **37**(2), 313–31 (2013)
17. Murphy, K., et al.: Evaluation of registration methods on thoracic CT: the EMPIRE10 challenge. IEEE Trans. Med. Imaging **30**(11), 1901–1920 (2011)
18. Papież, B.W., Heinrich, M.P., Fehrenbach, J., Risser, L., Schnabel, J.A.: An implicit sliding-motion preserving regularisation via bilateral filtering for deformable image registration. Med. Image Anal. **18**(8), 1299–311 (2014)
19. Papież, B.W., Szmul, A., Grau, V., Brady, J.M., Schnabel, J.A.: Non-local graph-based regularization for deformable image registration. In: MICCAI RAMBO, pp. 199–207 (2017)
20. Reinhardt, J.M., Ding, K., Cao, K., Christensen, G.E., Hoffman, E.A., Bodas, S.V.: Registration-based estimates of local lung tissue expansion compared to xenon ct measures of specific ventilation. Med. Image Anal. **12**(6), 752–763 (2008)
21. Rueckert, D., Sonoda, L.I., Hayes, C., Hill, D.L., Leach, M.O., Hawkes, D.J.: Non-rigid registration using free-form deformations: application to breast MR images. IEEE Trans. Med. Imaging **18**(8), 712–21 (1999)
22. Schmidt-Richberg, A., Werner, R., Handels, H., Ehrhardt, J.: Estimation of slipping organ motion by registration with direction-dependent regularization. Med. Image Anal. **16**, 150–159 (2012)
23. Schnabel, J.A., Heinrich, M.P., Papież, B.W., Brady, S.M.: Advances and challenges in deformable image registration: From image fusion to complex motion modelling. Med. Image Anal. **33**(10), 145–148 (2016)

24. Szmul, A., Papież, B.W., Matin, T., Gleeson, F., Schnabel, J.A., Grau, V.: Regional lung ventilation estimation based on supervoxel tracking. In: Medical Imaging 2018: Image-Guided Procedures, Robotic Interventions, and Modeling, vol. 10576, pp. 10576-1–10576-7 (2018)
25. Szmul, A., Papież, B.W., Hallack, A., Grau, V., Schnabel, J.A.: Supervoxels for graph cuts-based deformable image registration using guided image filtering. J. Electron. Imaging **26**(6), 061607 (2017)
26. Wild, J.M., et al.: Automatic image registration of lung CT and hyperpolarized helium-3 MRI via mutual information of proton MRI. NMR Biomed. **24**(2), 130–134 (2011)
27. Yamamoto, T., et al.: Investigation of four-dimensional computed tomography-based pulmonary ventilation imaging in patients with emphysematous lung regions. Phys. Med. Biol. **56**(7), 2279–98 (2011)
28. Yin, Y., Hoffman, E.A., Lin, C.L.: Mass preserving nonrigid registration of CT lung images using cubic B-spline. Med. Phys. **36**(9), 4213–4222 (2009)
29. Zhang, Q., et al.: A patient specific respiratory model of anatomical motion for radiation treatment planning. Med. Phys. **34**(12), 4772–4781 (2007)

Rigid Lens – Locally Rigid Approximations of Deformable Registration for Change Assessment in Thorax-Abdomen CT Follow-Up Scans

Sonja Jäckle(✉)[ID] and Stefan Heldmann[ID]

Fraunhofer Institute for Medical Image Computing MEVIS, Lübeck, Germany
{sonja.jaeckle,stefan.heldmann}@mevis.fraunhofer.de

Abstract. A general problem of any deformable image registration method for change assessment is to find a good balance between computing a precise match and keeping locally differences. In this work we present the *rigid lens* concept dealing with this issue. The rigid lens is based on locally rigid approximation of locally precise deformations and can be used for interactive viewing and visualization of changes as well as for automatic change detection. We demonstrate the rigid lens in the context of oncological workup of thorax-abdomen CT follow-up scans and evaluate the concept for change assessment based on a study with 1492 manually annotated lesion in scans from more than 400 patients.

Keywords: Change assessment · Image registration · Local rigidity

1 Introduction

Image registration is one of the central tasks in medical imaging with a wide range of application. The overall goal is alignment of images by spatially mapping corresponding locations. Registration typically stands at the beginning of an image processing pipeline and once spatial correspondence has been established, it allows for subsequent local or even voxel-wise comparison or other local processing. Typical usage in medical imaging is navigation support, motion correction, propagation of information such as markers or segmentations, change detection and change analysis. Behind these examples, there are hidden two competing registration goals that generally cannot be reached simultaneously. While the first examples ask for local alignment as perfect as possible, the assessment of (in particular) morphological changes requires to keep local differences. Thus, finding the right balance is a challenging and application depending task that needs to be solved by every image registration method.

In this work we present an approach dealing with this issue in the context of software support for reading and analyzing thorax-abdomen CT scans that undergo an oncological workup. Here, accurate deformable image registration

© Springer Nature Switzerland AG 2018
D. Stoyanov et al. (Eds.): RAMBO 2018/BIA 2018/TIA 2018, LNCS 11040, pp. 272–283, 2018.
https://doi.org/10.1007/978-3-030-00946-5_27

can be used to compare follow-up scans by synchronized viewing, to link courser positions to the retrieval and to propagate findings from prior images in follow-up scans. On the other hand, if the registration keeps local differences, it can be used for subtraction imaging with baseline and warped follow-up scans to assist radiologists with the detection and quantification of changes, such as new lesions or tumor growth.

State-of-the-art deformable registration approaches try to achieve a reasonable trade-off between alignment quality and preservation of local changes. For example in a variational registration setting, this is typically steered by a so-called regularization parameter that weights image similarity versus smoothness of the computed mapping [2,5,9,12,16,21]. Also variational approaches were introduced for deformable registration that incorporate local rigidity. This is done either by adding an penalty term to the objective function to be minimized [8,10,11,17,18] or by forcing local rigidity as hard constraints [6,7,13,14]. However, all these methods have been proposed for modeling stiff tissue such as bone and they require prior knowledge about the regions that shall be kept rigid. In our setting we generally cannot assume to have such prior information available. Furthermore, utilizing these type of methods would be quite costly since we have to run a complete registration if we change the local region to be kept rigid. To this end, we follow the ideas of Dzyubachyk et al. [3]. The authors introduced an interactive method with focus on finding bone lesion in follow-up MRI scans. Therefore, the user selects a point of interest on a skeletal structure, the surrounding area of interest is segmented by region growing and a locally rigid transform is derived from a pre-computed whole-body deformable registration. The derived rigid transformation is then used for visual side by side comparison of follow-up MRI scans by a lens view, color-fusion, warped iso-contours and a quiver plot of the local deformation.

In this work we extend the ideas from [3] to CT follow-up imaging, change detection and subtraction imaging. We consider a generalized setting for taking full advantage of locally precise deformable registration. We also present a lens tool called *rigid lens* for visualizing, detecting and analyzing changes by locally rigid approximations of the deformation field. We give quantitative measures for rating and detection of changes and evaluate the rigid lens and its use for change detection and change assessment with a quantitative study based on 1492 annotated tumors in thorax-abdomen CT follow-up scans.

2   Method

Our idea follows the work presented in [3] and is inspired by common lens viewing tools for interactive inspection of changes and image fusion of aligned images where one image is shown in the background and another image is shown inside a lens region. We assume that we have given two registered images which we call reference and template image and the corresponding deformation vector field warping the template image onto the reference image. Then in principle we could use a common lens tool to inspect the reference and warped template.

If the registration produced a reasonable alignment we will not recognize significant morphological differences between inside and outside the lens, since local change have been removed by registration. In the extreme case of perfect alignment the warped image will look almost identical to the reference image. However, our idea is to compute a rigid approximation to the given non-rigid deformation restricted to the lens region. Then we use the obtained rigid mapping for warping the template and show the result inside the lens region. As a result we obtain a locally rigid registration valid for the particular position of the lens region with complete morphology from the template preserved. The concept of the rigid lens is illustrated in Fig. 1 and the details are given next in Sects. 2.1 and 2.2.

Besides using the rigid lens for interactive viewing, where users hovers with the rigid lens over the reference image, we are also interested in its use for change detection. The most simple extensions is to perform subtraction imaging between reference and rigid lens. However, we are also interested in deriving measures that can be used for automatic change detection. To this end, in Sect. 2.3 we present three measures based on the hypothesis that relevant changes alter shape, size or appearance of structures.

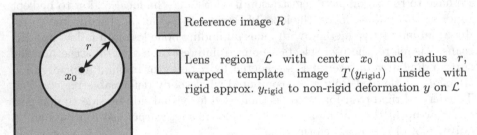

Reference image R

Lens region $\mathcal{L}$ with center x_0 and radius r, warped template image $T(y_{\text{rigid}})$ inside with rigid approx. y_{rigid} to non-rigid deformation y on $\mathcal{L}$

Fig. 1. Schematic overview of the rigid lens concept.

2.1   Modeling

Let $R, T : \mathbb{R}^3 \to \mathbb{R}$ denote the reference and template image, respectively, and let $\Omega \subset \mathbb{R}^3$ be a domain modeling the field of view of R. Then the goal of image registration is to find a deformation $y : \Omega \to \mathbb{R}^3$ that aligns the reference R and template T such that $R(x)$ and $T(y(x))$ are similar for $x \in \Omega$. For example common variational registration approaches compute y as a minimizer of an objective function of the type

$$\mathcal{D}(R, T(y)) + \alpha \mathcal{S}(y)$$

with so-called distance measure $\mathcal{D}$ that quantifies the similarity of reference R and warped moving image $T(y)$, smoother $\mathcal{S}$ that forces smoothness of the deformation and a regularization parameter $\alpha > 0$ that weights smoothness versus similarity. However, in the following we just assume that y is a non-rigid deformation produced by some registration algorithm and that reasonably well aligns R and T. Furthermore, for practical purpose we restrict ourselves to the discrete case. To this end, we assume the domain Ω is discretized by a uniform grid with resolution $h > 0$ and let Ω_h be the set of all cell-centered points. The idea of the rigid lens is to locally approximate y by a rigid transformation y_{rigid} on a lens region $\mathcal{L}$ defined as a neighborhood of a point x_0 and radius $r > h$:

$$\mathcal{L} \equiv \mathcal{L}_r(x_0) := \{x \in \Omega_h : \|x - x_0\|_2 \leq r\}.$$

For ease of notation, in the following we denote the lens region just by $\mathcal{L}$ always with the implicit understanding that $\mathcal{L}$ depends on center x_0 and radius r. Then we define y_{rigid} as rigid least squares solution, such that

$$\sum_{x \in \mathcal{L}} \|y(x) - y_{\text{rigid}}(x)\|^2 \overset{!}{=} \min. \tag{1}$$

Note that y_{rigid} depends on the lens region and center x_0, radius r, respectively, i.e., $y_{\text{rigid}}(x) \equiv y_{\text{rigid}}(\mathcal{L}; x) \equiv y_{\text{rigid}}(\mathcal{L}_r(x_0); x)$.

2.2 Algorithm

Least-squares-estimation of rigid transformations for fitting point clouds is a well-known problem in computer vision. Problem (1) is also known as Procrustes matching and tracing back to mid 1960's to the work of Whaba [20] and Schönemann [15]. Since then, various algorithms and methods have been proposed [4]. Dzyubachyk et al. [3] uses a unit quaternions based approach. Here we follow the work of Arun et al. [1] and Umeyama [19], that is based on the singular value decomposition which has shown to be the numerically most stable method [4]. For sake of completeness we give a sketch of the algorithm.

The rigid transformation can be parameterized by a rotation matrix $Q \in \text{SO}(3)$ and translation vector $b \in \mathbb{R}^3$, such that y_{rigid} can be written as $y_{\text{rigid}}(x) = Qx + b$ and above least-squares problem is equivalent to find Q, b such that

$$\sum_{x \in \mathcal{L}} \|y(x) - (Qx + b)\|^2 \overset{!}{=} \min \quad \text{s.t.} \quad Q^\top Q = I \text{ and } \det(Q) = 1. \tag{2}$$

First we compute mean and covariance of the point sets $\mathcal{L}$ and $y(\mathcal{L})$. We set

$$\mu_x := \frac{1}{|\mathcal{L}|} \sum_{x \in \mathcal{L}} x, \quad \mu_y := \frac{1}{|\mathcal{L}|} \sum_{x \in \mathcal{L}} y(x) \quad \text{and} \quad \Sigma_{xy} := \frac{1}{|\mathcal{L}|} \sum_{x \in \mathcal{L}} (x - \mu_x)(y(x) - \mu_y)^\top.$$

Next we compute the singular value decomposition $\Sigma_{xy} = UDV^\top$, with the diagonal matrix $D = \text{diag}(d_1, d_2, d_3)$ and singular values $d_1 \geq d_2 \geq d_3 \geq 0$. If $\text{rank}(\Sigma_{xy}) \geq 2$ then (2) has a unique solution

$$Q^* = USV^\top \quad \text{and} \quad b^* = \mu_y - Q^*\mu_x,$$

with diagonal matrix S defined as

$$S := \begin{cases} I, & \text{if } \det(U)\det(V) = 1, \\ \operatorname{diag}(1,1,-1), & \text{if } \det(U)\det(V) = -1. \end{cases}$$

Thus the solution y_{rigid} of (1) is given by

$$y_{\text{rigid}}(x) = Q^* x + b^*.$$

Note that from practical perspective we expect Σ_{xy} having full rank as this is the case iff $\mathcal{L}$ contains at least three (linear independent) points and the deformation y is invertible. Otherwise, either the lens region is degenerated or the registration results will most likely cause locally non-feasible deformations such as grid foldings.

2.3   Rigid Lens Measures for Change Detection

As mentioned above, we are interested in features for automatic change detection and visualization. Next we introduce three evident measures based on the hypothesis that relevant changes alter shape, size or appearance of structures. The first measure that we propose is the *average deformation difference* targeting changes in shape and size:

$$d_{\text{def}} = \frac{1}{|\mathcal{L}|} \sum_{x \in \mathcal{L}} \|y(x) - y_{\text{rigid}}(x)\|.$$

It estimates the degree of local rigidity of y and therefore provides information about local morphological changes w.r.t. lengths and angles. The second measure aims at detection of changes in size. We define the *average Jacobian* as

$$d_{\text{jac}} = \frac{1}{|\mathcal{L}|} \sum_{x \in \mathcal{L}} \det \nabla y(x).$$

Both measures d_{def} and d_{jac} are purely based on the computed deformation field only and do not take any image information into account, i.e., how the deformation affects the image appearance. To this end we propose the *relative intensity difference quotient* defined as

$$d_{\text{int}} = \frac{\sum_{x \in \mathcal{L}} |D(y_{\text{rigid}}, x) - D(y, x)|}{\sum_{x \in \mathcal{L}} D(y_{\text{rigid}}, x)}$$

with difference image $D(\phi, x) := |R(x) - T(\phi(x))|$. Clearly, d_{int} only makes sense in a mono-modal setting as ours and aims on subtraction imaging. However, under the assumption that the deformation y computed by non-rigid registration leads to better alignment than its locally rigid approximation y_{rigid} we expect that $D(y_{\text{rigid}}, x) \geq D(y, x)$. Therefore values of d_{int} are expected in the range $[0, 1]$ with $d_{\text{int}} \approx 1$ if y leads to almost perfect alignment, such that R and $T(y)$

are almost identical, and $d_{int} \approx 0$ if y and y_{rigid} produce basically the same warped images, i.e., $T(y)$ and $T(y_{rigid})$ are almost identical. Note, that d_{def}, d_{jac}, d_{int} are local averages depending on the location and size of the lens region $\mathcal{L} \equiv \mathcal{L}_r(x)$. Therefore, they can also be considered as point-wise measures at scale r, i.e., $d_{def} \equiv d_{def}(r, x)$, $d_{jac} \equiv d_{jac}(r, x)$ and $d_{int} \equiv d_{int}(r, x)$.

3 Results

We demonstrate the rigid lens and evaluate our measures for change detection on CT follow-up thorax-abdomen scans of cancer patients. The CT data used for our experiments was collected from patients referred from the oncology department at the Radboud University Medical Center, Nijmegen, the Netherlands. In total we used, 1263 thorax-abdomen CT scans of 487 patients from different scanners and protocols with slice thickness varying from 1 mm to 2 mm. Furthermore, we used 2898 annotations of tumors made by the radiologists during reporting for quantitative evaluation of the rigid lens measures. We implemented the rigid lens as an interactive application in MeVisLab (http://www.mevislab.de), where the user hovers the lens over a reference image. The rigid deformation is instantaneously calculated from the given non-rigid deformation and the locally rigid warped template image is displayed inside the lens region. All computations are performed in real time on a state-of-the-art off-the-shelf PC. The application was used for the computations and visualization of the results described below.

3.1 A Motivating Example

Our first example illustrates the rigid lens concept for interactive viewing with a deformation that almost perfectly aligns the images and removes relevant local changes. Figure 2 shows an example of a lens region with a kidney tumor inside. The tumor in the non-rigid deformed template matches nearly perfect the tumor in the reference, such that we cannot observe changes in the difference image. In contrast, with the rigid lens we can see significant tumor growth in the rigidly deformed template. The difference between non-rigid registered and rigidly deformed template are quite high, which is also reflected by the rigid lens measures: $d_{def} = 5.32$, $d_{int} = 0.67$, and $d_{jac} = 1.18$. The deformation in the lens region deviates 5.32 mm on average from the rigid deformation. This is also reflected by the Jacobian, that indicates volume growth of 18% in the lens region. Finally, our third measure d_{int} also takes a high value that indicates high intensity and appearance changes, respectively. Those high values are also visible in the intensity/deformation difference and Jacobian images shown in Fig. 2.

3.2 CT Follow-Up Registration

Now we look at thorax-abdomen CT follow-up scans, to demonstrate the utility of the proposed method. First we want to look on the visible effects and the qualitative information gain of the rigid lens in tumor regions. Afterwards we examine the quantitative benefit of the proposed algorithm in those regions.

Qualitative Study. The image top left of Fig. 3 shows the sagittal view of a CT abdomen scan with the considered tumor region, where we want to analyze

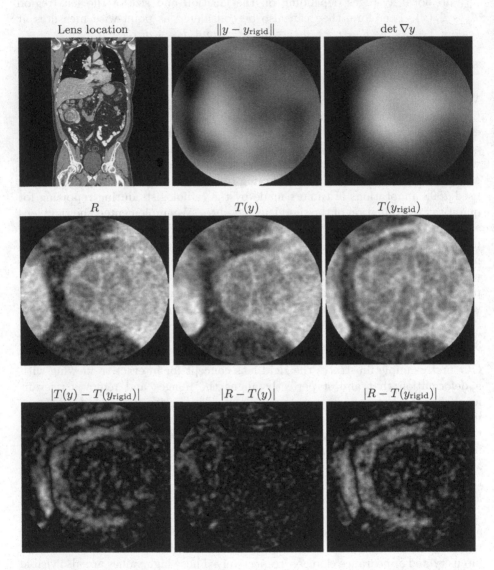

Fig. 2. CT abdomen scan with a rigid lens on a kidney tumor region: the image top left shows the coronal view of the reference image with the rigid template lens region. In the second row from left to right the lens region of the reference, the registered and rigid deformed template are displayed. The images of the last row show the intensity differences between the registered and the rigidly approximated and the difference image between the reference and the registered/rigid deformed template. The image top middle shows deformation differences between the registered and the rigidly approximated template and the image on the right shows the Jacobian of the deformation.

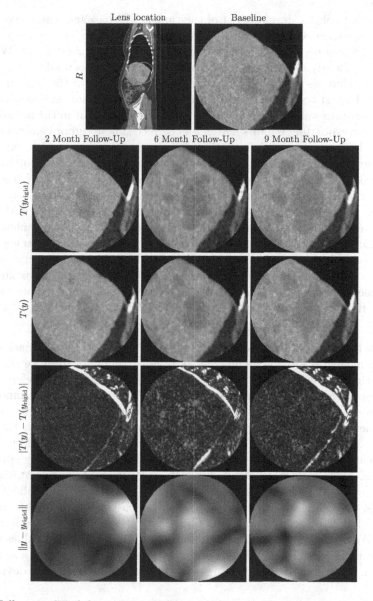

Fig. 3. Follow-up CT abdomen scan with a rigid lens on a liver tumor region: In the first row the sagittal view of the reference CT abdomen scan with the rigid template lens region and the lens region of the reference image are displayed. The rows from top to bottom show the rigidly approximated template region, the registered template region and intensity/deformation difference images between registered and rigid deformed template at the same position in the time follow-up template images.

the shape and volume development of the tumor. The baseline scan served as reference for registration with three follow-up scans token two, six, and nine month later. In the lens region a large and a small tumor can be recognized. With the rigid lens we clearly recognize how the tumors grow, whereas we do not recognize such tumor changes in the registered template images as in the rigid deformed region: In the first column the registration matches the tumor regions of the template image quite well to the ones of the reference image, but in the images token later the corresponding regions match less perfect. These tumor changes are also visible in the intensity and deformation difference between the registered and the rigid deformed template: In the first image we do not recognize high intensity and deformation changes in the tumor region, so the transformation of this region is quite rigid. In the images on the right we see more intensity and deformation differences in the tumor region, since the difference between the rigid deformed and registered tumor get higher. These observations fit to the calculated rigid lens measures listed in Table 1: We measured high deformation changes, which increase through the time follow-up images. Furthermore the intensity quotients are always on a high level and the average Jacobians indicates an expansion of the volume vector field. In summary we assessed a growing and expansion of the tumor in the lens region by approximating the deformation field rigidly.

Quantitative Study. In this experiment we do a quantitative evaluation of the rigid lens measures for change analysis of tumor regions. In total we considered 881 non-rigid follow-up registrations with the baseline image as reference and the corresponding follow-up images as templates. We used the tumor annotations (largest diameter and center) to define 1492 rigid lens regions and evaluated the average deformation difference, intensity difference and Jacobian in the region of interest. From in total 2898 annotations we only considered those with diameter $\geq$ 2cm to avoid statistics based on very small lens regions only containing few pixels. Furthermore, to avoid duplicate measurements in our statistics we used the annotations from the baseline scan for all corresponding follow-up registrations. Only in cases when no annotations at baseline are available, then the ones from follow-up scans were used. The results of our study are summarized in Table 2. We observe a large range of deformation differences with values ranging from 0.05mm to 16.13mm. We also observed intensity quotients on a significant high level. In average volume change d_{jac} is near 1, but standard deviation is

Table 1. Rigid lens measures to the corresponding follow-up data of Fig. 3. Each line shows the results of the corresponding template image.

Follow-up	d_{def}	d_{int}	d_{jac}
2 month	2.62	0.71	1.08
6 month	2.93	0.63	1.02
9 month	3.81	0.76	1.06

quite high $> 30\%$ indicating significant tumor growth or shrinkage. For better understanding we illustrate the meaning of $d_{\mathrm{jac}} \ll 1$ and $d_{\mathrm{jac}} \gg 1$ in Fig. 4.

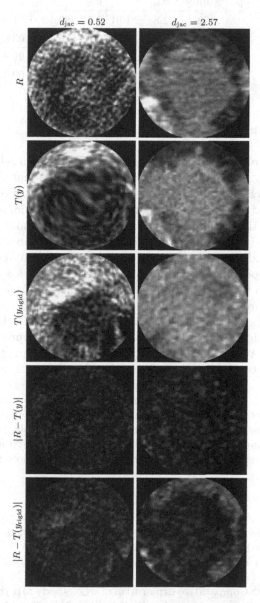

Fig. 4. Tumor regions with $d_{\mathrm{jac}} \ll 1$ and $d_{\mathrm{jac}} \gg 1$: In each column is from top to bottom the reference image, the original and rigid deformed template, and the absolute intensity differences between reference and original/rigid deformed template shown. We observed $d_{\mathrm{jac}} = 0.52$ in the first and $d_{\mathrm{jac}} = 2.57$ in the second column.

Table 2. Rigid lens measures of the quantitative study: Mean and standard deviation of the measured values are listed for each tumor type.

Tumor type	Number	d_{def}	d_{int}	d_{jac}
Liver	352	2.88 ± 1.91	0.52 ± 0.12	1.01 ± 0.34
Lung	157	2.65 ± 2.26	0.49 ± 0.14	1.03 ± 0.33
Other	983	3.27 ± 1.98	0.55 ± 0.14	0.99 ± 0.37
All	1492	3.11 ± 2.01	0.54 ± 0.14	1.00 ± 0.36

4   Conclusions

We proposed a simple approach for change assessment which is independent from any particular image registration method. We showed, that the rigid lens can be used to assess changes of volume, shape and appearance of structures. The benefits of the rigid lens are its interactive usage and its computationally cheap calculation in real time, yielding local rigid alignment without performing additional registration. Furthermore we introduced three measures for non-rigid local changes. We showed that the measures are generally able to indicate changes in shape, size and appearance. Finally we evaluated our tool for the assessment of tumor in follow-up CT scans and demonstrated the approach with a quantitative study. In future work, we aim to verify, that the rigid lens measures are sensitive to changes by correlating the results presented in Table 2 with ground-truth tumor growth. Furthermore, we aim to extent the approach for automatic change detection. Another interesting direction of research is the generalization of the rigid lens to comparison and change detection in multi-modal registration.

Acknowledgment. This research was supported by the AMI (Automation in Medical Imaging) project under the ICON program of the Fraunhofer Society, Germany. We gratefully acknowledge Bram van Ginneken and Colin Jacobs from the Diagnostic Image Analysis Group of Radboud University Medical Center, Nijmegen, the Netherlands for providing us data and for their value input in joint discussions.

References

1. Arun, K.S., Huang, T.S., Blostein, S.D.: Least-squares fitting of two 3-D point sets. IEEE Trans. Pattern Anal. Mach. Intell. **5**, 698–700 (1987)
2. Brown, L.G.: A survey of image registration techniques. ACM Computi. Surv. **24**(4), 325–376 (1992)
3. Dzyubachyk, O.: Comparative exploration of whole-body MR through locally rigid transforms. Int. J. Comput. Assist. Radiol. Surg. **8**(4), 635–47 (2013)
4. Eggert, D.W., Lorusso, A., Fisher, R.B.: Estimating 3-D rigid body transformations: a comparison of four major algorithms. Mach. Vis. Appl. **9**(5–6), 272–290 (1997)
5. Goshtasby, A.A.: Image Registration: Principles, Tools and Methods. Springer, London (2012). https://doi.org/10.1007/978-1-4471-2458-0

6. Haber, E., Heldmann, S., Modersitzki, J.: A computational framework for image-based constrained registration. Linear Algebr. Appl. **431**(3–4), 459–470 (2009)
7. König, L., Derksen, A., Papenberg, N., Haas, B.: Deformable image registration for adaptive radiotherapy with guaranteed local rigidity constraints. Radiat. Oncol. **11**(1), 122 (2016)
8. Loeckx, D., Maes, F., Vandermeulen, D., Suetens, P.: Nonrigid image registration using free-form deformations with a local rigidity constraint. In: Barillot, C., Haynor, D.R., Hellier, P. (eds.) MICCAI 2004. LNCS, vol. 3216, pp. 639–646. Springer, Heidelberg (2004). https://doi.org/10.1007/978-3-540-30135-6_78
9. Modersitzki, J.: Numerical Methods for Image Registration. Numerical Mathematics and Scientific Computation. Oxford University Press, Oxford (2004)
10. Modersitzki, J.: Image registration with local rigidity constraints. In: Horsch, A., Deserno, T.M., Handels, H., Meinzer, H.P., Tolxdorff, T. (eds.) Bildverarbeitung für die Medizin 2007, pp. 444–448. Springer, Heidelberg (2007). https://doi.org/10.1007/978-3-540-71091-2_89
11. Modersitzki, J.: FLIRT with rigidity - image registration with a local non-rigidity penalty. Int. J. Comput. Vis. **76**(2), 153–163 (2008)
12. Modersitzki, J.: FAIR: flexible algorithms for image registration, vol. 6. SIAM, Philadelphia (2009)
13. Reaungamornrat, S., Wang, A., Uneri, A., Otake, Y., Khanna, A., Siewerdsen, J.: Deformable image registration with local rigidity constraints for cone-beam CT-guided spine surgery. Phys. Med. Biol. **59**(14), 3761 (2014)
14. Ruthotto, L., Hodneland, E., Modersitzki, J.: Registration of dynamic contrast enhanced MRI with local rigidity constraint. In: Dawant, B.M., Christensen, G.E., Fitzpatrick, J.M., Rueckert, D. (eds.) WBIR 2012. LNCS, vol. 7359, pp. 190–198. Springer, Heidelberg (2012). https://doi.org/10.1007/978-3-642-31340-0_20
15. Schönemann, P.H.: A generalized solution of the orthogonal procrustes problem. Psychometrika **31**(1), 1–10 (1966)
16. Sotiras, A., Davatzikos, C., Paragios, N.: Deformable medical image registration: a survey. IEEE Trans. Med. Imaging **32**(7), 1153–1190 (2013)
17. Staring, M., Klein, S., Pluim, J.P.W.: Evaluation of a rigidity penalty term for nonrigid registration. In: Bartoli, A., Navab, N., Lepetit, V. (eds.) Workshop on Image Registration in Deformable Environments, pp. 41–50, September 2006
18. Staring, M., Klein, S., Pluim, J.P.W.: Nonrigid registration using a rigidity constraint. In: Reinhardt, J.M., Pluim, J.P.W. (eds.) Medical Imaging 2006: Image Processing. Proceedings of the SPIE, vol. 6144, pp. 355–364, March 2006
19. Umeyama, S.: Least-squares estimation of transformation parameters between two point patterns. IEEE Trans. Pattern Anal. Mach. Intell. **13**, 376–380 (1991)
20. Wahba, G.: A least squares estimate of satellite attitude. SIAM Rev. **7**(3), 409–409 (1965)
21. Zitová, B., Flusser, J.: Image registartion methods: a survey. Image Vision Comput. **21**, 977–1000 (2003)

Diffeomorphic Lung Registration Using Deep CNNs and Reinforced Learning

Jorge Onieva Onieva[✉] [iD], Berta Marti-Fuster, María Pedrero de la Puente, and Raúl San José Estépar[iD]

Applied Chest Imaging Laboratory, Department of Radiology,
Brigham and Women's Hospital, Harvard Medical School, Boston, MA, USA
{jonieva,rsanjose}@bwh.harvard.edu

Abstract. Image registration is a well-known problem in the field of medical imaging. In this paper, we focus on the registration of chest inspiratory and expiratory computed tomography (CT) scans from the same patient. Our method recovers the diffeomorphic elastic displacement vector field (DVF) by jointly regressing the direct and the inverse transformation. Our architecture is based on the RegNet network but we implement a reinforced learning strategy that can accommodate a large training dataset. Our results show that our method performs with a lower estimation error for the same number of epochs than the RegNet approach.

Keywords: Deep learning · Reinforced learning · Lung registration
Chest computed tomography · Diffeomorphism

1 Introduction

In this paper we address the problem of lung registration, with the aim of overlaying two chest CT scans from the same patient obtained during inspiration and expiration breath cycles. Numerous works have been published addressing lung registration in CT scans. Some of these methods competed in the EMPIRE10 Challenge [1], which evaluated registration methods on thoracic CT. Song *et al.* [2] proposed different configurations for their ANTS open source software package [3] to build diffeomorphic transformation models to perform a non-rigid image transformation that achieved good results in the challenge. Modat *et al.* [4] also achieved good results using a reformatted version of the Rueckert Free-Form Deformation algorithm [5] using the NiftyReg package. In 2013, Rühaak *et al.* [6] proposed a method based on minimizing the normalized gradient fields distance measure with curvature regularization.

This work has been funded by NIH NHLBI grants R01-HL116931 and R21HL140422. The Titan Xp used for this research was donated by the NVIDIA Corporation.

© Springer Nature Switzerland AG 2018
D. Stoyanov et al. (Eds.): RAMBO 2018/BIA 2018/TIA 2018, LNCS 11040, pp. 284–294, 2018.
https://doi.org/10.1007/978-3-030-00946-5_28

Deep learning has emerged in the last years as a powerful tool to solve different medical image problems [7–9], including lung registration. The use of strategies based on deep learning allows to register the images without the need of a dissimilarity metric, as the algorithm is optimized using just images saliency features. In this work, we used the RegNet architecture proposed by Sokooti *et al.* [10] to directly estimate a DVF using multiple resolution patches from a pair of input images. We focus on recovering the elastic diffeomorphic transformation. This is especially challenging in lung registration due to the large field displacement that takes places between the breathing cycle extremes.

The contributions of this work were twofold. First, we propose a new loss function that jointly estimates the direct and inverse diffeomorphic transformation. To train the algorithm, we obtained both fields using ANTs and visually validating the results. Second, we sequentially selected the data training patches more adequate for training using a reinforced learning strategy [11]. The reinforced learning strategy aims at selecting the most adequate training points allowing for a scalable approach in large training datasets.

2   Methods

2.1   Computation of Training Deformation Fields

We used 10 patients from the COPDGene cohort [12] to train our algorithm with inspiratory and expiratory high-resolution CT scanning. We tested the algorithm in another 5 different scans.

We registered the inspiration-expiration scans using ANTs [3] with the inspiration scan as the fixed image and the expiration scan as the moving one. We performed an initial affine registration using mutual information as the cost function. Then, a diffeomorphic B-spline registration was performed based on the Lagrangian diffeomorphic registration technique described in [13]. The parameters of the registration were optimized using Spearmint [14], a Bayesian optimization approach, using a publicly available reference dataset with corresponding landmarks [15].

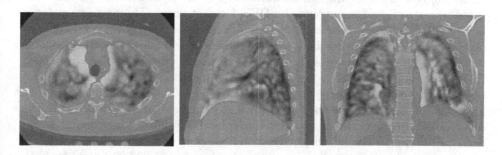

Fig. 1. Example of the DVF Jacobian for a test patient

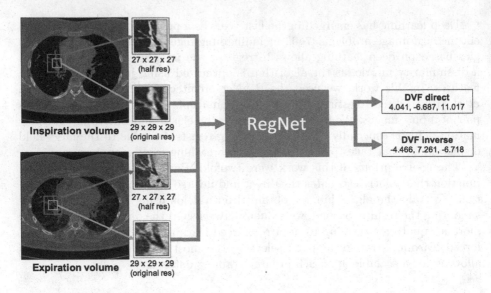

Fig. 2. Inspiratory-Expiratory registration regression network based on the RegNet architecture [10]

We focused on the registration of the lung area and ignored the rest of the image. To that end, we generated a lung mask using the segmentation method described in [16] as implemented in the Chest Imaging Platform. All the images were preprocessed to rescale them to an isometric spacing of $1 \times 1 \times 1$ mm. The DVFs and the lung masks reformatted to match the new resolution. The scans were visually assessed to ensure that the original registration and the lung masks were correct. We input into the CNN the inspiratory and the affined transformed expiratory images, as we were only interested in estimating the elastic part. Figure 1 shows an example of the Jacobian of the DFV for one of the used scans after applying our lung segmentation mask.

For all our experiments, we used the RegNet architecture proposed by Sokooti *et al.* [10] (Fig. 2). The original network takes as an input four 3D patches centered in a voxel, and it outputs the DVF for that voxel. The first two patches have a $29 \times 29 \times 29$ voxel size, and they are obtained at the original scan resolution (one of the patches belong to the fixed image, while the other belongs to the moving one). Analogously, we select another two patches (one from each image) with a $27 \times 27 \times 27$ voxel size, but these patches are obtained at the half resolution to capture a bigger context in the image. The main difference in our approach is that we performed additional experiments to obtain not only the direct DVF, but also the inverse diffeomorphic DVF (using the same architecture, just adding a second output vector).

To create our training dataset, we randomly selected 20,000 points for each scan that were within the bounds of the lung mask. For each point (voxel), we obtained the four patches that compound the network input, and stored both the direct DVF and the inverse DVF from the elastic component of the original transformation (network output). We used a total of 200,000 points to train/validate the algorithm. We followed a similar approach to create a test dataset with the 5 test scans. We randomly selected 5,000 voxels for each scan in bounds with the corresponding lung mask, for a total of 25,000 test data points.

2.2 Reinforced-Sequential Training

We evaluated different sequential training strategies as an alternative to a traditional learning approach, based on the concept of reinforced learning in machine learning [11]. Instead of training using all the data points in the training dataset, we split them into batches of $n = 5,000$ that were trained independently. We also reserved a fixed number of 3,000 points for validation in each epoch, which were common to all the sequences.

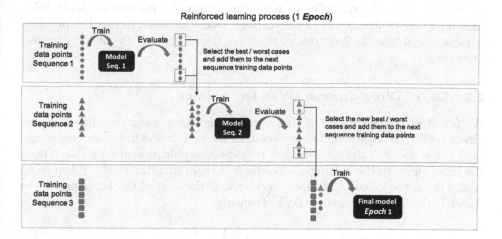

Fig. 3. Schema for the proposed reinforced learning workflow for one *Epoch*

We used an identical RegNet architecture, loss function and hyper parameters in all the sequences. The L2 loss error function is defined as:

$$L = \frac{1}{n} \sum_{i=1}^{n} (v_i - f(v_i))^2 \qquad (1)$$

where v_i is a ground truth vector of 3 coordinates containing the DVF for the voxel i, and $f(v_i)$ is the output of the CNN that contains the corresponding DVF prediction.

Every sequence begins with an initial learning rate of 0.0001, which is reduced by a factor of 0.8 whenever two consecutive epochs do not improve the validation loss. The training for a sequence is interrupted after 3 consecutive epochs with no improvement in the loss function for the validation data. A batch size of 40 and the default Keras library (v2.1.5) implementation of RMSprop optimizer are used to minimize the loss function L.

After training each sequence, we use the current state of the model to evaluate all the data points that were used in it, and select the best b and the worst w ones based on the loss function value. p_b and p_w are two hyperparameters that control the percentage of points used with respect to the total number of points n used in the sequence training. After each sequence we select the $b = n * p_b$ best points and the $w = n * p_w$ worst points of the current training (where $p, b\epsilon[0,1]$), and we keep them to be reused in the next sequence. By doing so, the method can reuse the data points that are thought to contain the most useful information for the current model. Therefore, $p = n - b - w$ new data points are added to the training dataset at the end of each sequence. The full process is represented in Fig. 3.

Since each sequence is trained independently and sequentially, there is a need to define a strategy to initialize the model weights at the beginning of each one of them. We tested three different strategies: continue with the last model state (like a regular training), use the best model that was found during the previous sequence, and use the best model that was found globally in all the previous sequences.

2.3   Use of Direct-Inverse DVFs for Training

We also tested the impact of training our algorithm using the diffeomorphic direct DVF (that contains the displacement for every voxel in the moving image to the closest one in the fixed image), the diffeomorphic inverse DVF (to go from the fixed image to the moving one) or both of them simultaneously. When using both DVFs, the value of the loss function L is the sum of the L2 error for the direct DVF and in the inverse DVF. Formally:

$$L = L_D + L_I \tag{2}$$

where L_D is the L2 loss function defined in Eq. 1 for the direct DVF and L_I is the L2 loss function for the inverse DVF. We compared the values of each one of the loss functions when using the different DVFs for the training.

3   Results

3.1   Evaluation of Reinforced-Sequential Training Strategies

We analyzed the performance of 5 different reinforced-sequential learning strategies, as described in the Sect. 2.2. Figure 4 shows the results of the validation loss value obtained during the first 3 *Epochs*. Note that in order to keep a consistent nomenclature and compare the results with a traditional learning approach, we define an *Epoch* like the moment where all the points in the training dataset have been used. It is important not to confuse it with each one of the regular epochs that happen during the training of each one of the sequences. Each reinforced learning *Epoch* is composed of around 60 sequential training steps, depending on the values of the hyperparameters p_b and p_w that are used to determine the number of data points to be reused in each sequence.

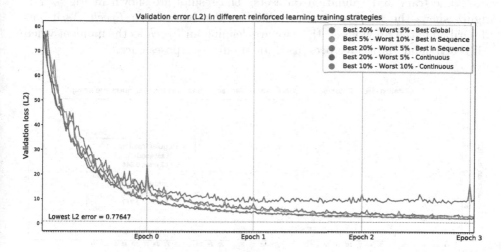

Fig. 4. Evaluation of reinforced-sequential training strategies

The figure shows that the variation of the hyperparameters p_b and p_w do not seem to have a big impact in the overall result, at least in the ranges that we tested ([0.05–0.2]). However, note how the strategy used to initialize the weights in each sequence can impact dramatically in the performance of the algorithm. Given the same values for p_b and p_w ($p_b = 0.2$ and $p_w = 0.05$), using the best model found for all the past sequences performed much worse than the other two strategies. A possible explanation for this behavior is that using this strategy may break the continuity in the learning process, leading to poor performance of the optimizers used during the training. We can also see that indeed the continuous model strategy seems to perform slightly better than the best model found in the previous sequence, although the differences are smaller. This may happen because, since the size of the training data used in each sequence is small compared to the overall training dataset size, and we also used pretty aggressive early stopping conditions, the best model found in a sequence should be very similar to the one found when the sequence stopped. Therefore, the effect of the break in continuity should be limited. In any case, we can conclude that using a continuous training strategy is the best candidate for the tested reinforced-sequential training approach.

The best strategy found was a continuous learning with $p_b = 0.2$ and $p_w = 0.05$, which reached an L2 validation error of 0.77647 after 34 *Epochs*.

3.2   Comparison of Reinforced-Sequential and Traditional Learning Strategies

We compared the learning process of one of the reinforced-sequential training (Continuous learning with $p_b = 0.2$ and $p_w = 0.05$) to traditional learning, using the same train and validation datasets. The results are shown in Fig. 5. The figure shows the L2 error in the validation dataset in each *Epoch*. As it was described in the previous section, we are defining an *Epoch* as the moment when all the training data have been used for training purposes once.

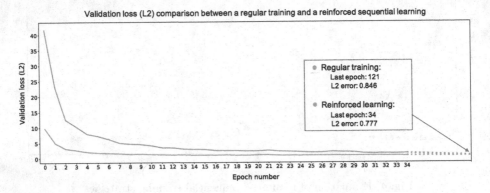

Fig. 5. Comparison of reinforced-sequential and traditional learning strategies

We can see how after very few *Epochs* (around 4–5), the loss error in the reinforced-sequential learning is already quite close to the best-achieved result, especially when compared to a regular training. This indicates that the use of the proposed reinforced-sequential strategy allows having a pretty good estimation of the algorithm performance with very few iterations over the training dataset. This may be particularly useful in a context where the data generation process is difficult but virtually unlimited.

Besides, the overall error after 34 *Epochs* in the best reinforced-sequential strategy was 0.77647, which is lower than a traditional learning after 121 epochs (0.846). These results suggest that our reinforced-sequential learning strategy may be used in different problems to increase the efficiency of other deep CNN algorithms.

Both algorithms were trained in the same hardware (using a Nvidia GEFORCE GTX 1080 Ti GPU). The total training time for the traditional training over 121 epochs was 2 days, 18:47:05 s, while the compared reinforced learning over 34 *Epochs* took 5 days, 1:13:35 s. The higher training time in the reinforced learning is due to the bigger number of iterations for every sequence as well as the extra time needed to evaluate the best/worst training data points after each sequence. The training time in reinforced learning could be reduced by selecting a higher number of training data points for each sequence.

3.3 Direct DVF and Inverse DVF in the Loss Function

We finally compared the performance of three regular trainings using different DVFs in the training loss function, evaluating the trained models in the test dataset. For evaluation purposes, we report the error distribution using the norm-2 Euclidean distance (in a mm scale) for the different DVFs used.

In the first training, we used the direct DVF to train the model and to evaluate the distance D in the test dataset. We did a second analog training but using the inverse DVF for training/testing. Finally, we trained a third model using an L2 loss function whose total value is the sum of the individual L2 losses for the direct and the inverse DVF respectively (as described in the Methods section).

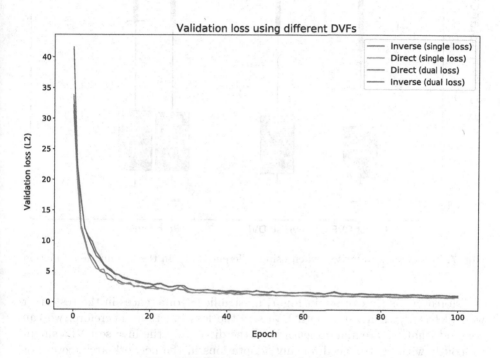

Fig. 6. Validation loss in full training

Figure 6 shows that the validation loss during the training of the direct DVF and the inverse DVF are very similar. However, when we look at the same metric in a training using a dual DVF loss, we can appreciate how the error is higher in the first epochs, but it ends up converging to a similar validation error in advanced phases of the training process. This indicates that the complexity of the problem increased (as we are predicting 2 fields instead of one), but after some epochs the network is able to perform predictions at a similar level than the single DVF training.

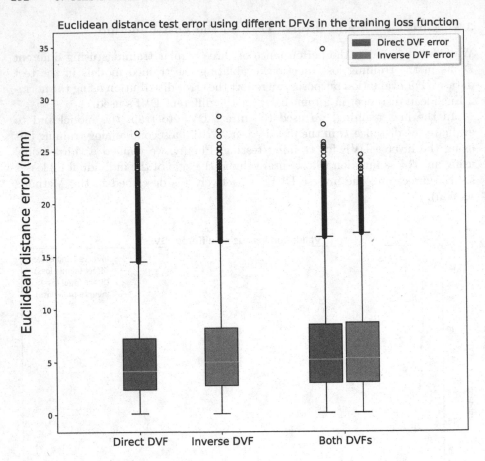

Fig. 7. Test error comparison when using different DVFs in the training loss function

Moreover, as we can see in Fig. 7, no significant differences in the test error were detected when using both DVFs in the loss function. Therefore, we can conclude that we are able to learn both the direct and the inverse DVFs simultaneously without the need for any adaptations in the network architecture or the training hyperparameters (learning rate, optimizer parameters, etc.).

4   Discussion

We proved the feasibility of using different training strategies to improve the accuracy of an algorithm based on deep CNNs, using the concepts of reinforced learning that have been applied to other tasks in the machine learning field. In the future, we will evaluate other strategies that can work in a more efficient way than the ones proposed since they could increase the total training time.

We evaluated the performance of our algorithm to study its convergence properties as well as the error when estimating just the direct and inverse DVF separately and jointly. Our results showed a lower error bound when the reinforced learning strategy was applied. We also showed that our diffeomorphic method can estimate both the direct and inverse DVF with an error that is similar to the one that is obtained when only estimating the direct or inverse DVF.

In the future, we will extend these strategies to bigger training datasets that can increase the generalization of the problem and reduce the total registration error.

References

1. Murphy, K., et al.: Evaluation of registration methods on thoracic CT: the EMPIRE10 challenge. IEEE Trans. Med. Imaging **30**(11), 1901–1920 (2011)
2. Song, G., Tustison, N.J., Avants, B.B., Gee, J.C.: Lung CT image registration using diffeomorphic transformation models. In: Medical Image Analysis for the Clinic: A Grand Challenge, pp. 23–32 (2010)
3. Avants, B.B., Tustison, N., Song, G.: Advanced Normalization Tools (ANTS). Insight J. **2**, 1–35 (2009)
4. Modat, M., McClelland, J., Ourselin, S.: Lung registration using the NiftyReg package. In: MICCAI2010 Workshop: Medical Image Analysis for the Clinic - A Grand Challenge, pp. 33–42 (2010)
5. Rueckert, D., Sonoda, L.I., Hayes, C., Hill, D.L.G., Leach, M.O., Hawkes, D.J.: Nonrigid registration using free-form deformations: application tobreast MR images. IEEE Trans. Med. Imaging **18**(8), 712–721 (1999)
6. Rühaak, J., Heldmann, S., Kipshagen, T., Fischer, B.: Highly accurate fast lung CT registration. In: SPIE Medical Imaging 2013: Image Processing, vol. 8669, pp. 86690Y-1–86690Y-9 (2013)
7. Litjens, G., et al.: A survey on deep learning in medical image analysis. Med. Image Anal. **42**, 60–88 (2017)
8. Miao, S., Wang, Z.J., Liao, R.: A CNN regression approach for real-time 2D/3D registration. IEEE Trans. Med. Imaging **35**(5), 1352–1363 (2016)
9. Eppenhof, K.A.J., Pluim, J.P.W.: Supervised local error estimation for nonlinear image registration using convolutional neural networks. In: Progress in Biomedical Optics and Imaging - Proceedings of SPIE, vol. 10133, February 2017
10. Sokooti, H., de Vos, B., Berendsen, F., Lelieveldt, B.P.F., Išgum, I., Staring, M.: Nonrigid image registration using multi-scale 3D convolutional neural networks. In: Descoteaux, M., Maier-Hein, L., Franz, A., Jannin, P., Collins, D.L., Duchesne, S. (eds.) MICCAI 2017. LNCS, vol. 10433, pp. 232–239. Springer, Cham (2017). https://doi.org/10.1007/978-3-319-66182-7_27
11. Kaelbling, L.P., Littman, M.L., Moore, A.W.: Reinforcement learning: a survey. J. Artif. Intell. Res. **4**, 237–285 (1996)
12. Regan, E.a., et al.: Genetic epidemiology of COPD (COPDGene) study design. COPD **7**(1), 32–43 (2010)
13. Avants, B.B., Epstein, C.L., Grossman, M., Gee, J.C.: Symmetric diffeomorphic image registration with cross-correlation: evaluating automated labeling of elderly and neurodegenerative brain. Med. Image Anal. **12**(1), 26–41 (2008)
14. Snoek, J., Larochelle, H., Adams, R.P.: Practical Bayesian optimization of machine learning algorithms. Adv. Neural Inf. Process. Syst. **25**, 2951–2959 (2012)

15. Castillo, R., et al.: A reference dataset for deformable image registration spatial accuracy evaluation using the COPDgene study archive. Phys. Med. Biol. **58**(9), 2861–2877 (2013)
16. Ross, J.C., et al.: Lung extraction, lobe segmentation and hierarchical region assessment for quantitative analysis on high resolution computed tomography images. In: Yang, G.-Z., Hawkes, D., Rueckert, D., Noble, A., Taylor, C. (eds.) MICCAI 2009. LNCS, vol. 5762, pp. 690–698. Springer, Heidelberg (2009). https://doi.org/10.1007/978-3-642-04271-3_84

Transfer Learning Approach to Predict Biopsy-Confirmed Malignancy of Lung Nodules from Imaging Data: A Pilot Study

William Lindsay, Jiancong Wang, Nicholas Sachs,
Eduardo Barbosa, and James Gee$^{(\boxtimes)}$

University of Pennsylvania, Philadelphia, PA 19103, USA
gee@upenn.edu

Abstract. The goal of this study is to train and assess the performance of a deep 3D convolutional network (3D-CNN) in classifying indeterminate lung nodules as either benign or malignant based solely on diagnostic-grade thoracic CT imaging. While prior studies have relied upon subjective ratings of malignancy by radiologists, our study relies only on data from subjects with biopsy-proven ground truth labels. Our dataset includes 796 patients who underwent CT-guided lung biopsy at one institution between 2012 and 2017. All patients have pathology-confirmed diagnosis (from CT-guided biopsy) and high-resolution CT imaging data acquired immediately prior to biopsy. Lesion location was manually determined using the biopsy guidance CT scan as a reference for a subset of 86 patients for this proof-of-concept study. Rather than training the network without a priori knowledge, which risks over fitting on small datasets, we employed transfer learning, taking the initial layers of our network from an existing neural network trained on a distinct but similar dataset. We then evaluated our network on a held out test set, achieving an area under the receiver operating characteristic curve (AUC) of 0.70 and a classification accuracy of 71%.

Keywords: Deep learning · Lung cancer · Machine learning

1 Introduction

1.1 Lung Cancer

Lung cancer is the leading cancer-related cause of death in the US and despite significant advances in treatment options, the five-year survival rate remains low at 18.6% [7]. This is partially explained by the fact that lung cancer has often progressed to an advanced stage by the time it becomes clinically noticeable to most patients. Multiple randomized studies investigating the survival benefit of lung cancer screening have been performed. Screening with plain chest radiographs and sputum cytology has proven questionably useful, but the pivotal National

© Springer Nature Switzerland AG 2018
D. Stoyanov et al. (Eds.): RAMBO 2018/BIA 2018/TIA 2018, LNCS 11040, pp. 295–301, 2018.
https://doi.org/10.1007/978-3-030-00946-5_29

Lung Screening Trial demonstrated a significant survival benefit of screening with low dose spiral computed tomography (CT) in high-risk patients. This study spurred a change in the United States Preventive Services Task Force screening guidelines, which now recommends annual low dose CT scans for patients with a high risk of lung cancer. Under these guidelines, 9 million Americans will receive a screening CT each year, resulting in 2.2 million positive test results [8], which will all require further evaluation. After a positive screening CT, the next step is a diagnostic, full resolution CT scan. If the radiologist finds this CT scan to be concerning, a CT-guided biopsy is performed.

1.2   Lung Biopsies

CT-guided lung biopsies are used to diagnose malignancy with pathologic certainty in patients with suspected lung cancer. Tissue is needed to confirm a diagnosis of lung cancer as well as to guide the application of targeted therapies. Although often necessary, CT-guided lung biopsies carry a risk of possible complications. Complications include pneumothorax, hemoptysis, pain, air embolism, and even death in rare cases. If lung nodules could be accurately classified into malignant vs. benign using exclusively non-invasive imaging data, biopsies could be avoided, sparing patients without malignancies the risk and cost of the biopsy.

1.3   Machine Learning in Lung Cancer Diagnosis

For nearly 30 years, physicians have sought to enhance their ability to accurately classify pulmonary nodules using predictive models [2]. In a study published in 1993, a Bayesian classifier was trained to classify solitary pulmonary nodules as benign or malignant based on hand-extracted clinical and radiographic features [4,5]. Even with a dataset of limited size, the investigators were able to train a model with an area under the curve (AUC) of 0.71. Various studies have also employed radiomics approaches, using handcrafted imaging features such as texture and entropy to predict for malignancy, with one such study achieving an AUC of 0.79 [6].

Recent advances in the field of computer vision, in particular the popularization of the convolutional neural network (CNN), have resulted in corresponding advances in the field of automated medical image analysis. In the field of lung nodule analysis specifically, multiple groups have presented impressive results. Chon et al. demonstrated that a deep learning approach could accurately detect pulmonary nodules from CT images employing a U-net architecture [1]. The interest pulmonary nodule classification peaked in 2017 when the popular "Kaggle Data Science Bowl" was focused on this topic. A public dataset from the Lung Image Data Consortium (LIDC) was made available and many groups submitted impressive solutions leveraging a variety of network architectures including U-net, AlexNet, and others [10].

All of these studies, however, relied on datasets without true ground truth labels. That is, the label of malignancy vs. non malignancy was based on subjective ratings of by radiologists, not on subjects with biopsy confirmed disease. Because of this, all of these models are limited in performance to what an actual radiologist can achieve today. A natural extension of these methods would be application to a dataset with ground truth labels provided by biopsies.

1.4   Transfer Learning

Because a large open dataset containing both ground truth pathology data and CT imaging data does not yet exist, we turned to transfer learning as a possible solution [9]. In transfer learning, a network is trained on one dataset and then fine-tuned using another dataset. In our case, we chose to train a network using an open dataset from the Lung Image Data Consortium of subjects with and without lung nodules containing CT imaging data along with subjective radiologists ratings of suspicious nodules. We then fine-tuned this network to predict pathologically-confirmed lung cancer, using a smaller dataset of patients with pathologically confirmed lung cancer diagnoses.

2   Methods

2.1   Dataset

Our dataset consists of 796 patients who underwent CT-guided lung biopsy at one institution between 2012 and 2017 to evaluate suspicious pulmonary nodules. All patients had pathology-confirmed diagnosis (from CT-guided biopsy) and high-resolution CT imaging data acquired immediately prior to biopsy. Lesion location was manually determined using the biopsy guidance CT scan as a reference for a subset of 86 patients for this proof of concept study. The median nodule size was 2.1 cm.

A random selection of 65 patients was used as the training set. The remaining 21 patients were reserved solely for testing and performance assessment.

In the training set, 72% of subjects had biopsies showing malignancy, while 28% of patients were shown to have benign disease. In the testing set, 72% were malignant, while 28% were benign.

Given the 3D location of nodule, the images were re-sampled to 1 mm × 1 mm × 1 mm resolution and a 64 × 64 × 64 cube volume around the center of nodule was then cropped. Visual inspection on the cropped volume was performed to ensure the inclusion of the full nodule. Examples of cropped volumes are shown in Fig. 1 below.

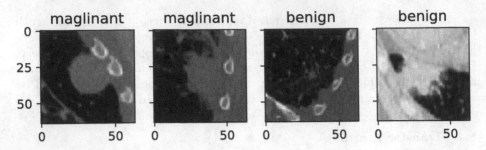

Fig. 1. Example 2D slice of a thoracic CT scan showing malignant and benign (non-malignant) lesions.

2.2 Network Construction

Rather than training the network without a priori knowledge, which risks over fitting on small datasets, we employed transfer learning, taking the initial layers of our network from an existing neural network trained on a distinct but similar dataset. In our case, we first identified an existing 3D-CNN to identify nodules from thoracic CT data that was trained on an open dataset from the LIDC [3]. Using the final batch pooling layer from the existing network, we then added three new untrained layers (spatial pooling, dense, and softmax) and re-trained the network using our training set employing dropout and batch normalization. This final 3D-CNN network was evaluated using the test set. The network schematic is shown in Fig. 2.

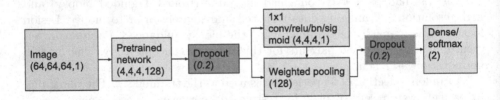

Fig. 2. A diagram showing our transfer learning methodology.

To reduce the model's parameters, we applied a simple weighted spatial pooling of the pretrained feature vector. Next, a voxel-wise importance map is regressed out with a conv/relu/bn/sigmoid sandwich and is used to weighted average the feature vector spatially, resulting in a single feature vector of 128 features. This layer is followed by a dense layer, a softmax classification layer and standard binary cross entropy loss. Our dataset contains much more malignant cases than benign. To counter class imbalance, class weight of 10:1 (benign to malignant) weight is added to the loss function. We use a standard Adam optimizer with learning rate 1e−3. Two drop out layers with keep rate 0.8/drop rate 0.2 are added to the network to counter overfitting. We use batch size 10

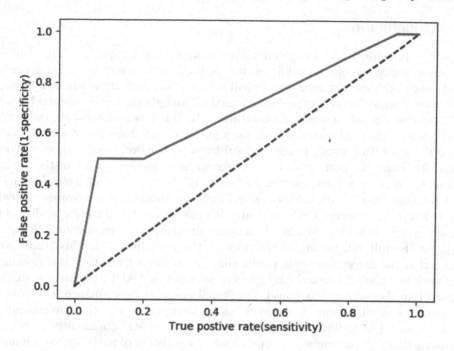

Fig. 3. Receiver Operating Characteristic Curve for fine tuned network.

and run the training for 2000 steps. Empirically this is enough for the network to reach convergence.

3   Results

When validated on a held out test set, our classifier achieved and AUC of 0.70 and a classification accuracy of 71%. The Receiver Operating Characteristic Curve can be seen in Fig. 3. Examples of incorrectly classified nodules can be seen in Fig. 4

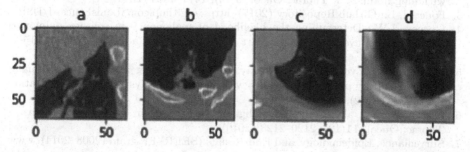

Fig. 4. Examples of mis-classified labels. (a), (b) are true malignant nodules labeled by the network as benign. (c), (d) are true benign nodules labeled by the network as malignant.

4   Conclusion

Machine learning based image analysis methods have the potential to significantly enhance radiology workflows, reduce the occurrence of missed diagnoses and false positives, and improve survival rates for lung cancer patients. However, creation of larger, more comprehensive medical image datasets is required before clinically acceptable models can be trained. In this proof of concept study, we demonstrate that a network trained on a publicly available dataset can be fine-tuned, even with a small number of subjects, to a more specific classification task. Although the performance of our model does not reach state-of-the-art in terms of classification accuracy or AUC, we believe that the inclusion of ground truth labels based on pathology is novel and an important step towards clinical adoption of lung cancer CAD software. We are currently extracting additional imaging and pathology data from our larger dataset, and a more complete analysis on the full 796 patients is planned in the near future. In this study, we hope that the larger sample size will allow us to further fine-tune our existing network and allow for meaningful gains in accuracy and AUC. Ultimately, single institution datasets will not lead to optimal classifier performance. Given the importance of diagnosing lung cancer at an early stage and the government's new screening guidelines, we strongly advise the medical community to begin construction of a comprehensive open dataset consisting of pathology and imaging data. Furthermore, radiologists don't makes clinical diagnoses using solely on imaging data. They often correlate their imaging finding with additional clinical data such as the patient's smoking history, demographics, and co-morbid conditions. We hope to expand our dataset to include additional clinical features from the patient's electronic medical record, with a goal of creating a workflow-integrated CAD solution for lung cancer screening.

References

1. Chon, A., et al.: Deep convolutional neural networks for lung cancer detection. Technical report, Stanford University (2017)
2. Deppen, S.A., et al.: Predicting lung cancer prior to surgical resection in patients with lung nodules. J. Thorac. Oncol. **9**(10), 1477–1484 (2014)
3. Foucard, L.: Github Repository (2017). https://github.com/LouisFoucard/DSB17
4. Gurney, J.W.: Determining the likelihood of malignancy in solitary pulmonary nodules with Bayesian analysis. Part II. Application. Radiology **186**(2), 415–22 (1993)
5. Gurney, J.W., Lyddon, D.M., McKay, J.A.: Determining the likelihood of malignancy in solitary pulmonary nodules with Bayesian Analysis. Part II. Application. Radiology **186**(2), 415–422 (1993)
6. Hawkins, S., et al.: Predicting malignant nodules from screening CT scans. J. Thorac. Oncol. **11**(12), 2120–2128 (2016)
7. Surveillance, Epidemiology, and End Results (SEER) Program (2008–2014). www.seer.cancer.gov
8. Lokhandwala, T., et al.: Costs of diagnostic assessment for lung cancer: a medicare claims analysis. Clin. Lung Cancer **18**(1), e27–34 (2017). https://doi.org/10.1016/j.cllc.2016.07.006

9. Yosinski, J., Clune, J., Bengio, Y., Lipson, H.: How transferable are features in deep neural networks? In: Advances in Neural Information Processing Systems, NIPS 2014, vol. 27. NIPS Foundation (2014)
10. Zhao, X., Liu, L., Qi, S., Teng, Y., Li, J., Qian, W.: Agile convolutional neural network for pulmonary nodule classification using CT images. Int. J. Comput. Assist. Radiol. Surg. 13(4), 585–95 (2018)

Convolutional Neural Network Based COPD and Emphysema Classifications Are Predictive of Lung Cancer Diagnosis

Charles Hatt[1,2]([⊠]), Craig Galban[2], Wassim Labaki[3], Ella Kazerooni[2,3], David Lynch[4], and Meilan Han[3]

[1] Imbio LLC, Ann Arbor, USA
charleshatt@imbio.com
[2] Department of Radiology, University of Michigan, Ann Arbor, USA
[3] Department of Internal Medicine, Division of Pulmonary and Critical Care, University of Michigan, Ann Arbor, USA
[4] Department of Medicine, Division of Radiology, National Jewish Health, Denver, USA

Abstract. Lung cancer is a leading cause of mortality and morbidity for patients suffering from Chronic Obstructive Pulmonary Disease (COPD). Both the presence of visually assessed emphysema on CT scans and abnormal pulmonary function tests are associated with the development of lung cancer. Based on recent results showing that convolutional neural networks (CNNs) applied to CT scans can predict spirometrically-defined COPD ($\frac{FEV_1}{FVC} < 0.7$), we hypothesized that CNN-based classification of COPD and emphysema is predictive of lung cancer development in the National Lung Cancer Screening (NLST) cohort. We trained spirometric COPD and visual emphysema CNN classifiers using data from the COPDGene study. The classifiers were then used to generate COPD and emphysema scores (CS_{CNN} and ES_{CNN}, respectively) on 7347 CT scans from the NLST study. Cox proportional hazards regression was used to model the effects of CS_{CNN}, ES_{CNN}, age, body mass index, education, gender, smoking pack-years, and years since smoking cessation on lung cancer diagnosis. It was found that, individually, both CS_{CNN} and ES_{CNN} were statistically significant predictors (p < 0.000 and p < 0.000, respectively) of lung cancer diagnosis hazard.

Keywords: CNN · COPD · Lung cancer screening · Survival analysis

1 Introduction

Chronic Obstructive Lung Disease (COPD), an inflammatory lung disease resulting in pulmonary airflow obstruction, is projected to be the fourth leading cause of death in the world by 2030 [1]. COPD is typically diagnosed using spirometry (i.e. pulmonary function tests, PFTs), with a forced expiratory volume in 1 second to forced vital capacity ratio ($\frac{FEV_1}{FVC}$) less than 70% being considered a COPD

© Springer Nature Switzerland AG 2018
D. Stoyanov et al. (Eds.): RAMBO 2018/BIA 2018/TIA 2018, LNCS 11040, pp. 302–309, 2018.
https://doi.org/10.1007/978-3-030-00946-5_30

diagnosis [1]. Emphysema, a sub-type of COPD that involves the thinning and destruction of the alveoli, is one of the diseases comprising COPD. Emphysema presence and severity is typically assessed by visual reading of thoracic computed tomography (CT) scans.

Lung cancer has been shown to be associated with spirometrically defined COPD (sCOPD), with Young et al. reporting a two-fold increase in lung cancer incidence among patients in the National Lung Cancer Screening Trial (NLST) who had COPD [2]. The presence of visually assessed emphysema on CT scans is also associated with lung cancer diagnosis, as a meta-analysis conducted by Smith et al. showed that the presence vs. absence of visual emphysema on CT resulted in a lung cancer diagnosis odds ratio of 3.50 [3].

It is therefore possible that using PFT and/or CT imaging data may allow for more accurate lung cancer risk stratification, which could improve lung cancer screening inclusion criteria and/or be used to help motivate patients to quit smoking [5]. Unfortunately, PFTs and visual assessment of emphysema are not always available due to the associated costs. In addition, visual assessment of emphysema is subjective and thus suffers from high intra and inter-reader variability [6].

It was recently shown that Convolutional Neural Networks (CNNs) can be used to train end-to-end CT-based classifiers of clinical COPD outcomes [7] such as GOLD stage, exacerbation frequency, and mortality. Based on these results, we hypothesized these techniques could used to improve lung cancer risk modeling without the need for PFTs or visual assessment of emphysema.

In this work, we present a CT-based CNN classification workflow for assessment of sCOPD and visual emphysema and show that classification results produced by the CNNs are predictive of lung cancer diagnosis hazard in the NLST cohort.

2   Methods

2.1   Data

The CNNs were trained using image and clinical data from the Genetic Epidemiology of COPD (COPDGene) study [8]. CT scans from the baseline image collection and 5-year follow-up were available for training and validation. Only scans reconstructed using a smooth kernel (GE Standard, Siemens B31f, or Philips B) were used in this study.

The CNN models trained on COPDGene data were applied to CT scans from the NLST. We processed low-dose CT scans from the NLST that were reconstructed with a Siemens B30f, GE Standard, Philips B, or Toshiba FC10 kernel, and that had a slice thickness of 2.5 mm or less. After accounting for missing clinical data and failed image processing, this resulted in 7347 datasets. 2694 of these datasets had associated spirometry data.

2.2 CNN Architecture

Image Processing. High resolution CT volumes are too large to train and process on current graphics processing units (GPUs). Similar to [7], we developed a data reduction strategy that used a subset of image slices for training and processing. A set of 8 axial slices, each down-sampled from 512×512 to 256×256 pixels, were randomly sampled from equally sized "zones" of the lung and combined into a single image montage (Fig. 1).

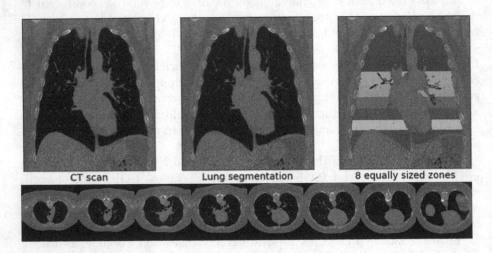

CT scan   Lung segmentation   8 equally sized zones

Fig. 1. Top: Image processing steps: segmentation and division of the lungs into 8 equally-sized zones. Bottom: 2048×256 pixel image montage used for training and classification. Each slice of the montage was randomly sampled from within it's corresponding zone

CNN Configuration. The CNN configuration is presented in Table 1. Both sCOPD and visual emphysema classifiers used this configuration for training and testing. The CNN was implemented in `PyTorch` and trained using stochastic gradient descent with a cross-entropy loss function, Nesterov momentum of 0.9, a learning rate of 0.001, and a batch size of 32.

Training. For the sCOPD classifier, subjects were classified as having COPD if they were in Global Initiative for Chronic Obstructive Lung Disease (GOLD) stage 1 or greater. GOLD stage 0 and PRISM subjects were classified as not having COPD. 3750 subjects were used for training. Due to the to use of random slices for processing each CT scan, data augmentation was used to increase the size of the training dataset from 3750 to 15000 by generating four different slice configurations for each subject. 5-year follow-up CT scans were used for training validation.

The emphysema classifier was trained using visual centrilobular emphysema classifications. A subset of the baseline COPDGene CT scans were visually scored by two analysts using the Fleischner Society classification system. Emphysema was classified as centrilobular (trace, mild, moderate, confluent, and advanced destructive emphysema), panlobular, and paraseptal (mild or substantial). A two-category classifier was generated that classified an image as having visual emphysema if it contained mild, moderate, confluent, or advanced destructive centrilobular emphysema, and no emphysema otherwise. Visual reads that were not agreed upon by both analysts were not used for training. A total of 875 subjects were used for training, resulting in 3500 training images after using the data augmentation strategy outlined above. 3500 datasets from different subjects were used for training validation.

Table 1. CNN configuration. conv3 $= 3 \times 3$ convolution. relu $=$ Rectified linear unit. maxpool $= 2 \times 2$ max-pooling. FC $=$ Fully-connected. dropout $= 50\%$ dropout.

input (256x2048x1)
(256x2048x1) >conv3 >relu >(256x2048x16) >conv3 >relu >(256x2048x16)
maxpool
(128x1024x16) >conv3 >relu >(128x1024x32) >conv3 >relu >(128x1024x32)
maxpool
(64x512x32) >conv3 >relu >(64x512x64) >conv3 >relu >(64x512x64)
maxpool
(32x256x64) >conv3 >relu >(32x256x128) >conv3 >relu >(32x256x128)
maxpool
(16x128x128) >conv3 >relu >(16x128x128) >conv3 >relu >(16x128x128)
maxpool
(16x128x128) >FC512 >relu >dropout >FC2
log softmax

CNN Validation and Testing. Following training, the CNN models were used to create sCOPD and emphysema classification probabilities (i.e. classification scores $CS_{CNN} \in (0, 1) \subset \mathbb{R}$, $ES_{CNN} \in (0, 1) \subset \mathbb{R}$, respectively) by taking the exponential of the model output. Classification scores were assigned to a binary category by thresholding at 0.5 (e.g. $CS_{CNN} > 0.5 \rightarrow$ sCOPD, $CS_{CNN} \leq 0.5 \rightarrow$ NO sCOPD). Validation and test accuracy was computed as the percentage of correct classifications.

The sCOPD classifier was further validated in a subset of NLST images (2694 subjects) with spirometry data available. Radiologist generated visual emphysema classification, however, was not available for the NLST datasets.

2.3 Statistical Analysis

Cox proportional hazard models were used to test the association between CS_{CNN} and ES_{CNN} and time-to-event of lung cancer diagnosis incidence.

Participants were censored at 6 years of follow-up. Regression models were adjusted for covariates known to be associated with cancer development including age, gender, body mass index, pack-years, and time since smoking cessation. Three models were generated: One with both CS_{CNN} and ES_{CNN} scores included as continuous variables, one with only the CS_{CNN} score included as a continuous variable, and one with only the ES_{CNN} score included as a continuous variable.

Kaplan-Meier curves were also generated for CS_{CNN} and ES_{CNN} classifiers for subjects that fell above and below the median classification scores within the NLST cohort (Fig. 2).

Both Cox proportional hazards regression and Kaplan-Meier analysis were implemented in `Python` using the `lifelines` package.

3   Results

3.1   Validation and Test Accuracy

Validation accuracy for the COPDGene cohort and test accuracy for the NLST cohort are shown in Table 2. The validation accuracy of the CS_{CNN} classifier was almost exactly the same as reported for test subset in [7]. It should also be noted that there was almost no decrease in the sCOPD classification accuracy when going from the COPDGene to the NLST scans, despite that fact that the patient cohorts and CT image acquisition and reconstruction parameters were different.

Table 2. Validation and test accuracy of the CS_{CNN} and ES_{CNN} classifiers

	Validation (COPDGene) accuracy	NLST test accuracy
sCOPD	77.7%	76.2%
Emphysema	79.8%	Not available

3.2   Statistical Analysis

Results for each Cox model are shown in Table 3. When CS_{CNN} and ES_{CNN} were not combined into a single model, both were statistically significant (p < 0.000) predictors of lung cancer diagnosis hazard. When combined in a single model, however, the statistical significance of the CS_{CNN} and ES_{CNN} classification scores decreased (to $p = 0.0195$ and $p = 0.0598$, respectively).

Table 3. Cox regression results. Statistically significant predictors are in bold.

	CS and ES		CS-only		ES-only	
	Hazard	p	Hazard	p	Hazard	p
CS_{CNN}	**1.7849**	**0.0195**	**2.46**	**0.0000**	-	-
ES_{CNN}	1.5934	0.0598	-	-	**2.3555**	**0.0000**
Age	**1.0632**	**0.0000**	**1.0651**	**0.0000**	**1.0660**	**0.0000**
BMI	0.9778	0.0625	**0.9723**	**0.0164**	0.9787	0.0745
Education	0.9935	0.6730	0.9931	0.6595	0.9935	0.6728
Gender	**0.7840**	**0.0237**	**0.7959**	**0.0334**	**0.7841**	**0.0237**
Pack-years	**1.0110**	**0.0000**	**1.0112**	**0.0000**	**1.0112**	**0.0000**
Quit-years	**0.9362**	**0.0000**	**0.9348**	**0.0000**	**0.9360**	**0.0000**
	Concordance	0.714	Concordance	0.711	Concordance	0.711

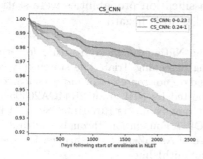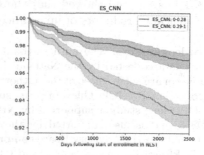

Fig. 2. Kaplan-Meier curves showing time to lung cancer diagnosis for subjects with CS_{CNN} and ES_{CNN} scores less than or greater than the median for the cohort. 0.23 and 0.28 are the median CS_{CNN} and ES_{CNN}, scores, respectively, in the NLST cohort.

4 Discussion and Conclusion

The relationship between objective quantitative CT-based assessment of emphysema (i.e. percent low-attenuation area, %LAA) and lung cancer has been shown to be either weak [9] or non-existent [3,10,11], despite an association between visual emphysema and lung cancer. In this work, we showed that CNN-based probability scores of spirometrically defined COPD and visual emphysema were both statistically significant predictors of lung cancer diagnosis hazard in the NLST cohort. An encouraging result of this work is that, although the sCOPD classifier was trained on full-dose CTs from the COPDGene study, the validation accuracy of the classifier decreased only 1.5% when applied to low-dose CTs from the NLST, which is evidence that the classifier was robust and not overfit to the training data.

The CNN architecture presented in this work uses only a subset of axial slices from a high-resolution CT image. A potential benefit of this architecture is that it might be possible to obtain accurate classification of sCOPD and/or emphysema from "incremental" CT scans (scans acquired with large spacing between slices), which when used in combination with low-tube currents, would allow for screening of COPD at very low x-ray doses. Another benefit of the image processing workflow is that, due to the use of random slices within lung zones, it may be possible to increase the accuracy of the classifier estimates by ensembling the results from multiple configurations.

A limitation of this preliminary work is that CNN models were only trained to classify COPD and emphysema as binary categories even though more granular data was available (e.g. GOLD 0–4 and Fleischner society emphysema classifications). Additionally, the variation in CNN scores obtained using different random slice configurations from the same image should be characterized to help understand the classification repeatability. Finally, a comparison with the performance of other quantitative CT-based COPD metrics (e.g. LAA-950 or Perc15) is of particular interest. Future work will focus on addressing these issues.

In conclusion, we trained CNNs to classify COPD and emphysema presence from CT images, and showed that the classification probabilities were statistically significant predictors of lung cancer diagnosis hazard.

Acknowledgements. The authors thank the National Cancer Institute for access to NCI's data collected by the National Lung Screening Trial. The statements contained herein are solely those of the authors and do not represent or imply concurrence or endorsement by NCI. This work was supported by NIH grant 2R44CA203050-02. The COPDGene study is supported by NIH Grant Numbers R01 HL089897 and R01 HL089856, and is also supported by the COPD Foundation through contributions made to an Industry Advisory Board comprised of AstraZeneca, Boehringer Ingelheim, Novartis, Pfizer, Siemens, Sunovion and GlaxoSmithKline.

References

1. Cruz, A.A.: Global surveillance, prevention and control of chronic respiratory diseases: a comprehensive approach. World Health Organization (2007)
2. Young, R.P., et al.: Airflow limitation and histology shift in the national lung screening trial. The NLST-ACRIN cohort substudy. Am. J. Respir. Criti. Care Med. **192**(9), 1060–1067 (2015)
3. Smith, B.M., Pinto, L., Ezer, N., Sverzellati, N., Muro, S., Schwartzman, K.: Emphysema detected on computed tomography and risk of lung cancer: a systematic review and meta-analysis. Lung Cancer **77**(1), 58–63 (2012)
4. National Lung Screening Trial Research Team: Reduced lung-cancer mortality with low-dose computed tomographic screening. New Engl. J. Med. **365**(5), 395–409 (2011)
5. McClure, J.B.: Are biomarkers a useful aid in smoking cessation? A review and analysis of the literature. Behav. Med. **27**(1), 37–47 (2001)
6. Bankier, A.A., De Maertelaer, V., Keyzer, C., Gevenois, P.A.: Pulmonary emphysema: subjective visual grading versus objective quantification with macroscopic morphometry and thin-section CT densitometry. Radiology **211**(3), 851–858 (1999)

7. González, G., et al.: Disease staging and prognosis in smokers using deep learning in chest computed tomography. Am. J. Respir. Crit. Care Med. **197**(2), 193–203 (2018)
8. Regan, E.A., et al.: Genetic epidemiology of COPD (COPDGene) study design. COPD J. Chronic Obstr. Pulm. Dis. **7**(1), 32–43 (2011)
9. Gierada, D.S., et al.: Quantitative CT assessment of emphysema and airways in relation to lung cancer risk. Radiology **261**(3), 950–959 (2011)
10. Wilson, D.O., et al.: Association of radiographic emphysema and airflow obstruction with lung cancer. Am. J. Respir. Crit. Care Med. **178**(7), 738–744 (2008)
11. Maldonado, F., Bartholmai, B.J., Swensen, S.J., Midthun, D.E., Decker, P.A., Jett, J.R.: Are airflow obstruction and radiographic evidence of emphysema risk factors for lung cancer?: a nested case-control study using quantitative emphysema analysis. Chest **138**(6), 1295–1302 (2010)

Towards an Automatic Lung Cancer Screening System in Low Dose Computed Tomography

Guilherme Aresta[1,2(✉)], Teresa Araújo[1,2], Colin Jacobs[5], Bram van Ginneken[5], António Cunha[1,3], Isabel Ramos[4], and Aurélio Campilho[1,2]

[1] INESC TEC, 4200 Porto, Portugal
guilherme.m.aresta@inesctec.pt
[2] Faculty of Engineering of University of Porto, 4200-465 Porto, Portugal
[3] University of Minho and Alto-Douro, 5001-801 Vila Real, Portugal
[4] Faculty of Medicine of University of Porto, 4200-319 Porto, Portugal
[5] Radboud University Medical Center, 6525 Nijmegen, The Netherlands

Abstract. We propose a deep learning-based pipeline that, given a low-dose computed tomography of a patient chest, recommends if a patient should be submitted to further lung cancer assessment. The algorithm is composed of a nodule detection block that uses the object detection framework YOLOv2, followed by a U-Net based segmentation. The found structures of interest are then characterized in terms of diameter and texture to produce a final referral recommendation according to the National Lung Screen Trial (NLST) criteria. Our method is trained using the public LUNA16 and LIDC-IDRI datasets and tested on an independent dataset composed of 500 scans from the Kaggle DSB 2017 challenge. The proposed system achieves a patient-wise recall of 89% while providing an explanation to the referral decision and thus may serve as a second opinion tool to speed-up and improve lung cancer screening.

Keywords: Computer aided diagnosis · Lung cancer
Low dose computed tomography images · Screening · Deep learning

1 Introduction

Lung cancer is the deadliest type of cancer worldwide in both men and women [1] but early diagnosis significantly increases patient survival rate. In fact, the National Lung Screen Trial (NLST) showed that annual screening of lung cancer risk groups with low-dose chest computed tomography (LDCT) via manual analysis of scans by experts reduces lung cancer mortality by 20% [2]. However, LDCT screening is challenging because (i) the process is prone to errors due to factors such as interobserver variability and (ii) the equipment and personnel costs of these programs inhibit their application on developing countries, where tobacco consumption is difficult to control [3]. To address the problem of lung

© Springer Nature Switzerland AG 2018
D. Stoyanov et al. (Eds.): RAMBO 2018/BIA 2018/TIA 2018, LNCS 11040, pp. 310–318, 2018.
https://doi.org/10.1007/978-3-030-00946-5_31

cancer detection we propose a second opinion system that helps to reduce the overall screening burden by indicating if a patient should or not be referred for follow-up. The framework is composed of an initial nodule detection step, nodule segmentation and finally a scan-wise decision based on the NLST criteria for positive screens and thus provides an interpretable justification of its decision.

Lung nodule detection is a mandatory step for the automatic referral pipeline. Deep learning has become the standard technique to complete this task, with the leaderboard of LUNA16[1] nodule detection challenge being mainly composed of these kind of approaches [4]. The most common pipeline is to detect candidates by slice or 3D-wise via an object detection framework such as Faster-R CNN [5] followed by a 3D convolutional neural network (CNN) for false-positive (FP) reduction and these systems achieve detection sensitivities greater than 0.80 with 0.125 FP/scan or greater than 0.90 with 1 FP/scan. Then, nodule segmentation is used for characterizing the detected abnormalities. The most common approach for nodule segmentation is to use intensity (or HU) and shape features [6], but CNNs can also be applied for 3D nodule segmentation and achieve Sorensen-Dice coefficients close to 0.8 [7].

Despite the advances on both nodule detection and segmentation, automatic patient referral is little explored. Recently, Kaggle[2] hosted a challenge aimed at the development of algorithms for predicting if a patient should be referred for follow-up after screening. The training set is composed of 1398 training scans with labels at the scan level. It is widely known that the majority of the scans originated from the NLST trial, but the exact origin of each anonymized scan has not been disclosed by Kaggle. In this challenge, the best methods used deep learning approaches with an initial candidate detection followed by an expected malignancy prediction that allow to achieve an overall log loss of 0.39–0.41.

We move beyond the nodule detection task and aim at tackling the more complex lung cancer screening pipeline. Our contribution to the state-of-the-art is a single step nodule detection algorithm followed by a segmentation and field-knowledge classification step that allows a near-human scan-wise abnormality detection performance for scan referral. The next section describes the developed algorithms and the datasets used for validation. Section 3 discusses the performance of the proposed system. Finally, Sect. 4 summarizes our study.

2   Method

Our system was designed to follow the standard clinician pipeline of NLST [2], where radiologists were instructed to refer a patient for follow-up if any non-calcified nodule with diameter $d > 4\,mm$ was found. With that in mind, our system is composed of 3 main steps (see Fig. 1) (i) nodule detection via YOLOv2 (Sect. 2.2) that focuses on nodules with $d > 4\,mm$, (ii) nodule segmentation for measurement and characterization via U-Net (Sect. 2.3) and (iii) scan-wise referral indication based on the NLST guidelines (Sect. 2.4).

---

[1] https://luna16.grand-challenge.org/home/.
[2] https://www.kaggle.com/c/data-science-bowl-2017.

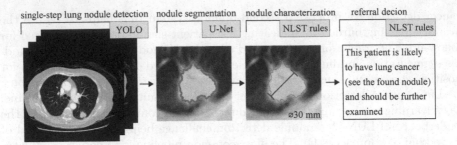

Fig. 1. Pipeline of the proposed lung cancer referral system.

2.1 Datasets and Technical Details

The nodule detection network is trained on the LUNA16 dataset [4], which contains 888 scans from the LIDC-IDRI dataset [8]. The LIDC-IDRI contains 1012 LDCT scans with variable slice thickness and nodule voxel-wise annotations from up to 4 different expert radiologists. The LUNA16 contains the information of 1186 nodules' centroids and diameter (no voxel-wise data) with an agreement level 3 or higher, as well as the centroid of non-nodule lesions of diagnostic interest. For the nodule detection step, we train in subsets 1–9 (20% validation) and test on the 89 scans of subset 0. The test set has 112 nodules, from which 80 have $d > 4$ mm. The nodule segmentation system is trained on LIDC-IDRI with an agreement level 1 or higher and multiple segmentations are combined via logical OR. We train on 1400 axial view 64×64 pixels (approx. 51×51 mm) patches, validate on 300 and test on 570 samples. We experimentally set the segmentation threshold at 0.5 by analysis of the results on the validation set.

We tested our screening system on 500 randomly selected scans from the 1st stage of the Kaggle dataset. The scans are labeled according to future cancer presence (123 cases) or low cancer risk (377 cases). All datasets are anonymized and there is no access to relevant patient metadata. Unless stated otherwise, we consider the HU interval $[-1000, 400]$ for our experiments.

Experiments were performed on a Intel Core i7-5960X @3.00 GHz, 32 Gb RAM, $2 \times$ GTX1080 desktop. The framework was developed on Python 3.5 and Keras 2.0.4. The YOLOv2 implementation is based on[3]. Both YOLOv2 and U-Net were trained with optimizer Adam (learning rate 1e–4) and we used real time data augmentation by randomly applying translations, zooms, edge sharpening, blurring and brightness and contrast alterations to the training data.

2.2 YOLOv2 for Lung Nodule Detection

Our framework uses YOLOv2 [9], an end-to-end 2D object detection network, to perform lung nodule detection without the need for a FP reduction step (refer to Fig. 2 for an example). Specifically, the network divides the input image in a grid

---

[3] https://github.com/experiencor/basic-yolo-keras.

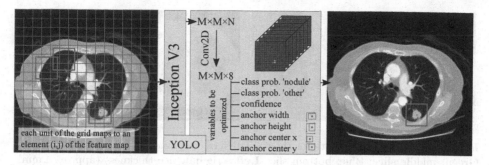

Fig. 2. Schematic representation of the YOLO framework applied to lung nodule detection. We consider a single anchor size for the optimization of the network.

and predicts, for each grid element, how likely there is a nodule there. Let our input image be divided in blocks of size defined by the network architecture. Each block can contain a nodule, which bounding box we impose to be 35×35 mm (51×51 pixels) to fit the largest nodules in the dataset. The model works as follows: (1) the InceptionV3 [10] network is used for extracting a $M \times M \times N$ feature map, F, where M is the spatial grid size and N is the number of feature maps from the input image; (2) F is convolved into a $M \times M \times 7$ new tensor, Y. Each element $m_{i,j,k} \in Y_k$ has a direct correspondence with a block from the input image and each of the 7 feature maps corresponds to a variable of the respective bounding $box_{i,j}$ to be optimized. The maps are responsible for controlling the probability of the box belonging to the 'nodule' or 'other' (non-nodule) classes ($p_{i,j}(\text{nodule}) = \sigma(m_{i,j,1})$), how likely there is a nodule on that block (confidence$_{i,j} = \sigma(m_{i,j,3})$), the box width/height ($\hat{w}_{i,j} = we^{m_{i,j,4}}$, $\hat{h}_{i,j} = he^{m_{i,j,5}}$) and the box center ($\hat{x}_{i,j} = x_{i,j} + \sigma(m_{i,j,6})$, $\hat{y}_{i,j} = y_{i,j} + \sigma(m_{i,j,7})$), where σ is a sigmoid function. The entire network can be trained end-to-end by minimizing the following loss function:

$$\mathcal{L}_{\text{YOLO}} = \mathcal{L}_1(x,y) + \mathcal{L}_2(w,h) + \mathcal{L}_1(\text{confidence}) + \mathcal{L}_2(\text{class}) \qquad (1)$$

where $\mathcal{L}_1$ is the squared error and $\mathcal{L}_2$ is the log loss function. In the end, only the boxes with high confidence and class probability are kept, as depicted in Fig. 2.

Since Inception V3 is pre-trained with RGB images, we train our model with images of the axial slice containing the nodule centroid together with one slice above and one slice below (2.5D). This strategy provides extra context to the network and has already been successful for lung nodule detection [11]. However, preliminary experiments led us to conclude that the selection of the non-central slices greatly hinders the nodule detection performance of YOLOv2. Namely, since all datasets show variable inter-scan slice thickness, the usage of the two immediate adjacent slices may provide a poor and irregular depth information. Instead, we retrieve slices from an approximate distance of 2 mm. This improved the system's performance by almost 20% since it allows blood vessels, natural

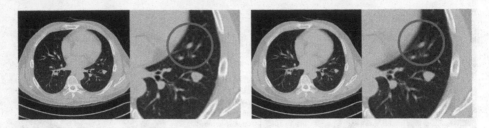

Fig. 3. Influence of slice depth for the reduction of confounders in 2.5D. Red: top slice; Green: middle slice; Blue: bottom slice **Left**: original slice thickness (approx. 1 mm); **Right**: with approximately 2 mm slice thickness both small and large blood vessels are more visible in the red and blue channels. (Color figure online)

nodules' confounders in the axial plane, to be better distinguished from the structures of interest (see Fig. 3) without compromising the model's speed.

Training Details. Having in account the goal of our system, we opt for a very low value of FP/scan, close to 0.25, and thus higher risk of nodule detection failure because (i) detecting one nodule per scan (assumed to be lung cancer representative) is enough for referral and (ii) a large number of FP can lead to non-proper scan referral and thus unnecessary medical procedures. Based on these assumptions, we adopt a training scheme that achieves high scan-wise referral recall and specificity rates with a low number of FP detections.

First, we train the detection module using 512×512 2.5D axial images that contain $d > 3$ mm nodules and use it for finding nodule candidates on all 2.5D axial images of the training scans. The resulting 2D predictions are combined to 3D nodule locations having in account the intra and inter-axial slice distance. Specifically, candidates are merged if there is more than 80% area overlap in the 2 adjacent slices. These 3D candidates integrate a second dataset composed of (1) all nodules from the training data with diameter ≥ 4 mm and (2) a set of nodules' confounders composed of FP predictions with probability higher than 0.5 and all nodules with $d < 4$ mm. YOLOv2 is then retrained from scratch so that the weights can adapt to the two class problem, thus significantly reducing the final number of FP detections. This framework avoids the need for a second classifier for FP reduction and thus extra training-related parameter tuning. Similarly to the training step, scan-wise predictions are made by merging depth-wise the candidates that resulted from sliding the model over the scan.

2.3   U-Net for Nodule Segmentation

We segment the found nodules via an adaptation of U-Net [12]. Our model has 5 contracting steps, a 1×1 bottle neck and a higher number of feature maps on the expansive part. Also, Batch Normalization is performed at each convolutional layer for regularization. We use the soft intersection over union (IoU) as loss

$$IoU = \frac{\sum S \circ \hat{S}}{\sum (S + \hat{S}) - \sum S \circ \hat{S}} \qquad (2)$$

where S and $\hat{S}$ are the ground truth and the segmentation prediction $\in [0, 1]$.

2.4   Rule-Based Classification

Finally, we perform a referral decision based on the guidelines of NLST. Specifically, a decision tree is used for indicating if a patient should be referred for further examination or not. First, scans where no nodule candidates are detected are considered as negatives. From the remaining, a scan is considered pathological if there is at least a nodule candidate with $d > 4\,mm$ and less than 50% of calcified area. The nodule diameter d is the equivalent diameter of our segmentation, thus the diameter of a perfect sphere with an equal volume as the volume of our segmentation. The calcified area is computed by calculating the total area of all volumes above a threshold of 70 HU.

3   Experimental Results and Discussion

Our pipeline is composed of a novel single-step nodule detection system, followed by U-Net for segmentation and a final referral decision based on the NLST guidelines. Table 1 compares the performance of our system with the the top-3 methods from LUNA16. A nodule is considered detected (TP) if the distance to the prediction centroid is less than the nodule radius and hits on non-nodule lesions are not considered as FP. Also, note that we only consider nodules of $d > 4\,mm$, instead of $d > 3\,mm$, since these are the ones with relevance for screening. Even though it is not possible to state that our system is as good as other approaches because the detection-per-radius performance is not publicly available, the achieved recall is satisfactory for a 2.5D single-step nodule detection framework that requires less model-related parameter tuning and computation power than other state-of-the-art methods. Furthermore, our nodule detection achieves a scan-wise recall (*i.e.*, finding at least one of the nodules in a scan) of 0.90, increasing to 0.95 if only nodules of $d > 4\,mm$ are considered.

U-Net achieves an average test IoU of 0.63 ± 0.02 and Sorensen-Dice coefficient of 0.79 ± 0.15, which is line with the state-of-the-art performance. Moreover, the

Table 1. Nodule detection accuracy of the top-3 from LUNA16 (Feb 2018) for 0.25 false-positive per scan and ours for nodules of diameter $d > 4\,mm$.

Name	PAtech	JianPeiCAD	FONOVACAD	ours $d > 4\,mm$
Recall	0.921	0.940	0.932	0.926

estimated diameter error is of 1.89 ± 3.20 mm, with greater errors occurring at the largest nodules. This means that the system is capable of providing a robust measurement that does not compromise the NLST rule-based decision.

Figure 4 shows examples of nodules and the respective segmentation predicted by our method on the independent NLST dataset. As depicted in Fig. 4A–B, we are capable of detecting nodules of different sizes and challenging textures and still provide a good segmentation. Furthermore, in Fig. 4B we show examples of calcified structures being correctly detected due to the field knowledge-based threshold on the soft tissue HU window.

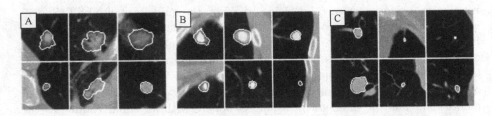

Fig. 4. Examples of predicted detections and segmentations on the NLST dataset (51×51 mm). **A**: nodules that contributed for a correct patient referral; **B**: benign and non-relevant lesions; **C**: false-positive and missed lesions.

In terms of referral, we evaluate our system in terms of scan sensitivity and specificity to ease the comparison with the specialists from NLST. We do not compare with Kaggle solutions because our method does not produce a referral probability and thus log loss computation is not possible. Our screening pipeline achieves a cancer detection sensitivity of 89.4%, which is in line with the findings of the NLST study. This suggests that the proposed system is successfully locating, measuring and applying the decision criteria to relevant abnormalities as depicted in Fig. 4A–B. For comparison purposes, NLST specialists were capable of successfully detecting 93.8% of the cancer cases by manual inspection of LDCT scans using the same radius-based criteria [2].

Despite its high sensitivity, our system is still not robust enough for unsupervised cancer screening. Namely, detecting FP, as showed in Fig. 4C, combined with the simplistic diameter decision which, although diagnostic relevant, is not sufficient to perform cancer prediction because our specificity is only 23.8%. This is in line with the NLST study, where 96.4% of the cancer cases referred for follow-up were actually FP detections. Instead, our method is to be used as an independent observer during the screening process since, unlike end-to-end deep learning approaches such as the Kaggle solutions, it has a human understandable reasoning behind the referral decision, *i.e.*, the clinician can verify the structure that the model considered to be of interest for the decision process. This means that our FP predictions can be easily checked by the expert during the screening.

4 Conclusions

We propose and validate a second opinion computer-aided lung cancer screening system that achieves high patient referral sensitivity. Despite its high performance, the decision based on the NLST criteria does not allow the system to be robust in terms of cancer risk prediction. Future research should thus focus on the development of advanced methods capable of characterizing nodules using a single or multiple time-points and predict nodule malignancy accordingly.

Ultimately, the high performance and explainability of our approach makes it an objective second-opinion system for clinicians to use during the screening process and can contribute to further increase the early detection of lung cancer.

Acknowledgements. Guilherme Aresta is funded by the FCT grant contract SFRH/BD/120435/2016. Teresa Araújo is funded by the FCT grant contract SFRH/BD/122365/2016. This study is associated with project NLST-375 and LNDetector, which is financed by the ERDF - European Regional Development Fund through the Operational Programme for Competitiveness - COMPETE 2020 Programme and by the National Fundus through the Portuguese funding agency, FCT - Fundação para a Ciência e Tecnologia within project POCI-01-0145-FEDER-016673.

References

1. Siegel, R.L., Miller, K.D., Jemal, A.: Cancer statistics, 2018. CA A Cancer J. Clin. **68**(1), 7–30 (2018)
2. The National Lung Screening Trial Research Team: Reduced lung-cancer mortality with low-dose computed tomographic screening. New England J. Med. **365**(5), 395–409 (2011)
3. Torre, L.A., Siegel, R.L., Ward, E.M., Jemal, A.: Global cancer incidence and mortality rates and trends-an update. Cancer Epidemiol. Biomark. Prev. **25**(1), 16–27 (2016)
4. Setio, A., Traverso, A., de Bel, T.: Validation, comparison, and combination of algorithms for automatic detection of pulmonary nodules in computed tomography images: The LUNA16 challenge. Med. Image Anal. **42**, 1–13 (2017)
5. Ren, S., He, K., Girshick, R., Sun, J.: Faster R-CNN: towards real-time object detection with region proposal networks. IEEE Trans. Pattern Anal. Mach. Intell. **39**(6), 1137–1149 (2017)
6. Messay, T., Hardie, R.C., Tuinstra, T.R.: Segmentation of pulmonary nodules in computed tomography using a regression neural network approach and its application to the lung image database consortium and image database resource initiative dataset. Med. Image Anal. **22**(1), 48–62 (2015)
7. Wang, S., Zhou, M., Liu, Z., et al.: Central focused convolutional neural networks: developing a data-driven model for lung nodule segmentation. Med. Image Anal. **40**(3), 172–183 (2017)
8. Armato, S.G., McLennan, G., Bidaut, L.: The Lung Image Database Consortium (LIDC) and Image Database Resource Initiative (IDRI): a completed reference database of lung nodules on CT scans. Med. Phys. **38**(2), 915 (2011)
9. Redmon, J., Farhadi, A.: YOLO9000: Better, faster, stronger. In: Proceedings of 30th IEEE Conference on Computer Vision and Pattern Recognition, CVPR 2017, pp. 6517–6525 (2017)

10. Szegedy, C., Liu, W., Jia, Y., et al.: Going deeper with convolutions. In: 2015 IEEE Conference on Computer Vision and Pattern Recognition (CVPR), pp. 1–9. IEEE, 7–12 June 2015

11. Ding, J., Li, A., Hu, Z., Wang, L.: Accurate pulmonary nodule detection in computed tomography images using deep convolutional neural networks, pp. 1–9. arXiv, June 2017

12. Ronneberger, O., Fischer, P., Brox, T.: U-Net: convolutional networks for biomedical image segmentation. In: Navab, N., Hornegger, J., Wells, W.M., Frangi, A.F. (eds.) MICCAI 2015. LNCS, vol. 9351, pp. 234–241. Springer, Cham (2015). https://doi.org/10.1007/978-3-319-24574-4_28

Automatic Classification of Centrilobular Emphysema on CT Using Deep Learning: Comparison with Visual Scoring

Stephen M. Humphries[✉], Aleena M. Notary, Juan Pablo Centeno, and David A. Lynch

National Jewish Health, Denver, CO 80206, USA
humphriess@njhealth.org

Abstract. The presence and severity of emphysema, scored visually on computed tomography (CT) using a classification system developed by the Fleischner Society, is a clinically significant index of disease severity. Since visual assessment can be subjective and is time consuming, our purpose was to evaluate the potential of a deep learning method for automatic grading of emphysema. The study cohort included 8213 subjects enrolled in the COPDGene study. Baseline CT and visual scores on 2500 subjects were used to train a deep learning model for classification of centrilobular emphysema according to the Fleischner system. The model was then used to predict emphysema scores on 5713 subjects not included in the training set. Predictions were compared with visual emphysema scores, pulmonary function tests (PFTs), smoking history and St. George Respiratory Questionnaire (SGRQ). Agreement between visual emphysema scores and those generated automatically was moderate (weighted $\kappa = 0.60$, $p < 0.0001$). Emphysema scores predicted by the deep learning model showed significant associations with PFTs, smoking history and SGRQ, similar to those seen in comparison with visual scores.

Keywords: Computed tomography · Emphysema · Deep learning

1 Introduction

Chronic obstructive pulmonary disease (COPD), the third leading cause of death in the U.S., is a heterogeneous group of lung disorders, including a range of patterns of emphysema, chronic bronchitis, and non-emphysematous obstruction

This work was supported by grants R01HL089897 and R01HL089856 from the National Heart, Lung, and Blood Institute. The Genetic Epidemiology of COPD (COPDGene) project is also supported by the COPD Foundation through contributions made to an industry advisory board representing AstraZeneca, Boehringer Ingelheim, Novartis, Pfizer, Siemens, Sunovion, and GlaxoSmithKline.

© Springer Nature Switzerland AG 2018
D. Stoyanov et al. (Eds.): RAMBO 2018/BIA 2018/TIA 2018, LNCS 11040, pp. 319–325, 2018.
https://doi.org/10.1007/978-3-030-00946-5_32

due to small-airway disease [7]. CT plays an important role in assessment of COPD. While quantitative image analysis techniques such as lung densitometry are able to detect and quantify emphysema [13], visual assessment has remained necessary for complete characterization of emphysema patterns [7].

To facilitate data comparison in research and clinical trials, and to improve diagnostic accuracy, the Fleischner Society developed a structured system for visual classification of phenotypic abnormalities on CT in subjects with COPD [6]. The system provides a six point ordinal scale (absent, trace, mild, moderate, confluent, and advanced destructive) for grading the severity of centrilobular emphysema, the prototypical form of emphysema seen in cigarette smokers. This approach was applied in the COPDGene study where baseline CT scans were retrospectively visually scored by trained analysts. Visual scores for presence and severity of centrilobular emphysema were found to be significantly associated with genetic loci previously associated with COPD [5] and with increased mortality risk [7]. Visual assessment required substantial effort, however, with multiple analysts working nearly four years to score approximately ten thousand scans.

The purpose of this study was to assess the feasibility of a deep learning model for automatic emphysema classification on CT. We hypothesized that the Fleischner system, a structured scale developed by domain experts, would provide an effective supervisory signal for training. To develop a model capable of predicting subject-level scores from volumetric CT, which are difficult to process at full resolution due to memory constraints of graphics processing units (GPUs), we combined a convolutional neural network (CNN) architecture with a long short-term memory (LSTM) layer. LSTMs are a type of recurrent neural network capable of learning dependencies in sequence data. They have been used with some success to classify data such as frame sequences from video clips [1]. This enabled efficient prediction using features extracted from axial image sequences sampled over a lung volume. We tested the approach by comparing predictions with visual scores and clinical parameters including pulmonary function tests and Global initiative for Obstructive Lung Disease (GOLD) stage.

2   Methods

2.1   Study Population

COPDGene is a prospective and multicenter investigation focused on the genetic epidemiology of COPD (ClinicalTrials. gov: NCT00608764). All subjects underwent volumetric inspiratory and expiratory CT using a standardized protocol [9]. Inspiratory CT on 8213 subjects were included in this work. The cohort was partitioned so that scans and visual scores on 2500 subjects were used for training and data on the remaining 5713 subjects were reserved for testing. Distribution of emphysema scores in training data was n = 774, 435, 473, 431, 275, 112 for Fleischner scores 0, 1, 2, 3, 4, and 5, respectively. Additional variables including GOLD stage, Forced Expiratory Volume in the first second percent predicted (FEV1%pred), FEV1/Forced Vital Capacity ratio (FEV1/FVC),

St. George Respiratory Questionnaire (SGRQ) and smoking history (pack-years) were retrieved from the study database for the test partition. The SGRQ is a respiratory health-related quality of life questionnaire where higher scores correspond to greater impairment [15]. Quantitative CT emphysema score calculated as the percentage of lung voxels with intensity less than −950 Hounsfield Units (LAA-950) was also used for comparison in test subjects.

2.2 Visual Scoring

Each CT study had been retrospectively visually scored by two trained analysts using the scale 0 = absent, 1 = trace, 2 = mild, 3 = moderate, 4 = confluent, and 5 = advanced destructive [7]. Analyst agreement was assessed periodically throughout the study as good to excellent (weighted κ range 0.71–0.80). Analyst discordances larger than one point in score were adjudicated by a thoracic radiologist. Mean analyst score rounded down to the nearest integer was recorded as the final value.

2.3 Classification Algorithm

In an initial process, segmentation was performed on all CTs using an automatic lung segmentation function included in an open source library [11,12]. Using Python and PyTorch [8] we implemented a combined CNN-LSTM network architecture [1] designed to predict visual centrilobular emphysema score from a sequence of 25 axial images. Axial images were sampled at evenly-spaced intervals over the height of each lung segmentation volume, excluding the upper and lowermost 5 mm. Figure 1 represents the architecture of the CNN-LSTM model. Briefly, the components of the network include four blocks consisting of two dimensional (2D) convolutions, rectified linear unit (RELU) activation and max pooling. The four 2D convolutional layers have 32 6 × 6, 96 3 × 3, 256 3 × 3 and 384 3 × 3 filters, respectively. The first two max pooling layers have stride 3 and the second two max pooling layers have stride 4. The input images are fed through the CNN portion separately to extract features, which are concatenated into a sequence and passed to the LSTM layer followed by a dense layer before output. The loss function is negative log likelihood.

The model was trained using CT scans and visual centrilobular emphysema scores, expressed as integers 0–5, on 2500 subjects. Some data augmentation was used, including in-plane image translations and offsets in sampling of axial images.

2.4 Statistical Analysis

Weighted κ statistics between analysts visual scores and automatic scores were computed. Descriptive statistics between CNN-LSTM emphysema scores and demographic and clinical parameters were computed. One-way analysis of variance (ANOVA) was used to test for significant differences in FEV1%pred.,

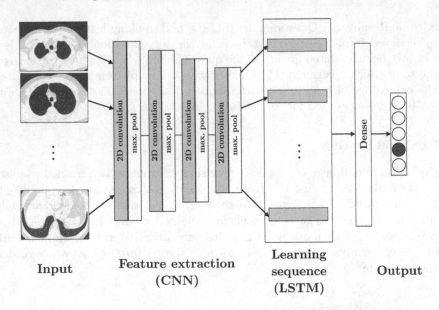

Fig. 1. The network combines CNN and LSTM architectures. 25 axial images sampled over the lung volume are separately processed by the CNN to extract features. These are concatenated into a sequence and passed to the LSTM layer, which learns representations of sequences that are useful for classification.

FEV1/FVC, SGRQ, LAA-950 and smoking history values stratified by emphysema severity scores. Chi-square tests of independence were used to compare centrilobular emphysema scores with GOLD stage. Statistical calculations were performed using R version 3.4.4 (2018-03-15). A p-value of <0.05 was considered statistically significant.

3   Results

Agreement between visual emphysema scores and those generated automatically by the CNN-LSTM was moderate (weighted $\kappa = 0.60$, $p < 0.0001$). Table 1 shows a confusion matrix comparing visual and automatic emphysema scores.

Table 2 shows comparison between visual emphysema score and clinical variables. ANOVA showed that more severe visual emphysema scores were significantly associated with diminished FEV1%pred and FEV1/FVC as well as increased SGRQ, LAA-950 and smoking pack-years ($p < 0.0001$). Chi-square test of independence examining the relationship between visual score and GOLD stage was significant, χ^2 (df $= 25$, n $= 5713$) $= 2716.4$, $p < 0.0001$. Similarly, Table 3 shows comparison between CNN-LSTM emphysema scores and clinical variables. ANOVA shows that more severe emphysema grades predicted by the CNN-LSTM were associated with more severe clinical measures. Chi-square test of independence examining the relationship between CNN-LTSM score and GOLD stage was also significant, χ^2 (df $= 25$, n $= 5713$) $= 3203.4$, $p < 0.0001$.

Table 1. Confusion matrix comparing visual emphysema scores with those predicted by the CNN-LSTM. Fleischner centrilobular emphysema scores are: 0 = absent, 1 = trace, 2 = mild centrilobular, 3 = moderate centrilobular, 4 = confluent, 5 = advanced destructive.

		CNN score					
		0	**1**	**2**	**3**	**4**	**5**
	0	895	700	385	40	3	0
	1	240	367	384	65	3	1
Visual score	**2**	87	174	589	253	20	0
	3	4	11	119	506	182	2
	4	0	1	5	113	332	57
	5	0	0	0	11	86	78

Table 2. Clinical variables according to visual emphysema score. FEV1%pred, FEV1/FVC, SGRQ, LAA-950 and pack-years are means (s.d.). GOLD data are number of subjects. Preserved Ratio Impaired Spirometry (PRISm) is defined as FEV1/FVC ratio ≥ 0.7.

	Visual emphysema score					
	0	**1**	**2**	**3**	**4**	**5**
n subjects	2023	1060	1123	824	508	175
FEV1%pred.	90.0(17.6)	83.8(19.5)	78.9(21.9)	66.7(24.1)	48.4(22.1)	40.2(21.1)
FEV1/FVC	.77(.08)	.73(.10)	.67(.12)	.57(.14)	.45(.13)	.39(.12)
SGRQ	17.3(19.0)	21.6(20.4)	24.7(21.5)	32.3(22.5)	41.2(20.6)	45.1(18.8)
LAA-950	2.5(3.1)	2.5(3.6)	3.9(5.0)	8.9(7.9)	22.0(11.3)	32.8(11.2)
Pack-yrs	35.1(19.5)	40.7(22.8)	46.9(24.0)	52.5(26.8)	26.8(55.9)	59.5(28.8)
GOLD Stage						
PRISm	303	177	112	42	7	0
0	1381	563	460	155	17	0
1	109	85	131	111	37	8
2	190	164	283	290	153	42
3	32	61	113	168	187	54
4	5	4	17	58	107	70

4   Discussion

The Fleischner Society visual scoring system is a clinically significant index of COPD severity that is associated with mortality risk. We have developed a CNN-LSTM model that is capable of automatic classification of centrilobular emphysema pattern on CT according to the Fleischner scale. In a group of 5713 test subjects, automatically scored emphysema patterns showed moderate agreement with visual scores and significant associations with GOLD stage, pulmonary function, SGRQ, LAA-950 and smoking pack-years. While agreement between visual and automatic emphysema scores in this test set is somewhat modest, similar statistical associations are seen when comparing visual and

Table 3. Clinical variables according to CNN-LSTM emphysema score. FEV1%pred, FEV1/FVC, SGRQ, LAA-950 and pack-years are means (s.d.). GOLD data are number of subjects.

	CNN-LSTM score					
	0	1	2	3	4	5
n subjects	1226	1253	1482	988	626	138
FEV1%pred.	91.4(16.1)	89.3(17.2)	81.9(20.7)	66.4(23.1)	49.0(21.2)	34.2(17.8)
FEV1/FVC	.78(.07)	.76(.08)	.70(.11)	.58(.14)	.46(.13)	.35(.10)
SGRQ	16.2(18.1)	18.4(19.6)	23.3(20.9)	31.7(22.6)	41.1(20.1)	47.9(17.1)
LAA-950	2.0(2.4)	2.5(2.9)	3.2(4.4)	8.1(7.6)	20.3(10.4)	38.5(8.5)
Pack-yrs	34.6(18.8)	38.2(20.9)	43.4(23.7)	52.7(27.0)	55.1(28.8)	55.8(25.4)
GOLD Stage						
PRISm	174	194	203	63	7	0
0	906	810	669	172	20	0
1	51	86	173	124	43	4
2	80	140	309	366	200	21
3	11	17	104	209	229	45
4	3	0	16	51	124	67

CNN-LSTM emphysema scores with other clinical parameters, suggesting that the CNN-LSTM learns to classify clinically significant features.

Deep learning has become the dominant approach in medical image analysis [16] for applications ranging from segmentation [10] and detection [14] to diagnosis [2]. One challenge when designing CNN architectures is to manage the total number of model parameters considering memory constraints of available GPUs. This is generally the case in applications using volumetric chest CT. Other researchers have shown that limiting model input to a small number (1–4) of relevant "canonical" slices, selected in pre-processing using anatomy detection methods, can be effective [3,4]. In the present study we instead used an LSTM architecture, which made it possible to limit the number of convolutional weights while still using 25 full-resolution axial images as input.

This study has some limitations. COPDGene uses a well-defined CT protocol and study images are very consistent. Performing both training and testing on images from this cohort may produce optimistic results. We also did not perform systematic comparisons of different CNN architectures. Future work will incorporate mortality and longitudinal assessment for further clinical validation.

5   Conclusions

A combined CNN-LSTM architecture provides an efficient model for subject-level prediction and can be trained to perform automatic classification of centrilobular emphysema on CT.

References

1. Donahue, J., et al.: Long-term recurrent convolutional networks for visual recognition and description. In: Proceedings of the IEEE Conference on Computer Vision and Pattern Recognition, pp. 2625–2634 (2015)
2. Esteva, A., et al.: Dermatologist-level classification of skin cancer with deep neural networks. Nature **542**(7639), 115 (2017)
3. González, G., et al.: Disease staging and prognosis in smokers using deep learning in chest computed tomography. Am. J. Respir. Crit. Care Med. **197**(2), 193–203 (2018)
4. González, G., Washko, G.R., San José Estépar, R.a.: Deep learning for biomarker regression: application to osteoporosis and emphysema on chest CT scans. In: SPIE Medical Imaging, vol. 10574 (2018)
5. Halper-Stromberg, E., et al.: Visual assessment of chest computed tomographic images is independently useful for genetic association analysis in studies of chronic obstructive pulmonary disease. Ann. Am. Thorac. Soc. **14**(1), 33–40 (2017)
6. Lynch, D.A., et al.: CT-definable subtypes of chronic obstructive pulmonary disease: a statement of the fleischner society. Radiology **277**(1), 192–205 (2015)
7. Lynch, D.A.: CT-based visual classification of emphysema: association with mortality in the COPDGene study. Radiology **288**, 859–866 (2018)
8. Paszke, A., et al.: Automatic Differentiation in PyTorch (2017)
9. Regan, E.A., et al.: Genetic epidemiology of COPD (COPDGene) study design. COPD J. Chronic Obstructive Pulm. Dis. **7**(1), 32–43 (2011)
10. Ronneberger, O., Fischer, P., Brox, T.: U-Net: convolutional networks for biomedical image segmentation. In: Navab, N., Hornegger, J., Wells, W.M., Frangi, A.F. (eds.) MICCAI 2015. LNCS, vol. 9351, pp. 234–241. Springer, Cham (2015). https://doi.org/10.1007/978-3-319-24574-4_28
11. Ross, J.C., et al.: Lung extraction, lobe segmentation and hierarchical region assessment for quantitative analysis on high resolution computed tomography images. In: Yang, G.-Z., Hawkes, D., Rueckert, D., Noble, A., Taylor, C. (eds.) MICCAI 2009. LNCS, vol. 5762, pp. 690–698. Springer, Heidelberg (2009). https://doi.org/10.1007/978-3-642-04271-3_84
12. Ross, J., Harmouche, R., Onieva, J., Diaz, A., Washko, G., Estepar, R.S.J.: Chest imaging platform: an open-source library and workstation for quantitative chest imaging. Am. J. Respir. Crit. Care Med. **191**, A4975 (2015)
13. Schroeder, J.D., et al.: Relationships between airflow obstruction and quantitative CT measurements of emphysema, air trapping, and airways in subjects with and without chronic obstructive pulmonary disease. Am. J. Roentgenol. **201**(3), W460–W470 (2013)
14. Setio, A.A.A., et al.: Pulmonary nodule detection in CT images: false positive reduction using multi-view convolutional networks. IEEE Trans. Med. Imaging **35**(5), 1160–1169 (2016)
15. Vestbo, J.: Evaluation of COPD longitudinally to identify predictive surrogate endpoints (ECLIPSE). Eur. Respir. J. **31**, 869–873 (2008)
16. Zhou, S.K., Greenspan, H., Shen, D.: Deep Learning for Medical Image Analysis. Academic Press, San Diego (2017)

On the Relevance of the Loss Function in the Agatston Score Regression from Non-ECG Gated CT Scans

Carlos Cano-Espinosa[1]([✉]) [iD], Germán González[2] [iD], George R. Washko[3],
Miguel Cazorla[1] [iD], and Raúl San José Estépar[4] [iD]

[1] Department of Computer Science and Artificial Intelligence,
University of Alicante, Alicante, Spain
cce1@alu.ua.es, miguel.cazorla@ua.es
[2] Sierra Research SL, Avda. Costa Blanca 132, Alicante, Spain
ggonzale@sierra-research.com
[3] Brigham and Women's Hospital, Pulmonary and Critical Care Medicine,
75 Francis Street, Boston, MA, USA
gwashko@bwh.harvard.edu
[4] Applied Chest Imaging Laboratory, Department of Radiology,
Brigham and Women's Hospital, Harvard Medical School, Boston, MA, USA
rjosest@bwh.harvard.edu

Abstract. In this work, we evaluate the relevance of the choice of loss function in the regression of the Agatston score from 3D heart volumes obtained from non-contrast non-ECG gated chest computed tomography scans. The Agatston score is a well-established metric of cardiovascular disease, where an index of coronary artery disease (CAD) is computed by segmenting the calcifications of the arteries and multiplying each calcification by a factor related to their intensity and their volume, creating a final aggregated index. Recent work has automated such task with deep learning techniques, even skipping the segmentation step and performing a direct regression of the Agatston score. We study the effect of the choice of the loss function in such methodologies. We use a large database of 6983 CT scans to which the Agatston score has been manually computed. The dataset is split into a training set and a validation set of $n = 1000$. We train a deep learning regression network using such data with different loss functions while keeping the structure of the network and training parameters constant. Pearson correlation coefficient ranges from 0.902 to 0.938 depending on the loss function. Correct risk group assignment measurements range between 59.5% and 81.7%. There is a trade-off between the accuracy of the Pearson correlation coefficient and the risk group measurement, which leads to optimize for one or the other.

This study was supported by the NHLBI awards R01HL116931, R01HL116473, and R21HL140422. We gratefully acknowledge the support of NVIDIA Corporation with the donation of the Titan Xp GPU used for this research.

D. Stoyanov et al. (Eds.): RAMBO 2018/BIA 2018/TIA 2018, LNCS 11040, pp. 326–334, 2018.
https://doi.org/10.1007/978-3-030-00946-5_33

Keywords: Loss functions · Agatston score · Regression Convolutional

1   Introduction

The Agatston score is a well-established metric used to measure the extent of coronary artery disease (CAD) in ECG-gated CT studies [1]. This biomarker is computed by measuring the volume and maximum intensity of the coronary artery calcifications (CAC) and adding the per-lesion score to learn a global index. The Agatston score is then used to classify subjects in five different clinically relevant risk groups, defined by the following ranges: $[0, 1]$, $(1, 100]$, $(100, 400]$, $(400, 1000]$, $(1000, \inf]$, as described [3].

Several works automate the computation of the Agatston following the same general pipeline: hearts are located using anatomy-based [9], atlas-based [7] or 2.5D object detection [4,11] strategies and a 3D Region of Interest (ROI) is extracted around the heart. Then, each CAC candidate is categorized as relevant or not using their relative position [16], texture and size features [6] or a combination of both [12,13]. Finally, the Agatston score is computed from the CACs. The latest work of [14,15] uses a deep-learning solution for CAC classification. This methodology uses a database of segmented CAC as the reference standard, where each voxel is labeled to indicate if it is part of a CAC or not, to train a lesion-based or a voxel-based classifier. In contrast, the work of [4] generates the inclusion and exclusion rules of the CACs by optimizing the global score directly.

The work of [5] uses a deep learning network for the regression of image-based biomarkers, and the work of [2] does so, specifically for the problem of Agatston from CT images. The latter approach minimizes the L2 cost function between the reference standard and the regressed Agatston score. While being attractive for its simplicity and achieving a similar Pearson correlation coefficient as other deep-learning based methods, it is inferior with respect to the classification of subjects to risk-groups. In this experimental work, we explore improvements to such methodology by analyzing the relevance of the cost-function of the regression network.

2   Materials and Methods

2.1   Database

COPDGene is a multi-center observational study designed to understand the evolution and genetic signature of COPD in smokers [10]. COPDGene contains a total of 10,000 pulmonary non-ECG gated CT Scans obtained with 16 detectors scanners. Subjects are both smokers and non-smokers, with ages between 45 and 80 years and 10 years of smoking history from non-hispanic white and non-hispanic African Americans ethnicities. The Agatston score was manually estimated in 6983 of such images, forming the database on which we train and evaluate the method.

We automatically select a region of interest (ROI) centered around the heart in each CT scan (Fig. 1), using the method of [4,11]. We use a prefixed ROI size to avoid the need of re-scaling the reference standard Agatston score. Each heart ROI is further normalized to a canonical size of $64 \times 64 \times 64$ voxels to enable their processing using a 3D convolutional neural network. The images are clamped to the range $[-500, 2000]$ HUs to highlight the lesions and discard lung structures. Mistakes in the automated location of the heart were eliminated by manual inspection, resulting in 6663 images that are divided between a training set ($n = 5663$) and a testing set ($n = 1000$).

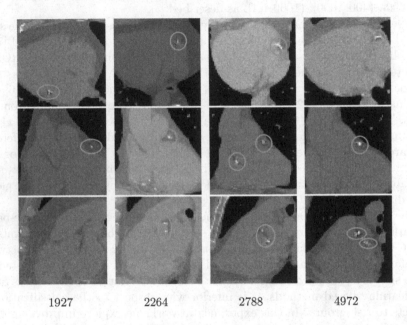

| 1927 | 2264 | 2788 | 4972 |

Fig. 1. Regions of Interest extracted around the heart. Each column corresponds to a case. Rows are the axial, coronal and sagittal planes that cross the central point of the ROI. Coronary Calcifications are identified by bright voxels found in the coronary arteries. They have highlighted with green circles. Numbers below each image correspond to the Agatston score value calculated using the full volumetric information. Please note that there are other bright voxels in the image that correspond to bone structure or calcifications that are not present in the coronary arteries. Such structures should be rejected by the algorithm. (Color figure online)

2.2   Data Augmentation

In our database, the number of cases in high-risk groups according to their Agatston score is lower than the number of cases in low-risk groups, as shown in Fig. 2. This poses challenges when training the regression network. We use

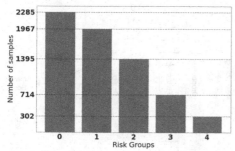

Group	Agatston Score range	subjects
0	$[0, 1]$	2285
1	$(1, 100]$	1967
2	$(100, 400]$	1395
3	$(400, 1000]$	714
4	> 1000	302

Fig. 2. Left: Distribution of database for each Risk Group, Right: Risk Groups Agatston score range as defined in [3].

a data augmentation technique to reduce such data imbalance. The technique generates an equalized number of cases per group by generating random displacements over the three axes, using a spherical probabilistic volume. Such is done to ensure that the new augmented sample is equidistant from the center of the heart in all directions. The data augmentation is done on-the-fly and to ensure reproducibility, the random seed of the data augmentation policy is fixed.

2.3 Convolutional Network

Due to its simplicity and for comparative purposes, we use the network proposed in [2] and depicted in Fig. 3. The network consists of three 3D convolutional-max-pooling blocks with rectified linear activation functions, followed by two fully connected layers that output the regression in a single neuron with linear activation. Dropout layers are present to prevent over-fitting. At test time, the negative regressions are clipped to 0, since the Agatston score is always positive. The optimizer used is the well known Adaptive Momentum optimizer [8], with an exponential decay rate.

Cost Functions: The convolutional network is optimized with respect to four different cost functions: mean square error of normalized values, absolute difference of normalized values, mean square error of the logarithmic scaled scores and absolute difference of the logarithmic scaled scores. The definition of the cost functions is shown in Table 1. We have chosen to optimize using linear and logarithmic cost functions because while the Agatston score is computed in a linear scale, its association to risk groups follows a loosely-logarithmic scale.

Categorization: We analyzed the performance of the network with respect to the direct risk group estimation for the subject in two manners: first, we assigned to each subject his risk group and regressed the group directly using the $L1$ norm as cost function. Second, we turned the regression network into a categorization one by substituting the last neuron for five neurons followed by

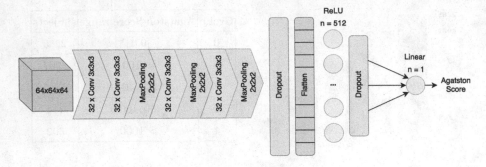

Fig. 3. Convolutional network diagram.

a softmax activation function and optimized the categorical cross entropy loss function.

2.4 Comparison Metrics

To evaluate the performance of the different cost functions, we use the well defined Pearson's correlation coefficient, the Spearman correlation coefficient and the risk-group accuracy (RGAcc), defined as the percentage of cases that correctly classified in their risk group.

3 Results

Table 1 shows the results obtained for the six defined loss functions. Better Pearson correlation coefficients are found when using linear cost functions instead of logarithmic ones. However, the RGAcc metric improves when using logarithmic cost functions. The Spearman correlation coefficient is higher in the logarithmic

Table 1. Loss function comparative results, Pearson 'ρ' and Spearman 's' correlation coefficients in linear and logarithmic scale, and Risk Group Accuracy '$RGAcc$'. 'Z' correspond to a normalization value, 5000 in this case. We have omitted 's' correlation coefficient in logarithmic scale since it is equivalent to 's' in linear scale due to the fact that a logarithmic transformation preserves ordering.

	Loss function	ρ	ρ (log)	s	RGAcc
(1)	$\frac{1}{n}\sum_{i=1}^{n}(\frac{y_i-x_i}{Z})^2$	0.932	0.664	0.843	55.2%
(2)	$\frac{1}{n}\sum_{i=1}^{n}\lvert\frac{y_i-x_i}{Z}\rvert$	0.938	0.657	0.903	59.5%
(3)	$\frac{1}{n}\sum_{i=1}^{n}(log(y_i+1)-log(x_i+1))^2$	0.902	0.620	0.949	78.2%
(4)	$\frac{1}{n}\sum_{i=1}^{n}\lvert log(y_i+1)-log(x_i+1)\rvert$	0.916	0.631	0.949	81.7%
(5)	Categorical cross entropy	N/A	N/A	N/A	75.7%
(6)	Categorical regression	N/A	N/A	N/A	81.1%

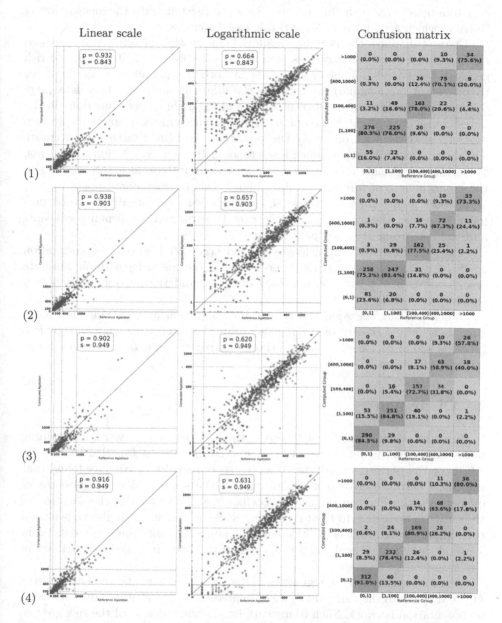

Fig. 4. Correlation results for the loss functions in Table 1. In each row, the first two plots represent the correlation plotted in linear and logarithmic scale respectively. Red dots were used for incorrect risk group result and blue dots depicted a correct group classification. The last plot shows the confusion matrix of risk groups, where the color of each cell represents the relative prevalence within the column. The numbers of the first column correspond to the loss functions described in Table 1. (Color figure online)

cost functions than in the linear ones. Such is consistent with the measurements RGAcc, which are higher in logarithmic cost functions.

Figure 4 displays the correlation plots between the reference standard and the computed Agatston score, as well as the concordance matrices of the risk groups. The correlation plots are made in both linear and logarithmic scales to provide a fair comparison between the different metrics. There is a large difference in performance between linear and logarithmic cost functions in the lowest range of the Agatston score, where the logarithmic cost functions produce more accurate results. Conversely, the logarithmic cost functions are less accurate with large Agatston scores, which leads to lower Pearson correlation coefficients. Since low-risk groups are more prevalent in the database as shown the Fig. 2, the logarithmic cost functions achieve better risk accuracy percentages.

In both logarithmic and linear scales, the mean absolute difference outperforms or equals the mean squared error for Pearson and Spearman coefficients and the risk group accuracy percentage.

The cost function that achieves a good trade-off between the correlation coefficient and the risk accuracy percentage is the mean logarithmic absolute error, with a $\rho = 0.916$ and accuracy of 81.7% and the maximum Spearman coefficient of 0.949.

When treating the Agatston risk group assignment as a classification problem, we achieve a RGAcc of 75.7% when using the categorical cross entropy loss function and of 81.1% when using a risk group regression with the mean average error loss function.

4   Discussion

In this work, we have shown that keeping the deep learning network, the training parameters and the data constant, the selection of the cost function has drastic effects on the performance of the Agatston score regression. We have found that the mean absolute error of the logarithm of the score achieves a good trade-off between the Pearson correlation coefficient and the correct classification of the subjects according to their risk group while achieving the highest Spearman correlation. Such result is of little surprise, since the risk groups are defined in a pseudo-logarithmic scale, and the errors of the linearly scaled network are in the lowest range.

As an alternative to the regression of the Agatston score and then assignment of the subjects to the risk groups, we have predicted the risk group directly using a classification network. Such framework breaks the ordering of the risk groups, and shows worse performance than the regression networks. When regressing the Agatston risk group directly, we achieve comparable, but lower, RGAcc than that obtained with our best Agatston score regression network. This comparison favor the Agatston score regression network, since it does not only provides the risk group but also quantifies the score itself.

One valid criticism of this work is the extreme simplicity of the network used. This has been chosen since (a) it achieves results comparable to the state of the art and (b) it is faster to train than deeper convolutional networks. Still, training time is of 600 s per epoch, and convergence is normally achieved around the 100th epoch, depending on the loss function. Such numbers are due to the 3D nature of the problem and the extension of the dataset.

The Pearson correlation coefficient is often referred in the literature as the figure of merit for biomarker regression methodologies. However, in our experiments, we have found that the Spearman correlation coefficient provides a more coherent view of the data as an aggregated statistic. Such is demonstrated with the data of Table 1, where the Spearman correlation relates more to the risk accuracy group than the Pearson correlation coefficient. The Pearson correlation coefficient depends on the per-case error, and high-valued cases can strongly bias the overall measurement. The Spearman correlation coefficient assess a monotonic relationship among variables, ignoring their absolute error. For cases such as the problem presented, it is more important to produce good rankings among the cases than minimizing the error on the Agatston score, and thus justifying Spearman's correlation as the preferred figure of merit.

References

1. Agatston, A.S., Janowitz, W.R., Hildner, F.J., Zusmer, N.R., Viamonte, M., Detrano, R.: Quantification of coronary artery calcium using ultrafast computed tomography. J. Am. Coll. Cardiol. **15**(4), 827–832 (1990)
2. Cano-Espinosa, C., Gonzlez, G., Washko, G.R., Cazorla, M., Estépar, R.S.J.: Automated Agatston score computation in non-ECG gated CT scans using deep learning. In: Proceedings of the SPIE: Medical Imaging 2018, February 2018
3. Erbel, R., Möhlenkamp, S., Kerkhoff, G., Budde, T., Schmermund, A.: Non-invasive screening for coronary artery disease: calcium scoring. Heart **93**(12), 1620–1629 (2007)
4. González, G., Washko, G.R., Estépar, R.S.J.: Automated Agatston score computation in a large dataset of non ECG-gated chest computed tomography. In: 2016 IEEE 13th International Symposium on Biomedical Imaging (ISBI), pp. 53–57. IEEE (2016)
5. Gonzlez, G., Washko, G.R., Estépar, R.S.J.: Deep learning for biomarker regression. Application to osteoporosis and emphysema on chest CT scans. In: Proceedings of the SPIE: Medical Imaging 2018, February 2018
6. Isgum, I., Prokop, M., Niemeijer, M., Viergever, M.A., van Ginneken, B.: Automatic coronary calcium scoring in low-dose chest computed tomography. IEEE Trans. Med. Imaging **31**(12), 2322–2334 (2012)
7. Isgum, I., Staring, M., Rutten, A., Prokop, M., Viergever, M.A., Van Ginneken, B.: Multi-atlas-based segmentation with local decision fusion—application to cardiac and aortic segmentation in CT scans. IEEE Trans. Med. Imaging **28**(7), 1000–1010 (2009)
8. Kingma, D., Ba, J.: Adam: a method for stochastic optimization. arXiv preprint arXiv:1412.6980 (2014)
9. Reeves, A.P., Biancardi, A.M., Yankelevitz, D.F., Cham, M.D., Henschke, C.I.: Heart region segmentation from low-dose CT scans: an anatomy based approach. In: Medical Imaging: Image Processing, p. 83142A (2012)

10. Regan, E.A., et al.: Genetic epidemiology of COPD (COPDgene) study design. COPD J. Chronic Obstr. Pulm. Dis. **7**(1), 32–43 (2011)
11. Rodriguez-Lopez, S., et al.: Automatic ventricle detection in computed tomography pulmonary angiography. In: 2015 IEEE 12th International Symposium on Biomedical Imaging (ISBI), pp. 1143–1146. IEEE (2015)
12. Shahzad, R., et al.: Vessel specific coronary artery calcium scoring: an automatic system. Acad. Radiol. **20**(1), 1–9 (2013)
13. Wolterink, J.M., Leiner, T., Takx, R.A., Viergever, M.A., Išgum, I.: An automatic machine learning system for coronary calcium scoring in clinical non-contrast enhanced, ECG-triggered cardiac CT. In: Medical Imaging 2014: Computer-Aided Diagnosis, p. 90350E. International Society for Optics and Photonics (2014)
14. Wolterink, J.M., Leiner, T., Viergever, M.A., Išgum, I.: Automatic coronary calcium scoring in cardiac CT angiography using convolutional neural networks. In: Navab, N., Hornegger, J., Wells, W.M., Frangi, A.F. (eds.) MICCAI 2015. LNCS, vol. 9349, pp. 589–596. Springer, Cham (2015). https://doi.org/10.1007/978-3-319-24553-9_72
15. Wolterink, J.M., Leiner, T., de Vos, B.D., van Hamersvelt, R.W., Viergever, M.A., Išgum, I.: Automatic coronary artery calcium scoring in cardiac CT angiography using paired convolutional neural networks. Med. Image Anal. **34**, 123–136 (2016)
16. Xie, Y., Cham, M.D., Henschke, C., Yankelevitz, D., Reeves, A.P.: Automated coronary artery calcification detection on low-dose chest CT images. In: Proceedings of SPIE, vol. 9035, p. 90350F (2014)

Accurate Measurement of Airway Morphology on Chest CT Images

Pietro Nardelli[1]([⊠])(iD), Mathias Buus Lanng[2], Cecilie Brochdorff Møller[2],
Anne-Sofie Hendrup Andersen[2], Alex Skovsbo Jørgensen[2],
Lasse Riis Østergaard[2], and Raúl San José Estépar[1](iD)

[1] Applied Chest Imaging Laboratory, Department of Radiology,
Brigham and Women's Hospital, Harvard Medical School, Boston, MA, USA
{pnardelli,rsanjose}@bwh.harvard.edu
[2] School of Medicine and Health, Aalborg University,
Fredrik Bajers Vej 7, 9220 Aalborg Øst, Denmark

Abstract. In recent years, the ability to accurately measuring and analyzing the morphology of small pulmonary structures on chest CT images, such as airways, is becoming of great interest in the scientific community. As an example, in COPD the smaller conducting airways are the primary site of increased resistance in COPD, while small changes in airway segments can identify early stages of bronchiectasis.

To date, different methods have been proposed to measure airway wall thickness and airway lumen, but traditional algorithms are often limited due to resolution and artifacts in the CT image. In this work, we propose a Convolutional Neural Regressor (CNR) to perform cross sectional measurements of airways, considering wall thickness and airway lumen at once. To train the networks, we developed a generative synthetic model of airways that we refined using a Simulated and Unsupervised Generative Adversarial Network (SimGAN).

We evaluated the proposed method by first computing the relative error on a dataset of synthetic images refined with SimGAN, in comparison with other methods. Then, due to the high complexity to create an in-vivo ground-truth, we performed a validation on an airway phantom constructed to have airways of different sizes. Finally, we carried out an indirect validation analyzing the correlation between the percentage of the predicted forced expiratory volume in one second (FEV1%) and the value of the Pi10 parameter. As shown by the results, the proposed approach paves the way for the use of CNNs to precisely and accurately measure small lung airways with high accuracy.

1 Introduction

In the last decade, several studies have been focused on the development of new algorithms to precisely locate small pulmonary structures, such as airways,

P. Nardelli and R. San José Estépar—This study was supported by the NHLBI awards R01HL116931, R01HL116473, and R21HL140422. The Titan Xp used for this research was donated by the NVIDIA Corporation.

D. Stoyanov et al. (Eds.): RAMBO 2018/BIA 2018/TIA 2018, LNCS 11040, pp. 335–347, 2018.
https://doi.org/10.1007/978-3-030-00946-5_34

on chest CT images. Once the structures are identified, the following step is represented by a quantitative measurement to extract geometrical properties, which may lead to improved diagnosis and new studies of lung disorders, as the morphology of the bronchial tree is commonly affected by inflammatory and infectious lung diseases. As an example, the smaller conducting airways are the structures most affected in patients with chronic obstructive pulmonary disease (COPD) [1], and the thickness of the airway wall (measured on CT) has been correlated to the severity and duration of asthma in different works [2,3]. For this reason, having a method that automatically analyzes airway walls thickness and lumen size is becoming of great interest for the scientific community.

On CT images, airways are often close to vessels and surrounded by parenchyma, and image resolution as well as noise artifacts often affect an accurate measurement. To perform airway wall thickness detection, the traditional approaches are based on non-parametric methods, which analyze the properties of the structure directly on the reconstructed CT signal. The most typical approach is the so-called full width at half max (FWHM) [4], which is based on the idea that the true edge of an ideal step function undergoing low-pass filtering is located at the FWHM location. An alternative popular approach to measure airway walls is the use of the zero crossing of the second order derivative (ZCSD) [5], which is used to characterize the signal transitions (i.e., lumen-to-wall and wall-to-parenchyma). More recently, a new approach for airway wall segmentation that starts from a coarse airway segmentation and implements an optimal graph construction method for wall segmentation was proposed [6]. However, all traditional methods suffer from over- and under-estimation errors when the structure size approaches the scanning resolution [7].

To overcome these issues, we propose to use a convolutional neural regressor (CNR) [8] approach, which uses a customized loss function to automatically and simultaneously measure airway wall thickness and airway lumen on small 2D patches extracted around the structure of interest. To the best of our knowledge, this approach has not yet been considered to solve problems such as measurement and analysis of the morphology of airways on CT images.

Since creating an accurate and reliable ground truth for small airway is quite a tedious and complicated task, to train the network we developed a synthetic model that aims at reproducing the main characteristics of airways with exact knowledge of the physical dimensions. The generated model is then refined using a Simulated and Unsupervised Generative Adversarial Network (SimGAN) [9].

New synthetic airway images are used for an initial validation to compute the relative error obtained by the proposed error. Then, as a further test, we created a synthetic phantom of airways with varying wall thicknesses. Finally, in order to prove the reliability of our approach, we performed an indirect validation on in-vivo cases in comparison to traditional methods through the correlation between the predicted FEV1% and the Pi10 parameter.

2   Materials and Methods

The proposed CNR algorithm used 2D patches of 32×32 pixels extracted from the structure of interest. These patches are then refined using SimGAN to resemble in-vivo patches better. In this section, we first introduce the creation and refinement of the synthetic patches. Then, the proposed CNR is described with the different training processes implemented. Finally, the validation methods are presented.

2.1   Synthetic Modeling of Airways

In order to generate reliable synthetic patches of airways, the main aspects of the structure of interest as well as the characteristics of the CT scanner with regard to resolution, PSF, and imposed noise have to be reproduced. Based on the knowledge that on reformatted axial plane airways have tangent vessels [10], each airway patch consisted of two bright ellipses (inner and outer walls) with a dark central zone (airway lumen) and zero, one or two tangent vessels, represented by bright ellipses rotated around the airway. The parameters to create the synthetic airways were randomly chosen based on physiological values and are reported in Table 1. Although the creation of a synthetic airway presents some limitations, we think that the proposed model represents an appropriate simulation that helps a neural network learn the main features of real airways. Also, using the multi-scale particle extraction method described in [11], 2D patches can be easily extracted along the airway's main axis, which is given by the first eigenvector of the Hessian matrix. For this reason, we do not consider 3D patches, which due to the different tubular profiles and a wide variation of 3D orientations that should be taken into account would increase the complexity of the modeling.

To reproduce the structure of the parenchyma, a Gaussian smoothing (with a standard deviation of 5) was applied to Gaussian distributed noise, to create some broadly correlated noise, which made a texture of multiple structures that

Table 1. Parameter ranges used for the creation of the airway model. All values were uniformly distributed within the specified ranges. LR stands for lumen radius.

Parameter	Parameter range
Lumen radius (LR)	0.5 to 6.0 (mm)
Airway wall thickness	0.1LR + 0.2 to 0.3LR + 1.5 (mm)
Number of vessels	0 to 2
Vessel radius (VR)	LR to LR + 0.8 (mm)
Skewness of reconstruction	−40 to 40 (degrees)
Airway Lumen Intensity	−1150 to −1050 (HU)
Airway Wall Intensity	−500 to −200 (HU)
Vessel Intensity	−50 to 50 (HU)

mimicked the parenchyma. Afterward, the correlated noise was altered to have a mean intensity of -900 HU and a standard deviation of 150. All values were empirically chosen.

All patches were created starting at a super-resolution of 0.05 mm/pixel in a sampling grid of 640×640 pixels. To obtain the final patch, the obtained images were first down-sampled to a resolution of 0.5 mm/pixel. Then, a PSF was simulated to mimic the blurring caused by the image reconstruction process. To this end, due to the small size of the patch, we assumed that the PSF can be approximated by means of a spatially locally invariant Gaussian function, as demonstrated in [12]. The standard deviation of the Gaussian filter was randomly chosen in an empirically determined range of 0.4 to 0.9 mm to simulate the differences in the PSF across CT scanners and manufacturers. Finally, a spatially correlated Gaussian noise was added to the image based on Gaussian distributed random noise smoothed with a Gaussian filter (with a standard deviation of 2), with the empirically determined mean of zero and standard deviation of 25. As a last step, the image is cropped to a 32×32 pixels grid.

2.2 SimGAN Refinement

Although the proposed generative model simulates reasonably well the geometrical aspects of the structure of interest, the generated patches still may present differences to patches extracted from real structures. For this reason, we implemented a SimGAN refinement, similar to the one described in [9], to improve the quality of the synthetic patches. SimGAN makes use of simulated and unsupervised learning by using a generative adversarial network (GAN) that consists of both a generator (refiner) and a discriminator. The purpose of the refining step is to trick the discriminator in deciding whether an image is a synthetic or real image.

For the implementation of this network, we pre-trained the refiner on synthetic images with 1000 steps and a batch size of 256, while the discriminator was pre-trained on real patches (extracted using the multi-resolution particles method described in [11], initialized with the technique of [13]) and refined patches, obtained from the pre-trained refiner, with 100 steps and a batch size of 256. The number of steps was the same as in [9]. Then, the adversarial training of the SimGAN network was trained for 10,000 steps, batch size of 256, and all parameters and loss function set as in [9]. An example of a generated synthetic airway is shown in Fig. 1.

2.3 Measurement of Airway Morphology

To extract both measurements for airways, we implemented a 9-layer 2D network, which consists of seven convolutional layers, five of which had stride 1 and two had stride 2, and two fully-connected layers (see Fig. 2). The network regresses the measure of the central structure in a patch 32×32 pixels, a size chosen to include enough neighborhood information for big structures, without losing specificity for small and thin features. To train the network, we used an

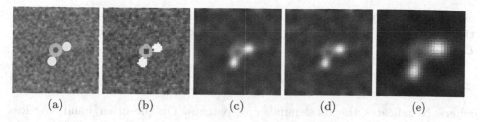

(a)   (b)   (c)   (d)   (e)

Fig. 1. Example of creation of a small synthetic airway patch (lumen: 0.7 mm, wall thickness: 1.25 mm). (a) The initial geometric model; (b) downsampling of the model; (c) blurring of the downsampled patch; (d) noise addition; (e) final synthetic airway (after applying SimGAN and cropping to obtain a 32 × 32 pixels patch).

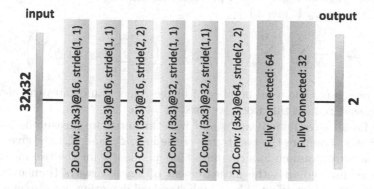

Fig. 2. Scheme of neural network used for measuring airways. The network is the same in both cases. The CNN for airways had 2 outputs (wall thickness and lumen)

Adam update ($\beta_1 = 0.9$, $\beta_2 = 0.999$, $\epsilon = 1e^{-08}$, decay $= 0.0$) with a specifically customized loss function that combines the absolute relative error and the precision of the measure to improve the network performance and stability (see Sect. 2.4).

The network was trained on a NVIDIA Titan X GPU machine, using the deep learning framework Keras [14] on top of TensorFlow [15], for 300 epochs at a learning rate of 0.001 and batch size of 64.

2.4 Customized Loss Function for Airway Morphology Measurement

When trying to accurately measure small airways with sizes at image resolution level, typical approaches usually have problems of under- or over-estimation. For this reason, in this paper we suggest the usage of a new loss function that combines the loss of the relative error over all images, $\mathcal{L}_\mu$, and the precision of the measure over 25 replicas of the same structure, $\mathcal{L}_\sigma$:

$$\mathcal{L}(\boldsymbol{y}, \widehat{\boldsymbol{y}}) = \mathcal{L}_\mu(\boldsymbol{y}, \widehat{\boldsymbol{y}}) + \lambda \cdot \mathcal{L}_\sigma(\boldsymbol{y}, \widehat{\boldsymbol{y}}) \tag{1}$$

where y is the true measure of a synthetic patch, $\widehat{y}$ is the measure predicted by the CNR, and λ defines the weight of $\mathcal{L}_\sigma$ with respect to $\mathcal{L}_\mu$. The definition of $\mathcal{L}_\mu$ is given by:

$$\mathcal{L}_\mu(y, \widehat{y}) = \sum_{i=1}^{N} \frac{|y_i - \widehat{y}_i|}{y_i} \tag{2}$$

where N indicates the total number of patches. On the other hand, the loss term for the precision, $\mathcal{L}_\sigma$, is computed over a number of replicas of the same geometric model (with fixed physical dimensions) to which varying PSFs are applied and a different number of airways and vessels are added with varying locations and rotations. This way, the network learns to accurately measure the structures of interest regardless of possible confounding factors inside the patch. The definition of $\mathcal{L}_\sigma$ is given by:

$$\mathcal{L}_\sigma = \frac{1}{N} \sum_{i=1}^{N} \left(\sum_{j=1}^{M} \left(y_{i,j} - \widehat{y}_{i,j} \right)^2 - \left(\frac{1}{M} \sum_{j=1}^{M} (y_{i,j} - \widehat{y}_{i,j}) \right)^2 \right) \tag{3}$$

where N represents the total number of images, and M indicates the number of replicas considered. In this work, we used M = 25.

Since for airways lumen radius and wall thickness are measured simultaneously, for this structure the two terms of the loss, $\mathcal{L}_\mu$ and $\mathcal{L}_\sigma$, are given by the sum of the corresponding loss computed independently for the two measures.

Since we noticed that the measurement of small airways (lumen less than 1.0 mm) was the most affected by a high standard deviation, we also empirically assigned a higher weight to the precision term of these structures so that they acquire more importance when computing the loss. Therefore, Eq. 1 becomes:

$$\mathcal{L}_a(y, \widehat{y}) = \mathcal{L}_\mu(y, \widehat{y}) + \lambda \cdot \left(\omega_l \cdot \mathcal{L}_{\sigma,l}(y, \widehat{y}) + \omega_{wt} \cdot \mathcal{L}_{\sigma,wt}(y, \widehat{y}) \right) \tag{4}$$

where $\lambda = 2.0$ has been empirically selected, l indicates the airway lumen, wt stands for wall thickness, and

$$\omega_l = \begin{cases} 1.5 & \text{if airway lumen} < 1.0 \text{ mm} \\ 1.0, & \text{otherwise} \end{cases} \tag{5}$$

and

$$\omega_{wt} = \begin{cases} 3.0, & \text{if wall thickness} < 1.0 \text{ mm} \\ 1.0, & \text{otherwise} \end{cases} \tag{6}$$

2.5   Training Set Definition

The training dataset consisted of 100,000 × 25 replicas of the same geometric model, to which varying PSFs were applied, and different additional vessels were added at varying locations and rotations. Therefore, a total of 2,500,000 training patches were used. Conversely, for the validation set we generated 1,000,000 patches (40,000 × 25 replicas).

The values of the parameters used for the creation of the images were randomly chosen in ranges that were empirically defined based on physiological measures of the structures of interest, as shown in Table 1. We trained the network using all images refined by SimGAN.

Finally, in order to help the network focus more on geometry than intensity values, during training, we applied a data augmentation that in addition to adding random noise it also randomly inverts intensity values inside the patches. Furthermore, we introduce a small random shift and random axes flipping to the patch to improve the learning of the network.

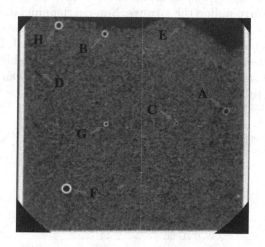

Fig. 3. An image taken from the CT scan of phantom showing the 8 tubes used for testing the CNR.

2.6   Experimental Setup

We evaluated the proposed approach for airway measurements on both synthetic and in-vivo cases. For the synthetic validation, we first generated a dataset of 200,000 patches (with random values chosen in the range of Table 1) that were used in three different experiments. First, we evaluated the accuracy of the algorithm by calculating the relative error (RE) between the CNR measurement and the ground truth defined by our geometrical model when varying lumen and the wall thickness size. To compare our results to the state-of-the-art methods, we also computed the absolute error obtained for airways with a wall thickness of 1.0 mm at the image resolution level (0.5 mm).

In order to demonstrate the ability of the method to accurately measure the structures of interest regardless of presence of noise and smoothness, as a second experiment we generated 100 images for each level of noise ($\sigma_n \in [0,40]$ HU) and for each level of Gaussian smoothing ($\sigma_s \in [0.4, 0.9]$ mm) and computed the mean RE (in percentage) across the 100 patches. We repeated the same experiment first fixing the wall thickness at 1.5 mm and considering three values of airway lumen (small: 0.5 mm; medium: 2.5 mm; large: 4.5 mm), and then fixing the airway lumen at 1.5 mm and using three wall thickness values (small: 0.5 mm; medium: 1.2 mm; large: 2.0 mm).

As a final test on synthetic images, we compared the proposed method for airway measurement to FWHM and ZCSD computing the mean RE (in percentage) on patches of different sizes.

As a further validation, we tested the performance of the algorithm on a CT airway phantom of known lumen size and wall thickness. The phantom was constructed using Nylon66 tubing inserted into polystyrene to simulate lung parenchyma surrounding the airways. Non-overlapping, 0.6 mm collimation images, 40 cm FOV, were acquired using a GE Siemens Sensation 64 CT scanner and reconstructed with a standard reconstruction kernel. Eight tubes with varying wall thickness and lumen diameter (reported in Table 2), as measured by a caliper, were studied. An image taken from the CT scan of the phantom showing the eight tubes is presented in Fig. 3.

Table 2. Wall thickness (WT) and lumen diameter (in mm) for the eight tubes of the synthetic phantom as measured by a caliper.

Tube	WT (mm)	Lumen (mm)
A	0.89	4.62
B	1.24	3.64
C	0.66	2.44
D	0.38	1.23
E	0.65	0.95
F	2.80	2.84
G	0.90	1.34
H	1.56	2.35

As a final experiment, since an accurate and reliable in-vivo ground-truth is very complicated to obtain, we performed an indirect validation by means of a physiological evaluation. To this end, we computed the Pi10 parameter with our approach and with ZCSD, and analyzed its correlation to FEV1% on 590 clinical cases, with airway particles extracted using [11]. Pi10 is a metric of airway thickness that is computed measuring the square root of the wall area across the whole airway tree and regressing the value at a hypothetical airway with an internal perimeter of 10 mm. The wall area is found by subtracting the area of the lumen from the airway area, while Pi is computed from the lumen radius.

3   Results

3.1   Synthetic Evaluation

Figure 4 shows the tendency of the RE for predictions obtained on the synthetic data when varying the lumen radius (Fig. 4a) and the wall thickness (Fig. 4b) of the airway. As expected, the error is small for airways with a large lumen (Fig. 4a), while it increases (with a tendency to under-estimate the measure) for lumens smaller than 1.0 mm, although it is always below a 10% RE. Regarding the wall thickness (Fig. 4b), a significant under-estimation error is obtained at sub-voxel levels (below the image resolution of 0.5 mm), while a tendency to over-estimation is obtained when the wall thickness is bigger than 2.0 mm.

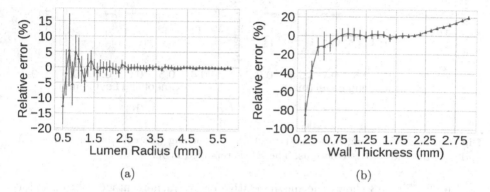

(a)   (b)

Fig. 4. Tendency of the relative error obtained with CNR when varying (a) airway lumen and (b) wall thickness.

On average, an absolute RE of 6.3% is obtained for airways with a wall thickness of 1.0 mm, while when the airway wall thickness is at the image resolution (0.5 mm) the absolute RE is at 13.09%. These REs are significantly lower than those previously reported in the literature for structures of similar sizes [5, 7].

Results obtained when fixing three values of airway lumen (0.5, 2.5, and 4.5 mm) and three values of wall thickness (0.5, 1.5, and 2.5 mm) and varying the level of noise and smoothing are presented in Fig. 5. As shown, for both measurements the RE is stable across the different levels of noise and smoothness. While for medium and large structures a very high accuracy is obtained (RE close to 0), the smallest structures (generated with airway lumen or wall thickness at the image resolution of 0.5 mm) are the one confusing the network the most determining also a bigger standard deviation. In all cases, the RE is stable when varying noise and smoothness, and the bias introduced by the CNR is small, with a little under-estimation for small structures, as expected. For small wall thicknesses (0.5 mm), when the smoothing level is low (<0.6 mm) a very small RE is obtained, while this error increases when applying higher levels of smoothing (>0.6 mm).

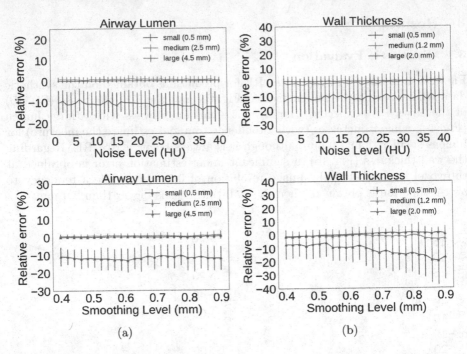

Fig. 5. Effect of varying noise (first row) and smoothing (second row) on lumen (a) and wall thickness (b) predictions. The RE is reported in %.

Finally, Table 3 shows the mean relative error (in percentage) obtained for different sizes of wall thickness using the proposed method in comparison to ZCSD and FWHM on the 200,000 testing patches. Three wall thickness intervals were chosen: lower than 0.7 mm, between 0.7 mm and 1.5 mm, and bigger than 1.5 mm. As shown, while traditional methods tend to have a very high relative error, especially for small airways, the proposed method yields a very high accuracy and outperforms them. Similar results were obtained for the airway lumen.

Table 3. Mean RE (in %) for the proposed method (CNR), FWHM, and ZCSD for the wall thickness (wt).

	wt ≤ 0.7 mm			0.7 mm < wt ≤ 1.5 mm			wt > 1.5 mm		
	CNR	FWHM	ZCSD	CNR	FWHM	ZCSD	CNR	FWHM	ZCSD
RE (%)	−7.6	−1153.9	−1034.2	1.04	−582.9	−895.6	0.28	−450.8	−200.3

3.2 Phantom Evaluation

The relative error obtained measuring the wall thickness of the eight tubes of the phantom using the proposed method (CNR) in comparison with traditional techniques are presented in Table 4. For completeness, the relative error obtained

Table 4. Mean RE (in %) obtained measuring the wall thickness (WT) on the eight phantom tubes using the proposed method (CNR) in comparison with FWHM and ZCSD. Smallest relative error is reported in bold. For completeness, the last column reports the relative error obtained measuring the lumen of the tubes with CNR (traditional methods only provide WT). All results are in %.

Tube	CNR WT	FWHM WT	ZCSD WT	CNR Lumen
A	**−2.5**	−115.1	−126.1	4.6
B	**17.5**	−25.9	−33.6	−6.3
C	−28.9	**−23.6**	−46.2	7.6
D	**−12.8**	−474.0	−79.0	10.4
E	**−13.0**	−4884.6	−20.5	9.8
F	**2.4**	−55.3	−59.8	−5.2
G	**5.4**	−18.06	−29.2	−7.8
H	**18.5**	−30.7	−40.3	−5.2

when measuring the lumen with CNR (not measured by traditional methods) is also reported. The proposed CNR has the lowest RE for all considered tubes, with the exception of tube C where FWHM gives the best result, and in general is able to well measure the wall thickness even for small and thin tubes, as in case of tube D. Although there is variance in the RE for the measurement of the wall thickness of all tubes, this variance is smaller than the one obtained using traditional methods, that for some tubes seem to really confounded. An important aspect to notice is the small RE obtained for all tubes when measuring the lumen radius with the proposed CNR.

3.3   In-Vivo Indirect Evaluation (FEV1% in Correlation to Pi10)

Table 5(a) shows the Pearson's correlation coefficient between FEV1% and the Pi10 metric computed with our approach and ZCSD in airway patches extracted from a real CT. The correlation coefficient between FEV1% and Pi10 calculated by ZCSD and CNR was −0.38 and −0.54, respectively, indicating a significantly higher correlation of the Pi10 computed by the CNR with FEV1%. This result suggests that the proposed method could potentially be used to accurately measure FEV1% in patients with COPD.

Table 5. Results from the indirect in-vivo analysis for airways. The Pearson's correlation coefficient for the correlation between the Pi10 computed with the ZCSD and SimGAN, and FEV1% is reported

	Correlation (CI)
ZCSD	−0.39 (−0.46, −0.32)
CNR	−0.60 (−0.65, −0.55)

4   Discussion and Conclusion

In this paper, a novel method to automatically measure and analyze the morphology of airways using deep learning on chest CT images is proposed. The use of a neural network in combination with SimGAN to refine the synthetic model and the proposed loss function represent the innovative aspects of this work.

Results from the validation on synthetic patches showed a low absolute relative error across all airway wall thicknesses and airway lumens. Although a direct comparison is not possible, considering the absolute relative error for airways of 1.0 mm, the presented method obtains a better performance (absolute relative error around 6%) than the method proposed in [16], where the wall thickness was measured on plastic tubes of 1.0 mm yield to an absolute relative error of approximately 10%. Also, a test for structures of different sizes and varying the level of noise and smoothing showed that the proposed method is not affected by noise or smoothing, and, as expected, only sizes at lower than the image resolution may determine a small increase of the prediction error. A comparison of two traditional algorithms shows that our method outperforms the state-of-the-art, especially for small and complex airways.

Finally, phantom-related results and indirect validation with in-vivo patches showed promising results, indicating the stability of the CNR in accurately measuring the wall thickness and lumen radius regardless of the varying starting conditions. This indicates that the method here proposed may potentially be used for future early diagnosis of lung disorders.

For future work, the creation of the synthetic model might be improved by reducing the level of approximation of the PSF and additive noise. Also, new refinement processes of the synthetic images, such as using CycleGAN [17], should be explored.

References

1. Hogg, J.C., McDonough, J.E., Suzuki, M.: Small airway obstruction in COPD: new insights based on micro-CT imaging and MRI imaging. Chest **143**(5), 1436–1443 (2013)
2. Awadh, N., Müller, N.L., Park, C.S., Abboud, R.T., FitzGerald, J.M.: Airway wall thickness in patients with near fatal asthma and control groups: assessment with high resolution computed tomographic scanning. Thorax **53**(4), 248–253 (1998)
3. Niimi, A., et al.: Airway wall thickness in asthma assessed by computed tomography: relation to clinical indices. Am. J. Respir. Crit. Care Med. **162**(4), 1518–1523 (2000)
4. Schwab, R.J., Gefter, W.B., Pack, A.I., Hoffman, E.A.: Dynamic imaging of the upper airway during respiration in normal subjects. J. Appl. Physiol. **74**(4), 1504–1514 (1993)
5. Estépar, R.S.J., Washko, G.G., Silverman, E.K., Reilly, J.J., Kikinis, R., Westin, C.-F.: Accurate airway wall estimation using phase congruency. In: Larsen, R., Nielsen, M., Sporring, J. (eds.) MICCAI 2006. LNCS, vol. 4191, pp. 125–134. Springer, Heidelberg (2006). https://doi.org/10.1007/11866763_16

6. Petersen, J., Nielsen, M., Lo, P., Saghir, Z., Dirksen, A., de Bruijne, M.: Optimal graph based segmentation using flow lines with application to airway wall segmentation. In: Székely, G., Hahn, H.K. (eds.) IPMI 2011. LNCS, vol. 6801, pp. 49–60. Springer, Heidelberg (2011). https://doi.org/10.1007/978-3-642-22092-0_5

7. Reinhardt, J.M., D'Souza, N., Hoffman, E.A.: Accurate measurement of intrathoracic airways. IEEE Trans. Med. Imaging 16(6), 820–827 (1997)

8. LeCun, Y., Bengio, Y., Hinton, G.: Deep learning. Nature 521(7553), 436 (2015)

9. Shrivastava, A., Pfister, T., Tuzel, O., Susskind, J., Wang, W., Webb, R.: Learning from simulated and unsupervised images through adversarial training. In: The IEEE Conference on Computer Vision and Pattern Recognition (CVPR), vol. 3, p. 6 (2017)

10. Weibel, E.R.: Morphometry of the Human Lung. Springer, Heidelberg (1965). https://doi.org/10.1007/978-3-642-87553-3

11. Kindlmann, G., San José Estépar, R., Smith, S., Westin, C.: Sampling and visualizing creases with scale-space particles. IEEE T. Vis. Comput. Gr. 15(6) (2009)

12. Schwarzband, G., Kiryati, N.: The point spread function of spiral CT. Phy. Med. Biol. 50(22), 5307 (2005)

13. Nardelli, P., Ross, J.C., Estépar, R.S.J.: CT image enhancement for feature detection and localization. In: Descoteaux, M., Maier-Hein, L., Franz, A., Jannin, P., Collins, D.L., Duchesne, S. (eds.) MICCAI 2017. LNCS, vol. 10434, pp. 224–232. Springer, Cham (2017). https://doi.org/10.1007/978-3-319-66185-8_26

14. Chollet, F., et al.: Keras (2015). https://keras.io

15. Abadi, M., et al.: Tensorflow: large-scale machine learning on heterogeneous distributed systems. arXiv preprint arXiv:1603.04467 (2016)

16. Nakano, Y., et al.: Computed tomographic measurements of airway dimensions and emphysema in smokers: correlation with lung function. Am. J. Respir. Crit. Care Med. 162(3), 1102–1108 (2000)

17. Zhu, J.Y., Park, T., Isola, P., Efros, A.A.: Unpaired image-to-image translation using cycle-consistent adversarial networks. arXiv preprint arXiv:1703.10593 (2017)

Author Index

Printed in the United States
By Bookmasters